Hypertrophic Cardiomyopathy—Current Challenges and Future Perspectives

Hypertrophic Cardiomyopathy—Current Challenges and Future Perspectives

Editors

Emanuele Monda
Francesco Pelliccia

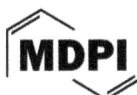

Basel • Beijing • Wuhan • Barcelona • Belgrade • Novi Sad • Cluj • Manchester

Editors

Emanuele Monda
University of Campania "Luigi Vanvitelli"
Naples, Italy

Francesco Pelliccia
Sapienza University
Rome, Italy

Editorial Office
MDPI
St. Alban-Anlage 66
4052 Basel, Switzerland

This is a reprint of articles from the Special Issue published online in the open access journal *Journal of Clinical Medicine* (ISSN 2077-0383) (available at: https://www.mdpi.com/journal/jcm/special_issues/Hypertrophic_Cardiomyopathy_HCM).

For citation purposes, cite each article independently as indicated on the article page online and as indicated below:

Lastname, A.A.; Lastname, B.B. Article Title. *Journal Name* **Year**, *Volume Number*, Page Range.

ISBN 978-3-0365-9849-9 (Hbk)
ISBN 978-3-0365-9850-5 (PDF)
doi.org/10.3390/books978-3-0365-9850-5

© 2024 by the authors. Articles in this book are Open Access and distributed under the Creative Commons Attribution (CC BY) license. The book as a whole is distributed by MDPI under the terms and conditions of the Creative Commons Attribution-NonCommercial-NoDerivs (CC BY-NC-ND) license.

Contents

About the Editors vii

Emanuele Monda, Giuseppe Limongelli and Francesco Pelliccia
Hypertrophic Cardiomyopathy—Current Challenges and Future Perspectives
Reprinted from: *J. Clin. Med.* **2023**, *12*, 6093, doi:10.3390/jcm12186093 1

Steven Lebowitz, Mariusz Kowalewski, Giuseppe Maria Raffa, Danny Chu, Matteo Greco, Caterina Gandolfo, et al.
Review of Contemporary Invasive Treatment Approaches and Critical Appraisal of Guidelines on Hypertrophic Obstructive Cardiomyopathy: State-of-the-Art Review
Reprinted from: *J. Clin. Med.* **2022**, *11*, 3405, doi:10.3390/jcm11123405 7

Marilena Melas, Eleftherios T. Beltsios, Antonis Adamou, Konstantinos Koumarelas and Kim L. McBride
Molecular Diagnosis of Hypertrophic Cardiomyopathy (HCM): In the Heart of Cardiac Disease
Reprinted from: *J. Clin. Med.* **2023**, *12*, 225, doi:10.3390/jcm12010225 31

Haobo Xu, Juan Wang, Shubin Qiao, Jiansong Yuan, Fenghuan Hu, Weixian Yang, et al.
Association of Types of Sleep Apnea and Nocturnal Hypoxemia with Atrial Fibrillation in Patients with Hypertrophic Cardiomyopathy
Reprinted from: *J. Clin. Med.* **2023**, *12*, 1347, doi:10.3390/jcm12041347 41

Francesca Girolami, Alessia Gozzini, Eszter Dalma Pálinkás, Adelaide Ballerini, Alessia Tomberli, Katia Baldini, et al.
Genetic Testing and Counselling in Hypertrophic Cardiomyopathy: Frequently Asked Questions
Reprinted from: *J. Clin. Med.* **2023**, *12*, 2489, doi:10.3390/jcm12072489 51

Niccolò Maurizi, Chiara Chiriatti, Carlo Fumagalli, Mattia Targetti, Silvia Passantino, Panagiotis Antiochos, et al.
Real-World Use and Predictors of Response to Disopyramide in Patients with Obstructive Hypertrophic Cardiomyopathy
Reprinted from: *J. Clin. Med.* **2023**, *12*, 2725, doi:10.3390/jcm12072725 61

Claire M. Lawley and Juan Pablo Kaski
Clinical and Genetic Screening for Hypertrophic Cardiomyopathy in Paediatric Relatives: Changing Paradigms in Clinical Practice
Reprinted from: *J. Clin. Med.* **2023**, *12*, 2788, doi:10.3390/jcm12082788 71

Felice Gragnano, Francesco Pelliccia, Natale Guarnaccia, Giampaolo Niccoli, Salvatore De Rosa, Raffaele Piccolo, et al.
Alcohol Septal Ablation in Patients with Hypertrophic Obstructive Cardiomyopathy: A Contemporary Perspective
Reprinted from: *J. Clin. Med.* **2023**, *12*, 2810, doi:10.3390/jcm12082810 79

Emyal Alyaydin, Julia Kirsten Vogel, Peter Luedike, Tienush Rassaf, Rolf Alexander Jánosi and Maria Papathanasiou
Sex-Related Differences among Adults with Hypertrophic Obstructive Cardiomyopathy Undergoing Transcoronary Ablation of Septal Hypertrophy
Reprinted from: *J. Clin. Med.* **2023**, *12*, 3024, doi:10.3390/jcm12083024 93

Francesco Santoro, Federica Mango, Adriana Mallardi, Damiano D'Alessandro, Grazia Casavecchia, Matteo Gravina, et al.
Arrhythmic Risk Stratification among Patients with Hypertrophic Cardiomyopathy
Reprinted from: *J. Clin. Med.* **2023**, *12*, 3397, doi:10.3390/jcm12103397 103

Andrea Ottaviani, Davide Mansour, Lorenzo V. Molinari, Kristian Galanti, Cesare Mantini, Mohammed Y. Khanji, et al.
Revisiting Diagnosis and Treatment of Hypertrophic Cardiomyopathy: Current Practice and Novel Perspectives
Reprinted from: *J. Clin. Med.* **2023**, *12*, 5710, doi:10.3390/jcm12175710 . . . . **117**

About the Editors

Emanuele Monda

Emanuele Monda is a cardiologist and PhD student at University of Campania "Luigi Vanvitelli" (Naples, Italy), with clinical and research interests in inherited and rare cardiac conditions. In recent years, he has been conducting research projects on this topic, resulting in the publication of more than 90 papers in international peer-reviewed journals. He is a fellow of the European Society of Cardiology (ESC), an active member of the Media Task Force of the ESC Council on Cardiovascular Genomics and an Associate Editor of Frontiers in Cardiovascular Medicine and Frontiers in Paediatrics.

Francesco Pelliccia

Dr. Francesco Pelliccia currently serves as an Associate Professor of Cardiology at the Department of Cardiovascular Sciences, Università Sapienza, Rome – Italy. He received his Doctorate of Medicine (M.D.) from the Università Sapienza, Rome – Italy, in 1989 and obtained his Philosophiae Doctorate (Ph.D.) in Cardiovascular Sciences from the Department of Cardiovascular and Neurological Sciences, University School of Cagliari, Cagliari – Italy, in 2008. His main scientific interests include interventional cardiology, takotsubo syndrome, MINOCA and hypertrophic cardiomyopathy. Dr. Pelliccia is currently a Fellow of the European Society of Cardiology and a Fellow of the American College of Cardiology. He currently serves as Associate Editor of the International Journal of Cardiology as well as Associate Editor of the *International Journal of Cardiology. Heart & Vasculature*.

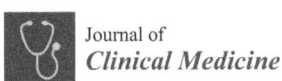

Editorial

Hypertrophic Cardiomyopathy—Current Challenges and Future Perspectives

Emanuele Monda [1,*], Giuseppe Limongelli [1] and Francesco Pelliccia [2]

1. Inherited and Rare Cardiovascular Diseases, Department of Translational Medical Sciences, University of Campania "Luigi Vanvitelli", 80131 Naples, Italy; limongelligiuseppe@libero.it
2. Department of Cardiovascular Sciences, Sapienza University, 00185 Rome, Italy; f.pelliccia@mclink.it
* Correspondence: emanuelemonda@me.com; Tel.: +39-3348607935

Hypertrophic cardiomyopathy (HCM) is a myocardial disorder characterized by left ventricular (LV) hypertrophy, which cannot be entirely attributed to loading conditions such as valve or congenital heart disease or hypertension [1,2]. This condition is relatively common, with a prevalence of 1:250–500 individuals, and is linked to increased rates of mortality and morbidity [2]. In recent years, the body of knowledge concerning the genetic underpinnings, natural history, risk assessment, and management of HCM has grown.

In this Special Issue, experts in the field delve into these topics through comprehensive reviews and original articles that explore the molecular basis, the role of genetic testing, risk stratification for sudden cardiac death (SCD), atrial fibrillation, and management of HCM. This Special Issue includes 10 articles, and we are delighted to introduce them to the readers of the Journal of Clinical Medicine.

1. Molecular Basis and Genetic Testing

In 40–60% of HCM cases, the disease is inherited as a Mendelian autosomal dominant condition with variable penetrance, associated with pathogenic variants in genes encoding proteins of the cardiac sarcomere [1]. An additional 5–10% of cases are caused by pathogenic variants in genes responsible for conditions mimicking the sarcomeric HCM phenotype [3], such as malformative syndromes (e.g., RASopathies) [4–6], storage diseases (e.g., Pompe disease, Fabry disease) [7], infiltrative conditions (e.g., cardiac amyloidosis) [8], and mitochondrial/neuromuscular conditions (e.g., Friedreich ataxia) [8–10]. Therefore, genetic testing plays a crucial role in identifying the underlying aetiology and guiding family screening and treatment [9].

In this Special Issue, the role of genetic testing in HCM is extensively discussed. Melas et al. describe the main genes implicated in the aetiology of HCM, define the role of diagnostic genetic panels (e.g., next-generation sequencing, whole-exome sequencing, and whole-genome sequencing), and introduce the potential of gene therapy in patients with HCM [10]. In contrast, Lawley et al. emphasize the importance of conducting clinical and genetic screening among paediatric family members of individuals with HCM [11]. Genetic testing should always be prescribed after comprehensive genetic counselling, which aims to educate patients and their families about the benefits and constraints of genetic testing, the genetic aspects related to the disease, and the potential for passing on the condition to their relatives [1]. In their comprehensive review, Girolami et al. address and deliberate on the most commonly posed questions by HCM patients, drawing on their extensive 20-year experience in genetic counselling [12].

2. Risk Stratification for Sudden Cardiac Death

SCD has historically been considered the most visible and tragic complication in patients with HCM [13]. Over the past two decades, several risk factors for SCD have been identified, leading to the development of various models and algorithms for the placement of implantable cardioverter-defibrillators (ICDs) in primary prevention [14]. The

Citation: Monda, E.; Limongelli, G.; Pelliccia, F. Hypertrophic Cardiomyopathy—Current Challenges and Future Perspectives. *J. Clin. Med.* 2023, 12, 6093. https://doi.org/10.3390/jcm12186093

Received: 14 September 2023
Accepted: 20 September 2023
Published: 21 September 2023

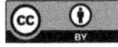

Copyright: © 2023 by the authors. Licensee MDPI, Basel, Switzerland. This article is an open access article distributed under the terms and conditions of the Creative Commons Attribution (CC BY) license (https://creativecommons.org/licenses/by/4.0/).

risk assessment for patients with HCM involves a comprehensive clinical evaluation, which includes clinical and family history, ECG, and imaging tests, with a focus on identifying major risk factors [1,2].

The risk stratification model proposed by the European Society of Cardiology guidelines on the management of cardiomyopathies suggests estimating the 5-year risk of SCD using the HCM-risk score and individualizing ICD implantation based on the estimated risk [1,15]. In contrast, the American College of Cardiology/American Heart Association recommends ICD placement in patients with at least one major risk factor associated with SCD [2,16]. Additionally, specific risk models have been proposed for paediatric patients [17,18].

In this Special Issue, Santoro et al. provide a comprehensive review that summarizes the risk factors associated with SCD in patients with HCM and discusses the different algorithms for ICD implantation [19].

3. Atrial Fibrillation

Atrial fibrillation (AF) is a prevalent cardiac rhythm disorder in HCM and is linked with increased morbidity and mortality [20]. Risk factors for AF in patients with HCM include advanced age, increased body mass index, disease severity, and left atrial enlargement [20].

Sleep apnoea is the most common type of sleep-disordered breathing. Its prevalence among patients with AF is approximately 50% and is likely related to the association between sleep apnoea and left atrial remodelling [21]. However, studies exploring the association between sleep apnoea and AF in HCM individuals are limited. Xu et al. aimed to investigate the association between obstructive sleep apnoea and central sleep apnoea and the prevalence of AF in this condition [22]. The authors observed that 56% of patients had obstructive sleep apnoea and 4% had central sleep apnoea. Additionally, both obstructive and central sleep apnoea were independently associated with AF, indicating the importance of considering sleep apnoea screening as part of AF management in individuals with HCM [22].

4. Pharmacological Treatment

The primary objectives of pharmacological treatment in HCM encompass the management of symptoms, lowering dynamic intraventricular gradients, addressing LV systolic dysfunction and HF, managing arrhythmias, and preventing cardioembolic events in patients with AF [23].

Beta-blockers are considered the first-line therapy for managing LV outflow tract (LVOT) obstruction [1,23,24]. For individuals experiencing persistent symptoms that are unresponsive or partially responsive to initial treatment, disopyramide may be considered as a secondary therapeutic option [1,23]. Nevertheless, information regarding the safety and effectiveness of disopyramide is limited to a small number of investigations. Maurizi et al. sought to assess the efficacy of disopyramide in addressing LVOT obstruction in HCM patients [25]. Among 118 patients treated with disopyramide, 28 (24%) showed a complete response (defined by reaching the New York Heart Association (NYHA) class I and an LVOT gradient <30 mmHg), 39 (33%) were incomplete responders (defined by a NYHA class >I and an LVOT gradient <30 mmHg), and 51 (43%) were non-responders (defined by no changes in NYHA class and an LVOT gradient >30 mmHg). NYHA class I/II was identified as an independent predictor of response to disopyramide treatment. Eighty patients (69%) showed prolonged QTc interval. However, no major drug-related adverse events were observed. The authors concluded that disopyramide can effectively reduce both LVOT gradients and symptoms in patients exhibiting less severe disease characteristics, all while maintaining a favourable arrhythmia safety profile [25].

Recently, an improved comprehension of the underlying causes of HCM has paved the way for the creation of treatments specifically designed to target the underlying substrate, emphasizing the need for an aetiological characterization of patients with HCM [26]. Thus,

Ottaviani et al. furnish a comprehensive overview of the present clinical approaches and delve into emerging therapeutic avenues for sarcomeric HCM, with particular attention to cardiac myosin inhibitors [27].

5. Invasive Strategies

Transaortic septal myectomy is considered as the preferred treatment choice for the majority of patients experiencing symptomatic LVOT obstruction that does not respond to medical treatment [2,28]. Myectomy yields instant and enduring elimination of the outflow obstruction and might contribute to atrial and ventricular reverse remodelling [29]. In cases where myectomy cannot be pursued, percutaneous alcohol septal ablation emerges as the most common alternative for addressing LVOT obstruction in HCM patients, with the advantage of shorter hospital stay with a risk of complications similar to myectomy when performed in high-volume centres [2,30]. The decision between myectomy and alcohol septal ablation is based on different variables, including age, comorbidities, centre experience, coronary artery anatomy, and patient preference, among others [2].

Lebowitz et al. provide a detailed review with the aim of discussing the indications of surgical myectomy and alcohol septal ablation, summarizing and comparing the novel techniques for the management of obstructive HCM and offering suggestions for the management of patients with complex presentations [31].

In addition, two different articles on the role of alcohol septal ablation are provided in this Special Issue. In their review, Gragnano et al. [32] provide a concise summary of the current evidence concerning alcohol septal ablation. In addition, they underscore the critical importance of assembling a multidisciplinary team of HCM experts comprising clinical and interventional cardiologists, along with cardiac surgeons who have substantial expertise in managing patients with obstructive HCM [32]. Furthermore, Alyaydin et al. investigate the differences related to sex among adults with HCM who undergo alcohol septal ablation. They observed that women tend to present at a more advanced age and with more severe symptoms and that the procedure is safe and effective for both sexes, with advanced age at the time of the intervention as an independent predictor of mortality [33].

The Editors hope that readers of this Special Issue will find it of interest.

Funding: The authors have not declared a specific grant for this research from any funding agency in the public, commercial, or not-for-profit sectors.

Conflicts of Interest: The authors declare no conflict of interest.

References

1. Arbelo, E.; Protonotarios, A.; Gimeno, J.R.; Arbustini, E.; Barriales-Villa, R.; Basso, C.; Bezzina, C.R.; Biagini, E.; Blom, N.A.; de Boer, R.A.; et al. 2023 ESC Guidelines for the Management of Cardiomyopathies. *Eur. Heart J.* **2023**, ehad194. [CrossRef] [PubMed]
2. Ommen, S.R.; Mital, S.; Burke, M.A.; Day, S.M.; Deswal, A.; Elliott, P.; Evanovich, L.L.; Hung, J.; Joglar, J.A.; Kantor, P.; et al. 2020 AHA/ACC Guideline for the Diagnosis and Treatment of Patients with Hypertrophic Cardiomyopathy: A Report of the American College of Cardiology/American Heart Association Joint Committee on Clinical Practice Guidelines. *Circulation* **2020**, *142*, e558–e631. [CrossRef] [PubMed]
3. Limongelli, G.; Monda, E.; Tramonte, S.; Gragnano, F.; Masarone, D.; Frisso, G.; Esposito, A.; Gravino, R.; Ammendola, E.; Salerno, G.; et al. Prevalence and Clinical Significance of Red Flags in Patients with Hypertrophic Cardiomyopathy. *Int. J. Cardiol.* **2020**, *299*, 186–191. [CrossRef] [PubMed]
4. Monda, E.; Prosnitz, A.; Aiello, R.; Lioncino, M.; Norrish, G.; Caiazza, M.; Drago, F.; Beattie, M.; Tartaglia, M.; Russo, M.G.; et al. Natural History of Hypertrophic Cardiomyopathy in Noonan Syndrome with Multiple Lentigines. *Circ. Genom. Precis. Med.* **2023**, *16*, 350–358. [CrossRef] [PubMed]
5. Lioncino, M.; Monda, E.; Verrillo, F.; Moscarella, E.; Calcagni, G.; Drago, F.; Marino, B.; Digilio, M.C.; Putotto, C.; Calabrò, P.; et al. Hypertrophic Cardiomyopathy in RASopathies: Diagnosis, Clinical Characteristics, Prognostic Implications, and Management. *Heart Fail. Clin.* **2022**, *18*, 19–29. [CrossRef]
6. Caiazza, M.; Rubino, M.; Monda, E.; Passariello, A.; Fusco, A.; Cirillo, A.; Esposito, A.; Pierno, A.; De Fazio, F.; Pacileo, R.; et al. Combined PTPN11 and MYBPC3 Gene Mutations in an Adult Patient with Noonan Syndrome and Hypertrophic Cardiomyopathy. *Genes* **2020**, *11*, 947. [CrossRef]

7. Rubino, M.; Monda, E.; Lioncino, M.; Caiazza, M.; Palmiero, G.; Dongiglio, F.; Fusco, A.; Cirillo, A.; Cesaro, A.; Capodicasa, L.; et al. Diagnosis and Management of Cardiovascular Involvement in Fabry Disease. *Heart Fail. Clin.* **2022**, *18*, 39–49. [CrossRef]
8. Lioncino, M.; Monda, E.; Palmiero, G.; Caiazza, M.; Vetrano, E.; Rubino, M.; Esposito, A.; Salerno, G.; Dongiglio, F.; D'Onofrio, B.; et al. Cardiovascular Involvement in Transthyretin Cardiac Amyloidosis. *Heart Fail. Clin.* **2022**, *18*, 73–87. [CrossRef]
9. Limongelli, G.; Adorisio, R.; Baggio, C.; Bauce, B.; Biagini, E.; Castelletti, S.; Favilli, S.; Imazio, M.; Lioncino, M.; Merlo, M.; et al. Diagnosis and Management of Rare Cardiomyopathies in Adult and Paediatric Patients. A Position Paper of the Italian Society of Cardiology (SIC) and Italian Society of Paediatric Cardiology (SICP). *Int. J. Cardiol.* **2022**, *357*, 55–71. [CrossRef]
10. Melas, M.; Beltsios, E.T.; Adamou, A.; Koumarelas, K.; McBride, K.L. Molecular Diagnosis of Hypertrophic Cardiomyopathy (HCM): In the Heart of Cardiac Disease. *J. Clin. Med.* **2022**, *12*, 225. [CrossRef]
11. Lawley, C.M.; Kaski, J.P. Clinical and Genetic Screening for Hypertrophic Cardiomyopathy in Paediatric Relatives: Changing Paradigms in Clinical Practice. *J. Clin. Med.* **2023**, *12*, 2788. [CrossRef] [PubMed]
12. Girolami, F.; Gozzini, A.; Pálinkás, E.D.; Ballerini, A.; Tomberli, A.; Baldini, K.; Marchi, A.; Zampieri, M.; Passantino, S.; Porcedda, G.; et al. Genetic Testing and Counselling in Hypertrophic Cardiomyopathy: Frequently Asked Questions. *J. Clin. Med.* **2023**, *12*, 2489. [CrossRef] [PubMed]
13. Maron, M.S.; Rowin, E.; Spirito, P.; Maron, B.J. Differing Strategies for Sudden Death Prevention in Hypertrophic Cardiomyopathy. *Heart* **2023**, *109*, 589–594. [CrossRef]
14. Monda, E.; Limongelli, G. Integrated Sudden Cardiac Death Risk Prediction Model For Patients with Hypertrophic Cardiomyopathy. *Circulation* **2023**, *147*, 281–283. [CrossRef] [PubMed]
15. O'Mahony, C.; Jichi, F.; Pavlou, M.; Monserrat, L.; Anastasakis, A.; Rapezzi, C.; Biagini, E.; Gimeno, J.R.; Limongelli, G.; McKenna, W.J.; et al. A Novel Clinical Risk Prediction Model for Sudden Cardiac Death in Hypertrophic Cardiomyopathy (HCM Risk-SCD). *Eur. Heart J.* **2014**, *35*, 2010–2020. [CrossRef]
16. Maron, M.S.; Rowin, E.J.; Wessler, B.S.; Mooney, P.J.; Fatima, A.; Patel, P.; Koethe, B.C.; Romashko, M.; Link, M.S.; Maron, B.J. Enhanced American College of Cardiology/American Heart Association Strategy for Prevention of Sudden Cardiac Death in High-Risk Patients with Hypertrophic Cardiomyopathy. *JAMA Cardiol.* **2019**, *4*, 644–657. [CrossRef]
17. Miron, A.; Lafreniere-Roula, M.; Steve Fan, C.-P.; Armstrong, K.R.; Dragulescu, A.; Papaz, T.; Manlhiot, C.; Kaufman, B.; Butts, R.J.; Gardin, L.; et al. A Validated Model for Sudden Cardiac Death Risk Prediction in Pediatric Hypertrophic Cardiomyopathy. *Circulation* **2020**, *142*, 217–229. [CrossRef]
18. Norrish, G.; Ding, T.; Field, E.; Ziółkowska, L.; Olivotto, I.; Limongelli, G.; Anastasakis, A.; Weintraub, R.; Biagini, E.; Ragni, L.; et al. Development of a Novel Risk Prediction Model for Sudden Cardiac Death in Childhood Hypertrophic Cardiomyopathy (HCM Risk-Kids). *JAMA Cardiol.* **2019**, *4*, 918–927. [CrossRef]
19. Santoro, F.; Mango, F.; Mallardi, A.; D'Alessandro, D.; Casavecchia, G.; Gravina, M.; Correale, M.; Brunetti, N.D. Arrhythmic Risk Stratification among Patients with Hypertrophic Cardiomyopathy. *J. Clin. Med.* **2023**, *12*, 3397. [CrossRef]
20. Philipson, D.J.; Rader, F.; Siegel, R.J. Risk Factors for Atrial Fibrillation in Hypertrophic Cardiomyopathy. *Eur. J. Prev. Cardiol.* **2021**, *28*, 658–665. [CrossRef]
21. Gami, A.S.; Pressman, G.; Caples, S.M.; Kanagala, R.; Gard, J.J.; Davison, D.E.; Malouf, J.F.; Ammash, N.M.; Friedman, P.A.; Somers, V.K. Association of Atrial Fibrillation and Obstructive Sleep Apnea. *Circulation* **2004**, *110*, 364–367. [CrossRef] [PubMed]
22. Xu, H.; Wang, J.; Qiao, S.; Yuan, J.; Hu, F.; Yang, W.; Guo, C.; Luo, X.; Duan, X.; Liu, S.; et al. Association of Types of Sleep Apnea and Nocturnal Hypoxemia with Atrial Fibrillation in Patients with Hypertrophic Cardiomyopathy. *J. Clin. Med.* **2023**, *12*, 1347. [CrossRef]
23. Iavarone, M.; Monda, E.; Vritz, O.; Calila Albert, D.; Rubino, M.; Verrillo, F.; Caiazza, M.; Lioncino, M.; Amodio, F.; Guarnaccia, N.; et al. Medical Treatment of Patients with Hypertrophic Cardiomyopathy: An Overview of Current and Emerging Therapy. *Arch. Cardiovasc. Dis.* **2022**, *115*, 529–537. [CrossRef] [PubMed]
24. Monda, E.; Lioncino, M.; Palmiero, G.; Franco, F.; Rubino, M.; Cirillo, A.; Verrillo, F.; Fusco, A.; Caiazza, M.; Mazzella, M.; et al. Bisoprolol for Treatment of Symptomatic Patients with Obstructive Hypertrophic Cardiomyopathy. The BASIC (Bisoprolol AS Therapy in Hypertrophic Cardiomyopathy) Study. *Int. J. Cardiol.* **2022**, *354*, 22–28. [CrossRef] [PubMed]
25. Maurizi, N.; Chiriatti, C.; Fumagalli, C.; Targetti, M.; Passantino, S.; Antiochos, P.; Skalidis, I.; Chiti, C.; Biagioni, G.; Tomberli, A.; et al. Real-World Use and Predictors of Response to Disopyramide in Patients with Obstructive Hypertrophic Cardiomyopathy. *J. Clin. Med.* **2023**, *12*, 2725. [CrossRef]
26. Monda, E.; Bakalakos, A.; Rubino, M.; Verrillo, F.; Diana, G.; De Michele, G.; Altobelli, I.; Lioncino, M.; Perna, A.; Falco, L.; et al. Targeted Therapies in Pediatric and Adult Patients with Hypertrophic Heart Disease: From Molecular Pathophysiology to Personalized Medicine. *Circ. Heart Fail.* **2023**, *16*, e010687. [CrossRef]
27. Ottaviani, A.; Mansour, D.; Molinari, L.V.; Galanti, K.; Mantini, C.; Khanji, M.Y.; Chahal, A.A.; Zimarino, M.; Renda, G.; Sciarra, L.; et al. Revisiting Diagnosis and Treatment of Hypertrophic Cardiomyopathy: Current Practice and Novel Perspectives. *J. Clin. Med.* **2023**, *12*, 5710. [CrossRef]
28. Pelliccia, F.; Limongelli, G.; Autore, C.; Gimeno-Blanes, J.R.; Basso, C.; Elliott, P. Sex-Related Differences in Cardiomyopathies. *Int. J. Cardiol.* **2019**, *286*, 239–243. [CrossRef]
29. Maron, B.J.; Dearani, J.A.; Smedira, N.G.; Schaff, H.V.; Wang, S.; Rastegar, H.; Ralph-Edwards, A.; Ferrazzi, P.; Swistel, D.; Shemin, R.J.; et al. Ventricular Septal Myectomy for Obstructive Hypertrophic Cardiomyopathy (Analysis Spanning 60 Years Of Practice): AJC Expert Panel. *Am. J. Cardiol.* **2022**, *180*, 124–139. [CrossRef]

30. Batzner, A.; Pfeiffer, B.; Neugebauer, A.; Aicha, D.; Blank, C.; Seggewiss, H. Survival After Alcohol Septal Ablation in Patients with Hypertrophic Obstructive Cardiomyopathy. *J. Am. Coll. Cardiol.* **2018**, *72*, 3087–3094. [CrossRef]
31. Lebowitz, S.; Kowalewski, M.; Raffa, G.M.; Chu, D.; Greco, M.; Gandolfo, C.; Mignosa, C.; Lorusso, R.; Suwalski, P.; Pilato, M. Review of Contemporary Invasive Treatment Approaches and Critical Appraisal of Guidelines on Hypertrophic Obstructive Cardiomyopathy: State-of-the-Art Review. *J. Clin. Med.* **2022**, *11*, 3405. [CrossRef] [PubMed]
32. Gragnano, F.; Pelliccia, F.; Guarnaccia, N.; Niccoli, G.; De Rosa, S.; Piccolo, R.; Moscarella, E.; Fabris, E.; Montone, R.A.; Cesaro, A.; et al. Alcohol Septal Ablation in Patients with Hypertrophic Obstructive Cardiomyopathy: A Contemporary Perspective. *J. Clin. Med.* **2023**, *12*, 2810. [CrossRef] [PubMed]
33. Alyaydin, E.; Vogel, J.K.; Luedike, P.; Rassaf, T.; Jánosi, R.A.; Papathanasiou, M. Sex-Related Differences among Adults with Hypertrophic Obstructive Cardiomyopathy Undergoing Transcoronary Ablation of Septal Hypertrophy. *J. Clin. Med.* **2023**, *12*, 3024. [CrossRef] [PubMed]

Disclaimer/Publisher's Note: The statements, opinions and data contained in all publications are solely those of the individual author(s) and contributor(s) and not of MDPI and/or the editor(s). MDPI and/or the editor(s) disclaim responsibility for any injury to people or property resulting from any ideas, methods, instructions or products referred to in the content.

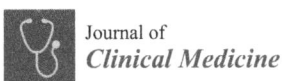

Journal of
Clinical Medicine

Review

Review of Contemporary Invasive Treatment Approaches and Critical Appraisal of Guidelines on Hypertrophic Obstructive Cardiomyopathy: State-of-the-Art Review

Steven Lebowitz [1,†], Mariusz Kowalewski [2,3,4,*,†], Giuseppe Maria Raffa [5], Danny Chu [6], Matteo Greco [5], Caterina Gandolfo [5], Carmelo Mignosa [5], Roberto Lorusso [2], Piotr Suwalski [3] and Michele Pilato [5]

Citation: Lebowitz, S.; Kowalewski, M.; Raffa, G.M.; Chu, D.; Greco, M.; Gandolfo, C.; Mignosa, C.; Lorusso, R.; Suwalski, P.; Pilato, M. Review of Contemporary Invasive Treatment Approaches and Critical Appraisal of Guidelines on Hypertrophic Obstructive Cardiomyopathy: State-of-the-Art Review. *J. Clin. Med.* 2022, 11, 3405. https://doi.org/10.3390/jcm11123405

Academic Editors: Emanuele Monda and Francesco Pelliccia

Received: 17 May 2022
Accepted: 10 June 2022
Published: 14 June 2022

Publisher's Note: MDPI stays neutral with regard to jurisdictional claims in published maps and institutional affiliations.

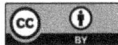

Copyright: © 2022 by the authors. Licensee MDPI, Basel, Switzerland. This article is an open access article distributed under the terms and conditions of the Creative Commons Attribution (CC BY) license (https://creativecommons.org/licenses/by/4.0/).

[1] University of Pittsburgh School of Medicine, Pittsburgh, PA 15213, USA; lebowitz.steven@medstudent.pitt.edu
[2] Cardio-Thoracic Surgery Department, Heart and Vascular Centre, Maastricht University Medical Centre (MUMC), 6200 MD Maastricht, The Netherlands; lorussobs@gmail.com
[3] Clinical Department of Cardiac Surgery, Central Clinical Hospital of the Ministry of Interior and Administration, Centre of Postgraduate Medical Education, 00-213 Warsaw, Poland; suwalski.piotr@gmail.com
[4] Thoracic Research Centre, Collegium Medicum, Nicolaus Copernicus University, Innovative Medical Forum, 87-100 Bydgoszcz, Poland
[5] Department for the Treatment and Study of Cardiothoracic Diseases and Cardiothoracic Transplantation, IRCCS-ISMETT, 90127 Palermo, Italy; graffa@ismett.edu (G.M.R.); sagreco@ismett.edu (M.G.); cgandolfo@ismett.edu (C.G.); cmignosa@ismett.edu (C.M.); mpilato@ismett.edu (M.P.)
[6] Department of Cardiothoracic Surgery, Division of Cardiac Surgery, University of Pittsburgh Medical Center Heart & Vascular Institute, University of Pittsburgh School of Medicine, Pittsburgh, PA 15213, USA; chud@upmc.edu
* Correspondence: kowalewskimariusz@gazeta.pl; Tel.: +48-502269249
† These authors contributed equally to this work.

Abstract: Background: Hypertrophic obstructive cardiomyopathy (HOCM) is a heterogeneous disease with different clinical presentations, albeit producing similar dismal long-term outcomes if left untreated. Several approaches are available for the treatment of HOCM; e.g., alcohol septal ablation (ASA) and surgical myectomy (SM). The objectives of the current review were to (1) discuss the place of the standard invasive treatment modalities (ASA and SM) for HOCM; (2) summarize and compare novel techniques for the management of HOCM; (3) analyze current guidelines addressing HOCM management; and (4) offer suggestions for the treatment of complex HOCM presentations. Methods: We searched the literature and attempted to gather the most relevant and impactful available evidence on ASA, SM, and other invasive means of treatment of HOCM. The literature search yielded thousands of results, and 103 significant publications were ultimately included. Results: We critically analyzed available guidelines and provided context in the setting of patient selection for standard and novel treatment modalities. This review offers the most comprehensive analysis to-date of available invasive treatments for HOCM. These include the standard treatments, SM and ASA, as well as novel treatments such as dual-chamber pacing and radiofrequency catheter ablation. We also account for complex pathoanatomic presentations and current guidelines to offer suggestions for tailored care of patients with HOCM. Finally, we consider promising future therapies for HOCM. Conclusions: HOCM is a heterogeneous disease associated with poor outcomes if left untreated. Several strategies for treatment of HOCM are available but patient selection for the procedure is crucial.

Keywords: hypertrophic obstructive cardiomyopathy; septal myectomy; alcohol septal ablation; left ventricle outflow tract obstruction; mitral valve surgery

1. Introduction

Hypertrophic cardiomyopathy (HCM) is the most common genetic heart disease, affecting about one in 200–500 people, but only a minority of cases (10–20%) are identified clinically [1,2]. It results from a genetic disorder with an autosomal dominant inheritance pattern caused by mutations in sarcomere proteins [3]. These mutations manifest phenotypically with myocardial hypertrophy and a small left ventricular cavity [3]. A subset of people with HCM have an obstructed left ventricular outflow tract (LVOT), which is the hallmark of hypertrophic obstructive cardiomyopathy (HOCM) [3]. One of the potential long-term effects of HOCM is heart failure (HF), and patients are at an increased risk of sudden cardiac death (SCD). Thus, intervention is critical in patients with advanced HOCM. The gold-standard treatment for HOCM is surgical septal myectomy (SM), in which a portion of the interventricular septum is removed to decrease LVOT obstruction (LVOTO) [4]. Alcohol septal ablation (ASA) is an alternative treatment for HOCM. This is a minimally invasive, intravascular procedure in which absolute alcohol is injected into the ventricular septal myocardial vasculature to induce necrosis of septal myocytes, thereby decreasing septal thickness and related LVOTO [5]. Although ASA is favorable in terms of invasiveness and recovery, SM is still considered the primary intervention for HOCM [5].

Importantly, there is a distinct advantage to invasive management over medical treatment of HOCM patients [6]. Indeed, more recently, other contributing factors in LVOTO were disclosed: the mitral valve (MV) and its subvalvular apparatus (SVA). It is noteworthy that in some patients with HOCM, the mechanism of LVOTO is entirely independent of septal hypertrophy. However, lengthened anterior mitral leaflet, bifid papillary muscles, and abnormal chordal attachment may also be causally associated with LVOTO [7]. Given this knowledge, treatment of the mitral valve and subvalvular apparatus should be considered along with SM where indicated [8].

Defining the appropriate treatment for HOCM might be challenging due to the extreme heterogeneity of the disease. SM with or without MV procedures and ASA are well recognized options for treatment [9]. The best approach, however, is still a matter of debate, and a patient-tailored approach represents a critical and necessary process.

2. Left Ventricular Outflow Tract Obstruction—Outcomes If Left Untreated

About two thirds of patients with HCM present with LV cavity obstruction, accounting for a diagnosis of HOCM [10]. Mechanisms of LVOTO in HCM are many, including isolated massive septal hypertrophy; systolic anterior motion (SAM) of the MV, in which the MV leaflet contacts the septum during systole; papillary muscle (PM) anomalies; and mitral leaflet anomalies [11]. Furthermore, these mechanisms may intervene in an isolated or associated fashion. The definition of LVOTO is dynamic outflow pressure >30 mmHg; this phenomenon is typically considered hemodynamically important when pressure >50 mmHg [11].

Patients with HCM and HOCM are at an increased risk of arrhythmogenic SCD [10]. This risk of SCD in HOCM does not have a correlation with LVOT gradient severity [1] and, therefore, is not only present in symptomatic individuals but also in those who are young and asymptomatic, including young athletes [8] in whom HCM is the most common cause of SCD [1]. Implantable cardioverter defibrillators (ICDs) are an effective treatment for terminating these potentially lethal ventricular arrhythmias. Complications related to the ICD implant, however, besides procedural complications [10], include inappropriate discharge and related anxiety and mental anguish. The decision to implant an ICD requires risk stratification. Risk factors for SCD include: patient history of ventricular fibrillation, sustained ventricular tachycardia, non-sustained ventricular tachycardia, or unexplained syncope; maximum left ventricular wall thickness >3 cm; abnormal blood pressure response during exercise; and family history of SCD in the setting of HCM [12]. Recently, late gadolinium enhancement on cardiac magnetic resonance imaging, a surrogate of myocardial fibrosis, apical aneurysms, and systolic dysfunction (LVEF < 50%), have been identified as significant risk factors for SCD [11].

The 2020 AHA/ACC guidelines offer the latest and, as yet most comprehensive description of SCD risk in patients with HCM. This document provides an algorithm for risk assessment, which helps to inform providers on the necessity of ICD implantation [13]. Prior to this, the 2014 ESC guidelines offered a formula which incorporates clinical variables to generate a risk score (SCD risk score > 6% is considered high and calls for ICD implantation) [11,12].

The superiority of invasive over medical treatment has been demonstrated. Indeed, Ball et al. analyzed 649 HOCM patients with resting LVOTO and compared invasively and conservatively treated groups. This study showed significantly lower mortality at 1-, 5-, and 10 years in the invasive group compared to the conservative cohort [14]. Therefore, patients with HOCM represent a unique opportunity to decrease the risk of SCD through septal reduction therapy. Although septal reduction has yet to be indicated for the reduction of SCD risk, a growing body of evidence supports that SM and ASA do decrease risk for SCD [10].

Heart failure is a known long-term outcome of untreated and refractory HOCM [10]. Patients treated with SM have a reduction in LVOTO and excellent long-term outcomes equivalent to the general population and superior to HOCM patients treated conservatively [4,15]. ASA is also a safe and effective treatment for HOCM, with good long-term survival compared to the general population and to those treated with SM [16,17].

The LVOT gradient itself may present an alternative method of risk stratification for patients with HOCM. This concept was observed in Lu et al.'s study, which stratified patient prognosis (using a composite adverse event rate) according to LVOT gradients. They found that patients with the best prognosis had a provoked LVOT gradient between 30–89 mm Hg, while a resting LVOT gradient >30 mm Hg was associated with the worst prognosis. Patients with a provoked LVOT gradient <30 mm Hg or >90 mm Hg fell into an intermediate risk category [18].

3. Invasive Management: Alcohol Septal Ablation

ASA is a minimally invasive procedure with a shorter recovery time compared to SM. These factors make it an attractive option for many HOCM patients without a clear indication for SM, such as requiring a concomitant MV procedure. Several studies have demonstrated the safety and efficacy of ASA; in one retrospective analysis of 952 patients who underwent ASA, Batzner et al. reported a 95.8% 5-year survival [19]. A separate, multinational study of 1275 ASA patients determined 1-, 5-, and 10-year survival to be 95%, 89%, and 77%, respectively [17].

Despite this promising data, ASA also carries significant risks. In a smaller study of 80 ASA patients, permanent pacemaker implantation was required in almost 10% of the treated patients, 10% required a re-do ASA and 2.5% went on to require SM, despite the initial procedure providing a significant reduction in septal thickness [20]. Batzner et al. demonstrated that 10.5% of patients required placement of a permanent pacemaker at the time of ASA, 1.9% required subsequent SM, and 5.1% required pacemaker placement after ASA [19]. Another study of 91 HOCM patients who underwent ASA found that approximately one in three patients had major complications, including cardiac death. Additionally, most complications were late, indicating the long-term risks associated with ASA [21].

The above-mentioned data are relevant in evaluating ASA for the treatment of HOCM, but other factors, including provider experience, must also be considered. A retrospective analysis by Veselka et al. addressed clinical experience as a determinant of ASA outcomes [22]. This study, including 1310 ASA patients at multiple clinical centers, analyzed differences between the first 50 patients ("first-50") and subsequent patients ("over-50") treated at each center. Significant findings between the first-50 and over-50 groups included a reduction in major cardiovascular adverse events from 21% to 12%. Additionally, the following significant outcomes were determined for the over-50 group: less major adverse events and cardiovascular mortality; less self-reported dyspnea of New York Heart Association (NYHA) class III and IV; less likelihood of having an LVOT gradient >30 mm Hg; and less likelihood of having a repeated septal reduction therapy [22]. Another study from the Mayo Clinic demonstrated the excellent outcomes of ASA at experienced centers, showing no significant difference in survival at a 5.7-year average follow-up compared to age- and sex-matched patients who underwent SM [16].

Age is yet another important factor to consider when discussing the safety of ASA for the treatment of HOCM. An analysis of 1197 patients with HOCM who underwent ASA aimed to elucidate outcomes between patients </= 50 years old ("young"), 51–64 years old ("middle-aged"), and >/= 65 years old ("older"); it was found that young patients had a significantly lower 30-day mortality and pacemaker implantation incidence than older patients. Additionally, young patients had a significantly reduced annual mortality rate compared to middle-aged and older patients [23].

Overall, available data suggest that ASA is a safe procedure, especially in younger patients, with a reduced length of recovery compared to myectomy. Significant drawbacks to discuss with patients, however, include the relatively high risk of permanent pacemaker implantation and re-intervention either via re-do ASA or the more invasive SM. Finally, any patient seeking treatment with ASA should be referred to a highly experienced center of clinical excellence for optimal outcomes. Evidence on ASA is further gathered in Table 1.

Table 1. Summary of the salient characteristics and results of studies on alcohol septal ablation for the treatment of hypertrophic obstructive cardiomyopathy discussed in this review.

Authors	Institution	N (Total)	Symptomatic Status Pre-ASA	N (Patients with Pre-ASA MR)	Average Pre-ASA LVOT Gradient (mm Hg)	Average Post-ASA LVOT Gradient (mm Hg)	Major Outcomes
Batzner et al. [19]	KWM Standort Juliusspital, Germany	952	698 patients NYHA Class III/IV	N/A	63.9 +/− 38.2	33.6 +/− 29.8	- Significant reduction in LVOT gradient - Estimated 5-year survival of 98.5% - 10.5% permanent pacemaker at time of ASA - 1.9% subsequent SM - 5.1% permanent pacemaker later on
Veselka et al. [17]	10 tertiary invasive European centers	1275	Average NYHA Class 2.9 +/− 0.5	N/A	67 +/− 36	16 +/− 21	- 30-day mortality of 1% - 1-, 5-, 10-year survival of 98%, 89%, 77% (respectively) - Independent predictors of all-cause mortality: pre-ASA age, septal thickness, and NYHA class; and LVOT gradient at last f/u - Significant improvement in NYHA class and LVOTG
Aguiar et al. [20]	Santa Maria Hospital, Lisbon, Portugal	80	74 patients NYHA class III/IV	26 (moderate MR)	96.3 +/− 34.6	27.1 +/− 27.4 (successful); 58.2 +/− 16.6 (unsuccessful)	- 6.3% minor complications; 2.5% major complications; 8.8% permanent pacemaker - 85.7% of patients achieved >50% reduction in LVOT gradient (successful) - 77% of patients with NYHA III/IV experienced reduction to NYHA I/II

Table 1. Cont.

Authors	Institution	N (Total)	Symptomatic Status Pre-ASA	N (Patients with Pre-ASA MR)	Average Pre-ASA LVOT Gradient (mm Hg)	Average Post-ASA LVOT Gradient (mm Hg)	Major Outcomes
ten Cate et al. [21]	Erasmus University Medical Center Rotterdam, Netherlands	91	91 patients NYHA class III/IV	MR grade 1.5 +/− 0.9	92 +/− 25	8 +/− 17	- 1-, 5-, 8-year survival of 96%, 86%, 67% (respectively) for ASA - 1-, 5-, 8-year survival of 100%, 96% 96% (respectively) for SM - ASA carried ~5-fold increased risk of composite cardiac death and aborted SCD compared to SM
Veselka et al. [22]	Euro-ASA Registry, 11 European Centers	1310	1098 patients NYHA class III/IV	N/A	73.9 +/− 41.8 ("first-50" group); 66.8 +/− 34.5 ("over-50" group)	20.8 +/− 27.5 ("first-50" group); 14.0 +/− 17.2 ("over-50" group)	- 30-day CV death rate of 2.1% for first-50, 0.4% for over-50 ($p = 0.01$) - 30-day pacemaker implantation rate of 15% for first-50, 9% for over-50 ($p < 0.01$) - Significantly greater rates of major adverse events and CV death in long-term f/u for first-50 group - Significantly greater rates of NYHA class III/IV, LVOT gradient > 30 mm Hg, and re-do septal reduction for first-50 group
Sorajja et al. [16]	Mayo Clinic, USA	177	177 patients NYHA class III/IV	N/A	70 +/− 40	85 +/− 16% reduction in LVOT gradient	- No significant difference in survival in ASA compared to general population and SM
Liebregts et al. [23]	7 tertiary invasive European centers	1197	NYHA class III/V by age group: 298 patients </= 50 years; 352 patients 51–64 years; 363 patients >/= 65 years	N/A	Age </= 50 years: 110 +/− 39; Age 51–64 years: 111 +/− 44; Age >/= 65 years: 121 +/− 47	Age </= 50 years: 26 +/− 31; Age 51–64 years: 27 +/− 35; Age >/= 65 years: 26 +/− 33	- Significantly lower mortality and ICD implantation in young vs. older patients - Similar adverse arrhythmic event rates among groups - Annual mortality rates of 1%, 2%, and 5% for young, middle-aged, and older patients, respectively ($p < 0.01$) - For young patients, age, residual LVOT gradient, and female sex were independent predictors of mortality

ASA, alcohol septal ablation; LVOT, left ventricle outflow tract; SM, surgical myectomy; MR, mitral regurgitation; SCD, sudden cardiac death; CV, cardiovascular; ICD, implantable cardioverter-defibrillator; N/A, not available.

4. Invasive Management: Surgical Myectomy

Surgical septal myectomy is considered the gold-standard treatment for HOCM [4]. Figure 1.

This technique is more invasive than ASA, as it most often involves median sternotomy. Once the heart is exposed, the operative technique involves removal of the hypertrophied portion of the muscular ventricular septum through an aortotomy in order to reduce the LVOTO. Figure 2.

Myectomy alone is associated with low operative mortality (<1%) and good long-term survival [24]. Septal approach without opening the aorta and approaching the IV septum through the mitral valve is a potential option (Figure 1).

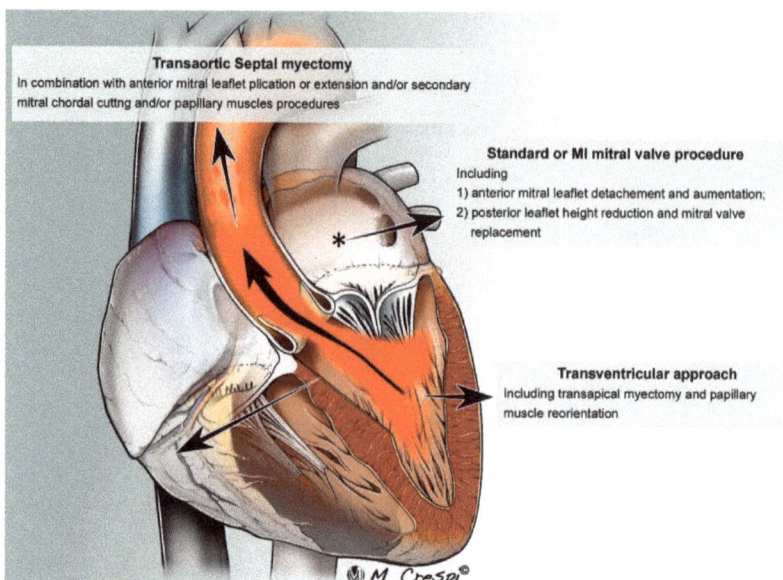

Figure 1. Summary of the proposed techniques for LVOT obstruction surgery. LA, left atrium. *—Conventional and minimally invasive mitral valve surgery approaches.

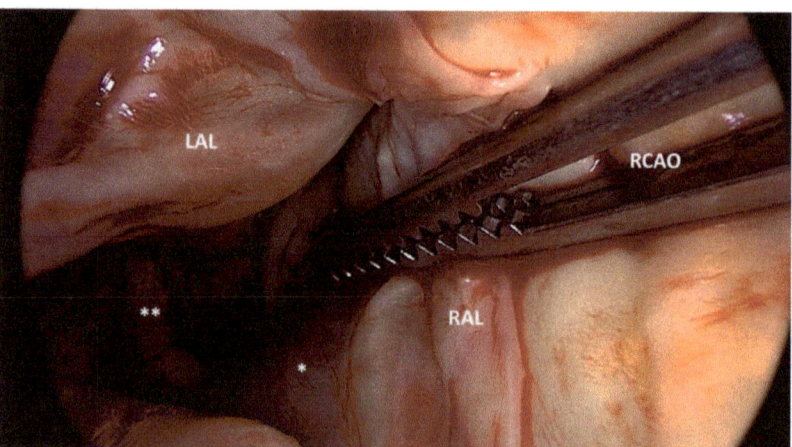

Figure 2. Surgical view of left ventricle outflow tract (LVOT) obstruction and the bulging of the interventricular septum (*) after left and right aortic valve leaflet retraction (LAL and RAL). RCAO: right coronary artery ostium. Jet lesions (**) produced by turbulence in the LVOT.

The safety and efficacy of SM have been extensively validated. In a retrospective study of 93 patients with HOCM who underwent myectomy in China, NYHA functional class was significantly decreased from an average of 3.09 to 1.12. Additionally, SAM of the anterior mitral leaflet (AML) was completely resolved in 98.9% of patients. Of note, SAM was present in all patients preoperatively. The LVOT gradient was also significantly reduced. In this cohort, 37 patients underwent concomitant operations with myectomy with no operative mortality [25]. These results indicate that SM, with or without concomitant operations, is safe and efficacious when performed at a dedicated and experienced referral center. In another study, Ommen et al. reported long-term results of HCM patients.

Patients were divided into three groups: those who underwent myectomy; those with LVOT obstruction who received conservative treatment; and those with non-obstructive HCM. Patients in the operative group did not have significantly different 1-, 5-, and 10-year survival compared to the non-obstructive group, nor compared to age- and sex-matched members of the general population. Additionally, operative patients had significantly better 1-, 5-, and 10-year survival compared to the conservatively treated HOCM group [4]. These findings demonstrate that SM is safe and that long-term outcomes are improved in HOCM patients who undergo myectomy compared to those treated conservatively.

A feared complication of HOCM is SCD and ventricular septal disruption. A retrospective study of 125 patients from the Mayo Clinic sought to determine the efficacy of SM in reducing fatal cardiac arrhythmia events. All patients in this study received ICD implantation and were divided into myectomy and non-myectomy groups. Among the myectomy group, only one patient experienced defibrillator discharge as opposed to 12 patients in the non-myectomy group ($p = 0.004$) over a follow-up period of about 4.5 years [26]. These results suggest that SM may reduce the likelihood of SCD in HOCM patients by reducing the rate of fatal cardiac arrhythmias after surgery.

Atrial fibrillation (AF) is a significant comorbidity in HCM, occurring in as many as 18% of patients [27]. In a recent study, Lapenna et al. sought to determine the feasibility of surgical ablation for refractory AF in HOCM patients undergoing concomitant cardiac procedures. Most patients underwent concomitant SM, while a smaller proportion of the 31-patient cohort underwent mitral valve repair or replacement. This study reported an operative mortality of 6% but a promising 7-year survival (87 +/− 6.1%). Moreover, they found that surgical ablation relieved AF at medium-term timepoints for a majority of patients, albeit also requiring medical therapy for satisfactory results [28].

It is also important to understand which patients may be poor candidates for SM. In a cohort of 503 SM patients, 19 (3.8%) were refractory to surgical intervention with a post-operative NYHA class of III-IV. While massive septal thickness ($\geq$30 mm) and younger age (<30 y.o.) were identified as predictors of suboptimal response to surgery [29] due to persistent or recurrent heart failure postoperatively, most young patients and those with massive hypertrophy experienced significant symptom relief and sustained clinical improvement from SM [29].

A wealth of data vouches for the efficacy and safety of SM. Patients who undergo this procedure have excellent short- and long-term outcomes. These include low operative mortality, decreased NYHA class, excellent long-term survival, and decreased event rates for arrhythmia. Thus, SM should be considered as the primary intervention for HOCM when performed by experienced operators. Table 2 summarizes the evidence on SM in the treatment of HOCM.

Table 2. Summary of the salient characteristics and results of studies on surgical myectomy for the treatment of hypertrophic obstructive cardiomyopathy discussed in this review.

Authors	Institution	N (Total)	Symptomatic Status Pre-SM	N (Patients with Pre-SM MR)	Average Pre-SM LVOT Gradient (mm Hg)	Average Post-SM LVOT Gradient (mm Hg)	Concomitant Procedure(s)	Major Outcomes
Wang et al. [25]	National Center for Cardiovascular Diseases, Beijing, China	93	80 patients NYHA class III/IV	32 (mild); 30 (moderate); 10 (moderately severe); 1 (severe)	91.76 +/− 25.08	14.78 +/− 14.01	10 MVR; 9 MVr; 6 AVR; 2 TV plasty; 18 CABG; 3 modified Maze; 2 cardiac tumor resection; 1 RVOT reconstruction; 12 multiple	- Significant reduction in NYHA Class - Complete resolution of SAM in 98.9% - Significant reduction in LVOT gradient - 0% operative mortality
Ommen et al. [4]	Mayo Clinic, USA	1337 (289 SM; 228 non-operative; 820 non-obstructive HCM)	348 patients NYHA III/IV (256 SM; 34 non-operative; 58 non-obstructive HCM)	71 (21 SM; 24 non-operative; 26 non-obstructive HCM)	29.2 +/− 39 (67.3 +/− 41 SM; 68.0 +/− 31 non-operative; 5.1 +/− 7 non-obstructive HCM)		64 patients	- 0.8% operative mortality - 1-, 5-, and 10-year post-SM survival similar to non-obstructive HCM and general population - Survival benefit for SM over non-operative
McLeod et al. [26]	Mayo Clinic, USA	125	48 patients NYHA III/IV (27 SM; 21 non-SM)	N/A	59 +/− 35 (SM group)	1 +/− 3 (SM group)	N/A	- 12 non-SM patients vs. 1 SM patient sustained ICD discharge to prevent SCD during f/u
Lapenna et al. [28]	Vita-Salute San Raffaele University, Milan, Italy	31	17 patients NYHA III/IV	12	56 +/− 31.8	N/A	Surgical ablation with SM (77%) and/or MVR/MVr (39%)	- 6% hospital mortality - 87 +/− 6.1% 7-year survival - 1- and 6-year arrhythmia control rates of 96 +/− 3.5% and 80 +/− 8.1% (respectively)
Wells et al. [29]	Tufts Medical Center, USA	503	503 patients NYHA III/IV	34	61 +/− 38	N/A	N/A	- 96% improvement to NYHA I/II - Non-responders to SM were younger with greater extent of septal hypertrophy

SM, surgical myectomy; LVOT, left ventricle outflow tract; MVR, mitral valve replacement; MVr, mitral valve repair; AVR, aortic valve replacement; CABG, coronary artery bypass grafting; RVOT, right ventricle outflow tract; SAM, systolic anterior motion; HCM, hypertrophic cardiomyopathy; SCD, sudden cardiac death; CV, cardiovascular; ICD, implantable cardioverter-defibrillator; N/A, not available.

5. Surgical Myectomy vs. Alcohol Septal Ablation: Meta-Analyses

To date, no randomized controlled trials have compared SM and ASA. However, several meta-analyses have made efforts to compare these procedures in a head-to-head fashion. The studies report, for the most part, roughly similar findings. They agree that SM and ASA provide similar: improvement in NYHA class [30–32]; in-hospital [31], short-term [32], and long-term [9,32–34] mortality; and rates of SCD [9,33,34]. Many of the meta-analyses also conclude that ASA is associated with significantly greater rates of permanent pacemaker implantation [9,31–34] and re-intervention [9,33,34]. Interestingly, the latest meta-analysis (Osman et al., 2019) reported significantly increased rates of peri-procedural mortality and stroke in patients who underwent SM [9]. The seven meta-analyses discussed in this review are described in Table 3.

Table 3. Meta-Analyses comparing septal reduction therapies (ASA and SM).

Authors	Year	N (Total)	N (ASA Patients)	N (SM Patients)	N (Studies Included)	Outcome
Zeng et al. [30]	2006	177	86	91	3	Both ASA and SM provide LVOT gradient- and clinical improvement, more PPM following ASA.
Alam et al. [31]	2009	351	183	168	5	Both procedures safe, slightly higher LVOT gradients following ASA.
Agarwal et al. [32]	2010	708	410	298	12	Higher LVOT gradients reduction following SM, similar safety and resolution of clinical symptoms.
Leonardi et al. [35]	2010	4094	2207	1887	27	Low rates of mortality and SCD after both ASA and SM; adjusted odds ratios for SCD lower in ASA;
Liebregts et al. [34]	2015	4804	2013	2791	24	Higher rates of PPM and reinterventions following ASA; no differences in long-term
Singh et al. [33]	2016	1824	805	1019	10	Higher rates of PPM and reinterventions following ASA; no differences in short and long-term
Osman et al. [9]	2019	8453	4213	4240	40	ASA associated with lower periprocedural mortality and stroke but higher rates of PPM and reintervention, no differences in long-term

ASA, alcohol septal ablation; SM, surgical myectomy; LVOT, left ventricle outflow tract; PPM, permanent pacemaker; SCD, sudden cardiac death.

The analyses conducted by Zeng et al. [30] and Alam et al. [31] included only three and five studies, respectively. Taking this into account, along with their relatively older publication dates, these meta-analyses may be considered less robust than their counterparts. Conversely, the meta-analysis by Osman et al. [9] is not only the latest, but also the largest (40 studies included with a total of 4240 patients) analysis to-date. This study asserts that ASA is associated with more ICD implantation and greater rates of re-intervention, whereas SM is associated with greater rates of peri-procedural mortality and stroke [9]. The former claim is supported by older literature [9,31,34], but the latter is novel and warrants further investigation.

Baseline patient characteristics must also be considered when comparing ASA and SM. Three of the meta-analyses found that patients who underwent SM were significantly younger than those who were treated with ASA [31,33,35]. After adjusting for baseline patient characteristics (LVOT gradient, age, sex, NYHA class, septal wall thickness, and risk factors for SCD), Leonardi et al. reported a lower odds ratio for the effect of ASA on all-cause mortality and SCD compared with SM [35]. These findings underscore the importance of considering factors that may affect which patients are selected for which procedure. For example, patients who undergo SM may have greater disease morbidity than those who opt for ASA, contributing to increased mortality in SM patients. Table 3 summarizes the data on previous meta-analyses comparing ASA vs SM for HOCM.

6. Alternative Invasive Treatment Options for HOCM

Dual-chamber (DDD) pacing has been considered as an alternative approach for the treatment of HOCM. Several studies have found that DDD pacing significantly reduces the LVOT gradient at immediate, short-term, and long-term time points [36–42]. Almost all of these studies, however, found that DDD pacing does not reduce the LVOT gradient below 30 mm Hg [37–41]. Additionally, Yue-Cheng et al. found that DDD pacing significantly reduces SAM at 1–4 years post-implantation [37].

Other important measures to consider are ventricular septal reduction; NYHA class and quality of life; and mitral regurgitation (MR). Several studies have found that DDD pacing offers no significant reduction in septal thickness [36,37,43]. Extensive evidence does suggest, however, that DDD pacing offers a significant reduction in NYHA class [36,38,39,41,42,44] and improvement in other quality of life scores [39–41,44]. Finally, Pavin et al. found that DDD pacing can significantly improve the degree of MR in select patients. The patients in this study whose MR was refractory to pacing also experienced minimal reduction in the LVOT gradient or had non-AML elongation abnormalities (including MV prolapse or annulus calcification) [45].

Despite promising evidence for the use of DDD pacing in HOCM, it remains inferior to SM and ASA. In a comparative study of 39 patients (20 SM; 19 DDD pacing), Ommen et al. found that SM is superior to DDD pacing in reducing LVOT gradient; providing symptomatic improvement; increasing exercise duration; and increasing maximal oxygen consumption [46]. Two studies comparing DDD pacing with ASA demonstrated that these therapies provide a similar reduction in LVOT gradient [43,44]. It was found, however, that ASA is superior in reducing NYHA class [42] and reducing septal thickness [43].

The data presented above suggest that DDD pacing is capable of reducing the LVOT gradient and SAM, as well as improving MR and NYHA class. Importantly, DDD pacing provides no significant reduction in septal thickness and is inferior to SM in improving hemodynamic and functional measures and to ASA in improving NYHA class and reducing septal thickness. Pending stronger evidence, there may be a role for DDD pacing in patients with HOCM for whom SM and ASA are contraindicated and who have mild LVOT gradients and limited septal hypertrophy.

Another novel approach to the treatment of HOCM is radiofrequency catheter ablation (RFCA). This is a percutaneous procedure in which radio waves (as opposed to alcohol, as in ASA) are used to create an area of necrosis in the ventricular septum. This may provide a more targeted approach than ASA, since limitations of the latter include anatomic variability of septal perforator arteries in 5–15% of patients [47], complete heart block, and induction of arrhythmia [48].

Studies have shown that RFCA is capable of significantly reducing the LVOT gradient and NYHA class at acute [49,50], medium-term [47,48,50], and long-term [48,50,51] time points. Liu et al. found that RFCA resulted in an initial increase in septal thickness followed by a significant decrease at 1, 3, and 6 months [50]. They also reported a significant reduction in MR [50]. Another study demonstrated a significant reduction in septal thickness at 6 months [47]. Important complications of RFCA have been reported in several studies, including transient pulmonary edema in one of seven patients [48] and complete AV block requiring permanent pacemaker implantation in four of nineteen patients [49].

Currently, there are not enough data to support the use of RFCA in the treatment of HOCM. The few small studies published on this subject, however, provide preliminary support for the safety and efficacy of RFCA. If future, larger studies support these early results, there may be a role for RFCA in the treatment of HOCM patients who are poor surgical candidates and have poor vascular anatomy that is incompatible with ASA. There are no comparative studies of RFCA and ASA, and inferences regarding safety in terms of arrhythmias or postoperative PPM implantation are vague.

7. The Mitral Valve

The mitral valve is classically implicated in the pathophysiology of HOCM via SAM of the AML. SAM can also occur, however, due to involvement of an elongated posterior mitral leaflet [52]. The mitral valve and subvalvular apparatus may contribute to HOCM through SAM-independent mechanisms. Figure 3.

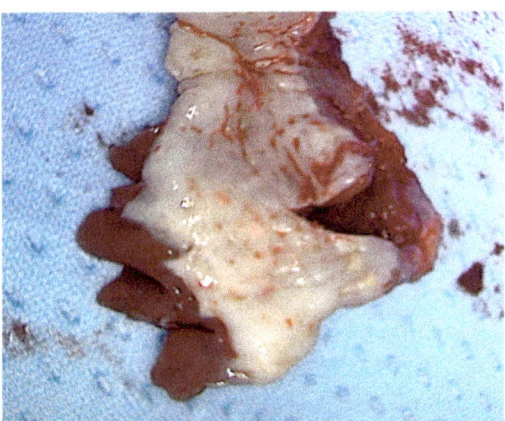

Figure 3. Specimen of interventricular septum showing endocardial fibrosis secondary to trauma caused by systolic anterior motion of the anterior leaflet of the mitral valve.

These anatomic abnormalities include abnormally long MV leaflets (anterior or posterior), bifid PM, and papillary muscle attachment directly to the mitral leaflet base. These anomalies can cause LVOTO even in the absence of septal hypertrophy [6]. Figure 4.

Surgical approaches to the treatment of the above-stated abnormalities include myectomy with concomitant MV replacement (MVR) or repair (MVr) with or without papillary muscle repositioning (Figure 5).

Many studies have validated the safety and efficacy of concomitant surgical reduction of MR with SM [52–61]. Given the inherent long-term effects of MVR (anticoagulation with a prosthetic valve, short life of a tissue valve), MVr may be favorable when possible. A prospective randomized study found that patients who underwent MVr with SM, as opposed to MVR with SM, had significantly greater overall survival at 2 years and less thromboembolic events; all other outcomes were similar [62]. Additionally, a quantitative meta-analysis of 23 studies found that MVr is superior to MVR in terms of reoperation and thromboembolic events. This meta-analysis concluded that MVr should be the first line treatment over MVR in HOCM patients with MR undergoing concomitant SM [63]. These studies fail, however, to address patients on an individual basis. In a retrospective study of 115 patients who underwent SM with either MVR (N = 48) or MVr (N = 67), Kaple et al. underscored the importance of anatomic variability in operative technique. They found that MVr is a durable method but note its limited use in patients with appropriate anatomical anomalies, such as long leaflets and degenerative MV pathology; such patients may comprise as much as half of the population of interest [64].

Some HOCM patients exhibit minimal septal hypertrophy (<18 mm); the primary mechanism of LVOTO in these patients is related to MV pathology. In these patients, myectomy is sometimes forgone in favor of MVR due to fear of iatrogenic ventricular septal defect (VSD) [65]. Two studies have demonstrated, however, that SM with or without concomitant MV intervention is safe in this population [65,66].

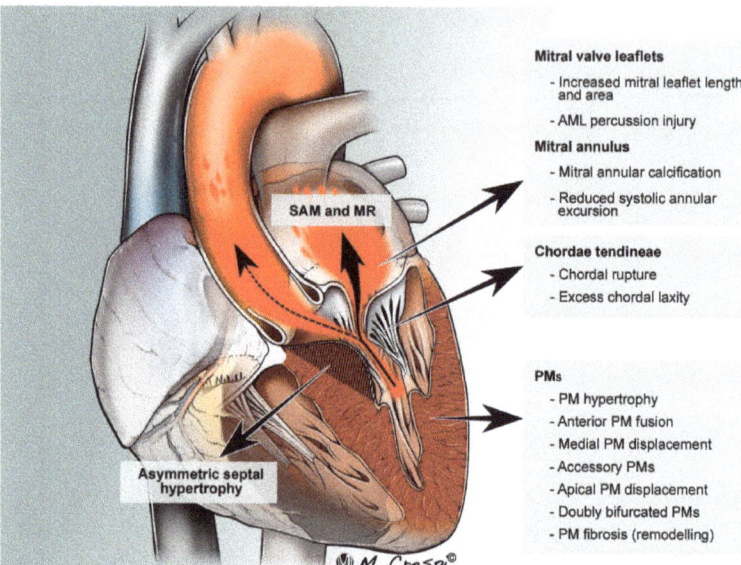

Figure 4. Pathophysiology of left ventricle outflow tract (LVOT) obstruction (dotted arrow) in hypertrophic obstructive cardiomyopathy. SAM: systolic anterior motion; MR: mitral regurgitation, MV, mitral valve; AML, anterior mitral leaflet; PM, papillary muscle; APM, anterior papillary muscle; MPM, medial papillary muscle. (from Silbiger J.J. et al. J Am Soc Echocardiogr 2016).

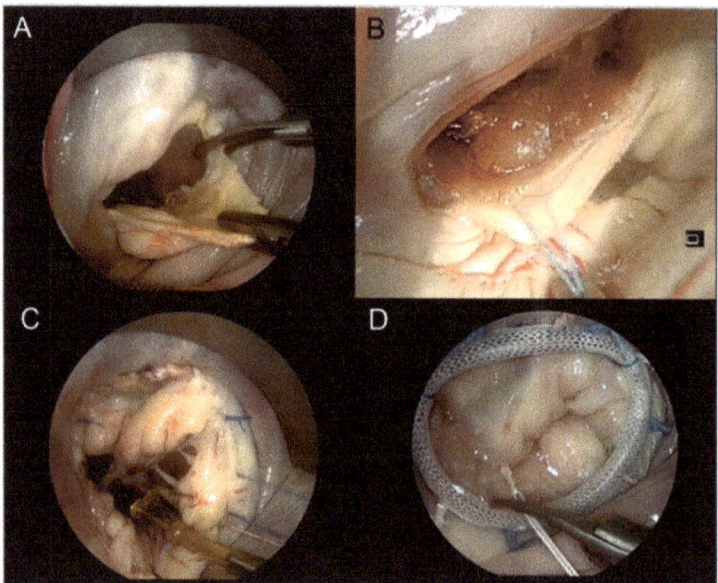

Figure 5. Minimally invasive HOCM surgery. Transmitral SM. Incision at the base of mitral leaflet (**A**); pull back suture placement to facilitate SM (**B**); mitral valve repair with loop-technique (**C**); completed mitral valve annuloplasty (**D**) concomitant to LVOTO repair.

It is important to consider MV anomalies when selecting between SM and ASA. Studies have found that SM with concomitant MV intervention is superior to ASA in reducing SAM and MR in appropriately selected patients [67,68]. Additionally, SM with concomitant MV intervention can be performed safely and efficaciously through a minimally invasive trans-mitral approach. Studies have demonstrated reduced SAM and LVOT gradients via these techniques [69,70]. Figure 5.

Myectomy with concomitant MVR or MVr is safe and efficacious and should be performed in patients with MR and/or MV anatomical anomalies contributing to HOCM. The choice of MVR versus MVr should be made on a patient-by-patient basis and consider the individual's anatomy. Anatomy favoring MVr includes lengthened MV leaflet(s), degenerative valve disease, and subvalvular morphologies including anomalous PM insertion and chordal attachment at the valve base [64]. This, again, underscores the importance of careful evaluation of preoperative imaging. MVr should be considered over MVR when possible due to the inherent implications associated with exogenous valves. In addition, mild septal hypertrophy does not necessarily preclude SM with or without concomitant MV intervention. These patients should be considered for the correct procedure on an individual basis without strict exclusion of SM due to fear of creating a VSD. In addition, in patients with intrinsic MV pathology, SM, with or without concomitant MV procedure, is favorable over ASA. It has also been demonstrated that minimally invasive options are safe when combining SM with MV intervention.

8. The Subvalvular Apparatus

Papillary muscle (PM) morphology can contribute as a mechanism of LVOTO in HOCM [71] and particularly in patients with a minor degree of septal hypertrophy (<15 mm) [72]. This may be readily identified via echocardiography and must be considered in preoperative evaluation [73]. Numerous studies have validated the safety and efficacy of SM with concomitant PM realignment, excision of anomalous PM, and cutting of abnormally thickened chordae tendinae [74–79]. Figure 6.

Ferrazi et al. have demonstrated that surgical treatment addressing septal hypertrophy and valvular defects is effective in decreasing LVOTO, thus relieving HF symptoms while also avoiding later MV replacement [74].

A prospective randomized study found that SM with concomitant subvalvular intervention was superior in terms of abolishing LVOTO and improving MR as compared to SM alone in patients with subvalvular pathology [80].

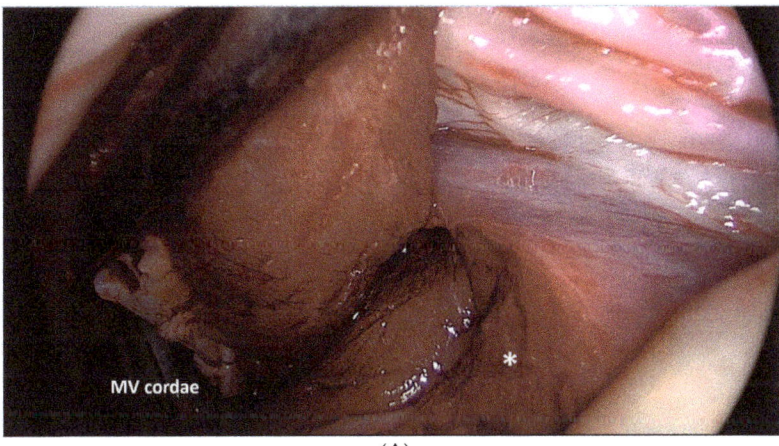

(A)

Figure 6. *Cont.*

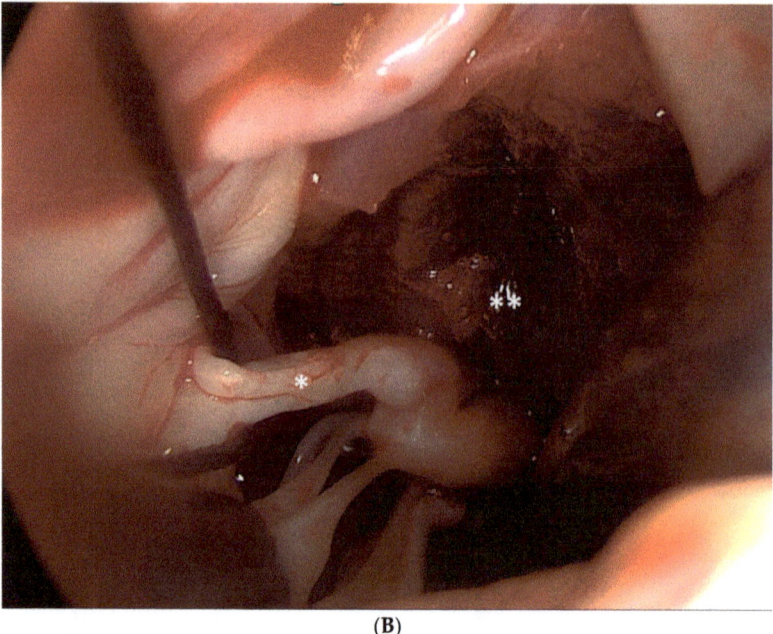

(B)

Figure 6. Surgical myectomy (*) was performed starting at the nadir of the right coronary sinus, and extended apically to achieve the exposure of the papillary muscles. MV: mitral valve (**A**). Surgical view of the diseased mitral valve secondary cordae (*) and papillary muscles (**) after myectomy. It is noteworthy that the bases of the papillary muscles are now visible (**B**).

Performing SM with a concomitant subvalvular procedure is a safe and efficacious operative strategy. Preoperative echocardiograms must be carefully evaluated to determine if subvalvular morphology requires intervention.

9. Mid-Ventricular and Apical Hypertrophy

Left ventricular hypertrophy (LVH) in HOCM is typically localized to the subaortic portion of the septum. Rarely, hypertrophy may be present in the mid-ventricular or apical septum [81]. Although rare, mid-ventricular obstruction is a very serious phenotype of HOCM as it has been identified as a predictor of adverse outcomes, including sudden death and potentially lethal arrhythmias [82].

Patients with mid-ventricular or apical hypertrophy often require unique operative approaches. The transapical approach is a relatively new operative technique that can be applied in cases of mid-ventricular and apical hypertrophy. A study of 113 patients with apical hypertrophy who underwent transapical myectomy reported acceptable mortality and survival and a 76% clinical improvement [83]. Several studies have found that patients with mid-ventricular obstruction can be safely and efficaciously treated with transapical myectomy, transaortic myectomy, or a combination of the two procedures. Findings included adequate survival and short- and long-term outcomes; improvement in NYHA class; and improvement in the LVOT gradients [84–86].

Patients with mid-ventricular and apical hypertrophy should be given special consideration. Use of transapical myectomy has provided a successful alternative to heart transplant in patients with apical hypertrophy. The transaortic approach can be extended for use in patients with mid-ventricular obstruction where applicable or can be combined with the transapical approach when obstruction extends distally.

10. ECMO and Other MCS

There is scant literature on the use of ECMO in the setting of HOCM. Case reports [87–89] demonstrate that in patients in hemodynamic crisis pre- and/or post-operatively, ECMO may be considered and used as bridging therapy until support can be withdrawn (Table 4).

Table 4. Salient characteristics and results of ECMO case reports discussed in this review.

Authors	Institution	Indication for ECMO	Outcomes
Husaini et al. [87]	Washington University School of Medicine, USA	Cardiogenic shock secondary to Takotsubo cardiomyopathy	V–A ECMO until patient stable enough for SM
Basic et al. [88]	Kerckhoff Heart and Thorax Center, Germany	Cardiogenic shock	ECMO until patient stable enough for SM with MVR
Williams et al. [89]	Prince Charles Hospital, Australia	Chronic thromboembolic pulmonary hypertension	ECMO pre- and post-operatively (pulmonary endarterectomy, SM, and MVR)

V–A ECMO, veno-arterial extracorporeal membrane oxygenation; SM, surgical myectomy; MVR, mitral valve replacement.

Several reports describe the use of mechanical circulatory support (MCS) systems in the setting of HOCM [90,91], mostly as a bridge-to-transplantation. These treatment strategies include percutaneous interventions with interatrial shunts, left atrial assist devices (LAADs), and ventricular assist devices (VADs) in various configurations [90], but the data is limited to single-heart transplantation excellence centres [92].

11. Guidelines

Several guidelines exist for the treatment of HOCM and fall into two categories: guidelines for cardiac pacing, and guidelines specifically addressing HCM. The 2008 ACC/AHA/ARS guidelines and 2013 ESC guidelines are the most recent to address pacing [93,94]. In regard to HOCM, both provide very similar recommendations. They agree that DDD pacing is not typically a stand-alone interventional treatment for HOCM, but is indicated in symptomatic patients who cannot be considered for or do not wish to undergo SM or ASA [93,94].

The most recent guidelines specifically addressing the treatment of HCM are the 2011 ACCF/AHA guidelines; the 2014 ESC guidelines; and the 2020 AHA/ACC guidelines [11],[13,95]. Each represents fairly comprehensive recommendations for the invasive treatment of HOCM. They each include recommendations for SM, ASA, and DDD pacing and advise considering anatomical variants such as MV and subvalvular apparatus involvement [11,95]. The 2014 and 2020 guidelines also include recommendations for the treatment of patients with mid-cavity or apical hypertrophy [11,13].

The 2020 AHA/ACC guidelines [13] represent the most comprehensive recommendations for the invasive management of HOCM. These guidelines are more current and slightly more comprehensive than the 2011 and 2014 guidelines [11,95]. When considering DDD pacing in HOCM, the 2021 ESC pacing guidelines [96] are the most current and specific to HOCM. In addition to pacing for the management of LVOTO, they provide guidance on pacemaker implantation following ASA and SM, as well as on cardiac resynchronization therapy in end-stage HCM. Figure 7 delineates a possible algorithm on poor surgical candidate management. Given the amount of literature that has only recently been published on the subject of HOCM, current guidelines may be insufficient to account for every scenario, warranting an update.

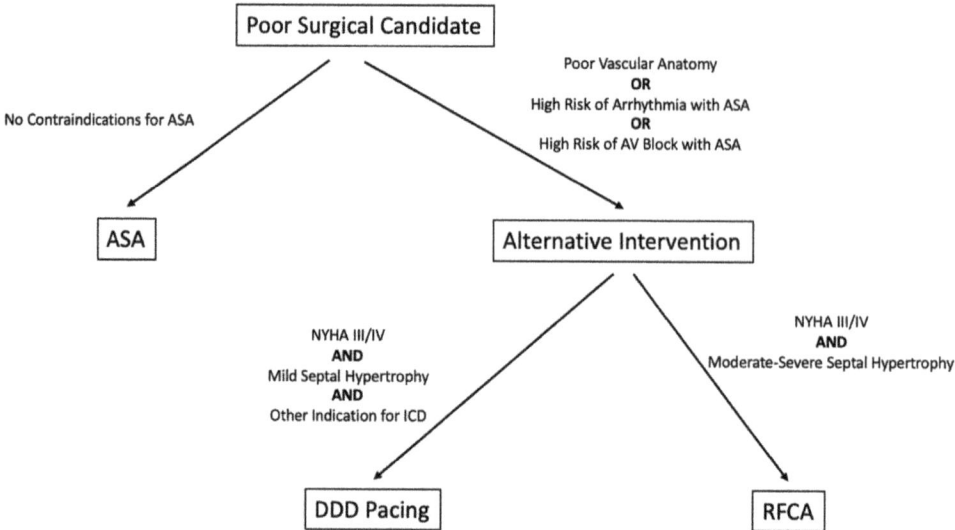

Figure 7. Proposed algorithm for alternative treatments when surgery is contraindicated. At this time, DDD pacing and RFCA are not indicated for the treatment of HOCM by any guidelines.

12. Genetics

HCM is a genetic disease associated with autosomal dominant inheritance of mutant sarcomere proteins [3]. As a genetic disease, there is much interest in the use of genetic testing to aid in risk stratification and disease management and in the use of gene therapy as a treatment modality.

Genetic testing is often performed on patients with HCM/HOCM and, in some cases, their asymptomatic relatives. Subsequent genetic counseling aids patients in family planning and can also aid providers in risk stratification. For example, certain mutations and complex genotypes are associated with greater risk and more severe phenotypes [97]. A retrospective analysis of 626 patients with HCM aimed to determine differences in genotype positive versus genotype negative patients. Positive status was associated with more non-sustained ventricular tachycardia, history of syncope, and greater LVH, and was a risk factor for all-cause mortality, cardiovascular mortality, heart failure mortality, and SCD and aborted SCD. Negative status was associated with a higher NYHA class and greater LVOT gradient [98].

Studies have yielded novel and important information on the genetics of HCM, such as the impact of environmental factors on phenotype [99]. Gene therapy is an attractive, potentially curative option for the treatment of HCM. Promising data have come from a study investigating the mutant MYCB3 gene associated with infant HF and death. This study has shown promise in murine models and in human pluripotent stem cell-derived cardiomyocytes using an AAV-9 vector which transfers functional MYCB3 to restore function [100].

The global COVID-19 pandemic has raised concerns regarding the effect of infection on the heart. Bos et al. demonstrated that cardiac tissue from HCM patients exhibits a five-fold greater expression of ACE-2 than control cardiac tissue. Since the SARS-CoV-2 virus uses the ACE-2 receptor for entry into host cells, up-regulation of this protein in HCM (and possibly in other heart diseases) may provide an explanation for cardiac patients demonstrating an increased risk of infection and poor outcomes in COVID-19 illness [101].

13. Medical Therapy

While critical appraisal of pharmacological treatments is far beyond the scope of this review [102], HOCM-associated hypercontractility is targeted by old and novel drugs alone or in combination with invasive approaches. Among them, beta-blockers and calcium channel blockers have for years been a mainstay of therapy to reduce dynamic LVOTO, improve symptoms, and prevent atrial and ventricular arrhythmias [11,103–106]. Disopyramide (an antiarrhythmic class IA agent) is often used on top of beta-blockers to improve symptoms and reduce intraventricular gradients in patients with LVOTO due to its negative inotropic effect [107].

Several emerging treatments are currently being tested in clinical trials; perhexiline, a potent carnitine palmitoyl transferase-1 (CPT-1) inhibitor, improves myocardial energetics in HCM [108], and has the potential to reduce LVH in HCM [NCT04426578]; ranolazine, a late sodium current inhibitor was tested in RESTYLE-HCM and associated with a reduction in 24-h burden of premature ventricular complexes in HOCM [109].

A recently published randomized, double-blind, placebo-controlled, phase 3 clinical trial assessed the use of mavacamten, a cardiac myosin inhibitor, for the treatment of HOCM. Olivotto et al. reported a significant improvement in NYHA class, exercise tolerance, LVOTO, and symptom scores in patients assigned to receive mavacamten over those in the placebo group [110]. Additionally, the VALOR-HCM trial showed that mavacamten improved symptoms and significantly reduced eligibility for SM among symptomatic patients with obstructive HCM who were candidates for SM on maximally tolerated medical therapy [111,112]. These landmark clinical trials pave the way for a novel medical treatment in patients with HOCM.

14. Minimally Invasive Surgery

Minimally invasive SM with or without concomitant MV intervention is an attractive option for patients as it provides the outcomes of SM with less surgical injury. Case reports have demonstrated success using minimally invasive approaches such as SM with aortic valve replacement through right mini-thoracotomy [113] and robotic SM with MVr in a patient with idiopathic hypertrophic subaortic stenosis [114]. Although the latter patient did not have per definition HOCM, this case demonstrated a successful operative technique that may be employed for SM.

A retrospective analysis compared 24 patients who underwent SM via right mini-thoracotomy with 26 patients who underwent traditional SM via sternotomy. The groups had similar aortic cross clamp times, post-operative pacemaker implantation rates, LVOT gradient reduction, and residual SAM [115]. Another retrospective analysis of 34 full sternotomy and 86 mini-sternotomy SM cases reported excellent results. Both groups had significant reductions in NYHA class, similar resting LVOT gradients at follow-up, similar median times on bypass, and similar major complication rates. The mini-sternotomy group had a slightly longer (39 min versus 35 min; $p = 0.017$) time while on cross clamp [116].

A recent, larger study reported outcomes for 51 HOCM patients who underwent right mini-thoracotomy for minimally invasive septal reduction. Jiang et al. report a significant reduction in LVOT gradient and septal thickness, as well as the abolishment of SAM and mitral regurgitation (or insignificant MR) for all patients [117]. These results further underscore the feasibility and safety of minimally-invasive surgery for septal reduction and MR for patients with HOCM.

15. MitraClip^{TM}

Percutaneous MV "edge-to-edge" repair using MitraClip^{TM} is a relatively new, minimally-invasive option for patients who are poor surgical candidates [118]. Some small studies have reported outcomes of MitraCip^{TM} use in HOCM patients. One study consisting of five HOCM patients who received the device reported reductions in SAM, LVOT gradient, MR, and NYHA class [119].

Despite little data existing on the use of percutaneous MV plication in HOCM patients, the results of small studies are impressive and indicate a role for the use of MitraClip^{TM} in the treatment of patients with HOCM who are, again, poor SM and ASA candidates.

16. Conclusions

Hypertrophic obstructive cardiomyopathy is a heterogeneous disease with different clinical presentations, albeit producing similar dismal long-term outcomes if left untreated. Several approaches are available for treatment of HOCM; alcohol septal ablation and surgical myectomy are safe and effective, but patient selection for the procedure is crucial. In the case of elevated operative risk, novel treatments are available and are currently being tested in the setting of HOCM.

Author Contributions: M.K., S.L. and G.M.R.: Conceptualization, Formal analysis, Methodology, Supervision, Validation, Writing—original draft; D.C., M.G., C.G., C.M., R.L. and P.S.: Data curation, validation, methodology, Writing—review & editing; M.P.: Conceptualization, Supervision, Validation. All authors have read and agreed to the published version of the manuscript.

Funding: This work was supported by the Italian Ministry of Health, Rome, Italy (Ricerca Corrente: RC 2022, Line 3A).

Institutional Review Board Statement: Not applicable.

Informed Consent Statement: Not applicable.

Data Availability Statement: Data underlying this article will be shared on reasonable request to the corresponding author.

Conflicts of Interest: The authors declare that the research was conducted in the absence of any commercial or financial relationships that could be construed as a potential conflict of interests.

References

1. Maron, B.J. Clinical Course and Management of Hypertrophic Cardiomyopathy. *N. Engl. J. Med.* **2018**, *379*, 655–668. [CrossRef] [PubMed]
2. Maron, B.J.; Rowin, E.J.; Casey, S.A.; Maron, M.S. How Hypertrophic Cardiomyopathy Became a Contemporary Treatable Genetic Disease with Low Mortality: Shaped by 50 Years of Clinical Research and Practice. *JAMA Cardiol.* **2016**, *1*, 98–105. [CrossRef] [PubMed]
3. Nishimura, R.A.; Seggewiss, H.; Schaff, H.V. Hypertrophic Obstructive Cardiomyopathy: Surgical Myectomy and Septal Ablation. *Circ. Res.* **2017**, *121*, 771–783. [CrossRef]
4. Ommen, S.R.; Maron, B.J.; Olivotto, I.; Maron, M.S.; Cecchi, F.; Betocchi, S.; Gersh, B.J.; Ackerman, M.J.; McCully, R.B.; Dearani, J.A.; et al. Long-term effects of surgical septal myectomy on survival in patients with obstructive hypertrophic cardiomyopathy. *J. Am. Coll. Cardiol.* **2005**, *46*, 470–476. [CrossRef]
5. Smedira, N.G.; Lytle, B.W.; Lever, H.M.; Rajeswaran, J.; Krishnaswamy, G.; Kaple, R.K.; Dolney, D.O.; Blackstone, E.H. Current effectiveness and risks of isolated septal myectomy for hypertrophic obstructive cardiomyopathy. *Ann. Thorac. Surg.* **2008**, *85*, 127–133. [CrossRef]
6. Yang, Y.J.; Fan, C.M.; Yuan, J.Q.; Qiao, S.B.; Hu, F.H.; Guo, X.Y.; Li, Y.S. Survival after alcohol septal ablation versus conservative therapy in obstructive hypertrophic cardiomyopathy. *Cardiol. J.* **2015**, *22*, 657–664. [CrossRef]
7. Patel, P.; Dhillon, A.; Popovic, Z.B.; Smedira, N.G.; Rizzo, J.; Thamilarasan, M.; Agler, D.; Lytle, B.W.; Lever, H.M.; Desai, M.Y. Left Ventricular Outflow Tract Obstruction in Hypertrophic Cardiomyopathy Patients without Severe Septal Hypertrophy: Implications of Mitral Valve and Papillary Muscle Abnormalities Assessed Using Cardiac Magnetic Resonance and Echocardiography. *Circ. Cardiovasc. Imaging* **2015**, *8*, e003132. [CrossRef]
8. Raffa, G.M.; Romano, G.; Turrisi, M.; Morsolini, M.; Gentile, G.; Sciacca, S.; Armaro, A.; Stringi, V.; Mattiucci, G.; Magro, S.; et al. Pathoanatomic Findings and Treatment During Hypertrophic Obstructive Cardiomyopathy Surgery: The Role of Mitral Valve. *Heart Lung Circ.* **2019**, *28*, 477–485. [CrossRef]
9. Osman, M.; Kheiri, B.; Osman, K.; Barbarawi, M.; Alhamoud, H.; Alqahtani, F.; Alkhouli, M. Alcohol septal ablation vs myectomy for symptomatic hypertrophic obstructive cardiomyopathy: Systematic review and meta-analysis. *Clin. Cardiol.* **2019**, *42*, 190–197. [CrossRef]
10. Rigopoulos, A.G.; Ali, M.; Abate, E.; Matiakis, M.; Melnyk, H.; Mavrogeni, S.; Leftheriotis, D.; Bigalke, B.; Noutsias, M. Review on sudden death risk reduction after septal reduction therapies in hypertrophic obstructive cardiomyopathy. *Heart Fail. Rev.* **2019**, *24*, 359–366. [CrossRef]
11. Authors/Task Force Members; Elliott, P.M.; Anastasakis, A.; Borger, M.A.; Borggrefe, M.; Cecchi, F.; Charron, P.; Hagege, A.A.; Lafont, A.; Limongelli, G.; et al. 2014 ESC Guidelines on diagnosis and management of hypertrophic cardiomyopathy: The Task Force for the Diagnosis and Management of Hypertrophic Cardiomyopathy of the European Society of Cardiology (ESC). *Eur. Heart J.* **2014**, *35*, 2733–2779. [PubMed]

12. Iwai, S. Sudden Cardiac Death Risk Stratification and the Role of the Implantable Cardiac Defibrillator. *Cardiol. Clin.* **2019**, *37*, 63–72. [CrossRef] [PubMed]
13. Writing Committee Members; Ommen, S.R.; Mital, S.; Burke, M.A.; Day, S.M.; Deswal, A.; Elliott, P.; Evanovich, L.L.; Hung, J.; Joglar, J.A.; et al. 2020 AHA/ACC Guideline for the Diagnosis and Treatment of Patients with Hypertrophic Cardiomyopathy: A Report of the American College of Cardiology/American Heart Association Joint Committee on Clinical Practice Guidelines. *Circulation* **2020**, *142*, e558–e631.
14. Ball, W.; Ivanov, J.; Rakowski, H.; Wigle, E.D.; Linghorne, M.; Ralph-Edwards, A.; Williams, W.G.; Schwartz, L.; Guttman, A.; Woo, A. Long-term survival in patients with resting obstructive hypertrophic cardiomyopathy comparison of conservative versus invasive treatment. *J. Am. Coll. Cardiol.* **2011**, *58*, 2313–2321. [CrossRef] [PubMed]
15. Woo, A.; Williams, W.G.; Choi, R.; Wigle, E.D.; Rozenblyum, E.; Fedwick, K.; Siu, S.; Ralph-Edwards, A.; Rakowski, H. Clinical and echocardiographic determinants of long-term survival after surgical myectomy in obstructive hypertrophic cardiomyopathy. *Circulation* **2005**, *111*, 2033–2041. [CrossRef]
16. Sorajja, P.; Ommen, S.R.; Holmes, D.R.; Dearani, J.A., Jr.; Rihal, C.S.; Gersh, B.J.; Lennon, R.J.; Nishimura, R.A. Survival after alcohol septal ablation for obstructive hypertrophic cardiomyopathy. *Circulation* **2012**, *126*, 2374–2380. [CrossRef]
17. Veselka, J.; Jensen, M.K.; Liebregts, M.; Januska, J.; Krejci, J.; Bartel, T.; Dabrowski, M.; Hansen, P.R.; Almaas, V.M.; Seggewiss, H.; et al. Long-term clinical outcome after alcohol septal ablation for obstructive hypertrophic cardiomyopathy: Results from the Euro-ASA registry. *Eur. Heart J.* **2016**, *37*, 1517–1523. [CrossRef]
18. Lu, D.Y.; Hailesealassie, B.; Ventoulis, I.; Liu, H.; Liang, H.Y.; Nowbar, A.; Pozios, I.; Canepa, M.; Cresswell, K.; Luo, H.C.; et al. Impact of peak provoked left ventricular outflow tract gradients on clinical outcomes in hypertrophic cardiomyopathy. *Int. J. Cardiol.* **2017**, *243*, 290–295. [CrossRef]
19. Batzner, A.; Pfeiffer, B.; Neugebauer, A.; Aicha, D.; Blank, C.; Seggewiss, H. Survival After Alcohol Septal Ablation in Patients with Hypertrophic Obstructive Cardiomyopathy. *J. Am. Coll. Cardiol.* **2018**, *72*, 3087–3094. [CrossRef]
20. Aguiar Rosa, S.; Fiarresga, A.; Galrinho, A.; Cacela, D.; Ramos, R.; de Sousa, L.; Goncalves, A.; Bernardes, L.; Patricio, L.; Branco, L.M.; et al. Short- and long-term outcome after alcohol septal ablation in obstructive hypertrophic cardiomyopathy: Experience of a reference center. *Rev. Port. Cardiol.* **2019**, *38*, 473–480. [CrossRef]
21. ten Cate, F.J.; Soliman, O.I.; Michels, M.; Theuns, D.A.; de Jong, P.L.; Geleijnse, M.L.; Serruys, P.W. Long-term outcome of alcohol septal ablation in patients with obstructive hypertrophic cardiomyopathy: A word of caution. *Circ. Heart Fail.* **2010**, *3*, 362–369. [CrossRef] [PubMed]
22. Veselka, J.; Faber, L.; Jensen, M.K.; Cooper, R.; Januska, J.; Krejci, J.; Bartel, T.; Dabrowski, M.; Hansen, P.R.; Almaas, V.M.; et al. Effect of Institutional Experience on Outcomes of Alcohol Septal Ablation for Hypertrophic Obstructive Cardiomyopathy. *Can. J. Cardiol.* **2018**, *34*, 16–22. [CrossRef] [PubMed]
23. Liebregts, M.; Faber, L.; Jensen, M.K.; Vriesendorp, P.A.; Januska, J.; Krejci, J.; Hansen, P.R.; Seggewiss, H.; Horstkotte, D.; Adlova, R.; et al. Outcomes of Alcohol Septal Ablation in Younger Patients with Obstructive Hypertrophic Cardiomyopathy. *JACC Cardiovasc. Interv.* **2017**, *10*, 1134–1143. [CrossRef]
24. Raffa, G.M.; Franca, E.L.; Lachina, C.; Palmeri, A.; Kowalewski, M.; Lebowitz, S.; Ricasoli, A.; Greco, M.; Sciacca, S.; Turrisi, M.; et al. Septal Thickness Does Not Impact Outcome After Hypertrophic Obstructive Cardiomyopathy Surgery (Septal Myectomy and Subvalvular Mitral Apparatus Remodeling): A 15-Years of Experience. *Front. Cardiovasc. Med.* **2022**, *9*, 853582.
25. Wang, S.; Luo, M.; Sun, H.; Song, Y.; Yin, C.; Wang, L.; Hui, R.; Hu, S. A retrospective clinical study of transaortic extended septal myectomy for obstructive hypertrophic cardiomyopathy in China. *Eur. J. Cardiothorac. Surg.* **2013**, *43*, 534–540. [CrossRef] [PubMed]
26. McLeod, C.J.; Ommen, S.R.; Ackerman, M.J.; Weivoda, P.L.; Shen, W.K.; Dearani, J.A.; Schaff, H.V.; Tajik, A.J.; Gersh, B.J. Surgical septal myectomy decreases the risk for appropriate implantable cardioverter defibrillator discharge in obstructive hypertrophic cardiomyopathy. *Eur. Heart J.* **2007**, *28*, 2583–2588. [CrossRef] [PubMed]
27. Siontis, K.C.; Geske, J.B.; Ong, K.; Nishimura, R.A.; Ommen, S.R.; Gersh, B.J. Atrial fibrillation in hypertrophic cardiomyopathy: Prevalence, clinical correlations, and mortality in a large high-risk population. *J. Am. Heart Assoc.* **2014**, *3*, e001002. [CrossRef] [PubMed]
28. Lapenna, E.; Pozzoli, A.; De Bonis, M.; La Canna, G.; Nisi, T.; Nascimbene, S.; Vicentini, L.; Di Sanzo, S.; Del Forno, B.; Schiavi, D.; et al. Mid-term outcomes of concomitant surgical ablation of atrial fibrillation in patients undergoing cardiac surgery for hypertrophic cardiomyopathydagger. *Eur. J. Cardiothorac. Surg.* **2017**, *51*, 1112–1118. [CrossRef]
29. Wells, S.; Rowin, E.J.; Boll, G.; Rastegar, H.; Wang, W.; Maron, M.S.; Maron, B.J. Clinical Profile of Nonresponders to Surgical Myectomy with Obstructive Hypertrophic Cardiomyopathy. *Am. J. Med.* **2018**, *131*, e235–e239. [CrossRef]
30. Zeng, Z.; Wang, F.; Dou, X.; Zhang, S.; Pu, J. Comparison of percutaneous transluminal septal myocardial ablation versus septal myectomy for the treatment of patients with hypertrophic obstructive cardiomyopathy—A meta analysis. *Int. J. Cardiol.* **2006**, *112*, 80–84. [CrossRef]
31. Alam, M.; Dokainish, H.; Lakkis, N.M. Hypertrophic obstructive cardiomyopathy-alcohol septal ablation vs. myectomy: A meta-analysis. *Eur. Heart J.* **2009**, *30*, 1080–1087. [CrossRef] [PubMed]
32. Agarwal, S.; Tuzcu, E.M.; Desai, M.Y.; Smedira, N.; Lever, H.M.; Lytle, B.W.; Kapadia, S.R. Updated meta-analysis of septal alcohol ablation versus myectomy for hypertrophic cardiomyopathy. *J. Am. Coll. Cardiol.* **2010**, *55*, 823–834. [CrossRef] [PubMed]

33. Singh, K.; Qutub, M.; Carson, K.; Hibbert, B.; Glover, C. A meta analysis of current status of alcohol septal ablation and surgical myectomy for obstructive hypertrophic cardiomyopathy. *Catheter. Cardiovasc. Interv.* **2016**, *88*, 107–115. [CrossRef]
34. Liebregts, M.; Vriesendorp, P.A.; Mahmoodi, B.K.; Schinkel, A.F.; Michels, M.; ten Berg, J.M. A Systematic Review and Meta-Analysis of Long-Term Outcomes after Septal Reduction Therapy in Patients with Hypertrophic Cardiomyopathy. *JACC Heart Fail.* **2015**, *3*, 896–905. [CrossRef]
35. Leonardi, R.A.; Kransdorf, E.P.; Simel, D.L.; Wang, A. Meta-analyses of septal reduction therapies for obstructive hypertrophic cardiomyopathy: Comparative rates of overall mortality and sudden cardiac death after treatment. *Circ. Cardiovasc. Interv.* **2010**, *3*, 97–104. [CrossRef]
36. Jurado Roman, A.; Montero Cabezas, J.M.; Rubio Alonso, B.; Garcia Tejada, J.; Hernandez Hernandez, F.; Albarran Gonzalez-Trevilla, A.; Velazquez Martin, M.T.; Coma Samartin, R.; Rodriguez Garcia, J.; Tascon Perez, J.C. Sequential Atrioventricular Pacing in Patients with Hypertrophic Cardiomyopathy: An 18-year Experience. *Rev. Esp. Cardiol.* **2016**, *69*, 377–383. [CrossRef]
37. Yue-Cheng, H.; Zuo-Cheng, L.; Xi-Ming, L.; Yuan, D.Z.; Dong-Xia, J.; Ying-Yi, Z.; Hui-Ming, Y.; Hong-Liang, C. Long-term follow-up impact of dual-chamber pacing on patients with hypertrophic obstructive cardiomyopathy. *Pacing Clin. Electrophysiol.* **2013**, *36*, 86–93. [CrossRef]
38. Jeanrenaud, X.; Goy, J.J.; Kappenberger, L. Effects of dual-chamber pacing in hypertrophic obstructive cardiomyopathy. *Lancet* **1992**, *339*, 1318–1323. [CrossRef]
39. Fananapazir, L.; Cannon, R.O., 3rd; Tripodi, D.; Panza, J.A. Impact of dual-chamber permanent pacing in patients with obstructive hypertrophic cardiomyopathy with symptoms refractory to verapamil and beta-adrenergic blocker therapy. *Circulation* **1992**, *85*, 2149–2161. [CrossRef]
40. Nishimura, R.A.; Trusty, J.M.; Hayes, D.L.; Ilstrup, D.M.; Larson, D.R.; Hayes, S.N.; Allison, T.G.; Tajik, A.J. Dual-chamber pacing for hypertrophic cardiomyopathy: A randomized, double-blind, crossover trial. *J. Am. Coll. Cardiol.* **1997**, *29*, 435–441. [CrossRef]
41. Galve, E.; Sambola, A.; Saldana, G.; Quispe, I.; Nieto, E.; Diaz, A.; Evangelista, A.; Candell-Riera, J. Late benefits of dual-chamber pacing in obstructive hypertrophic cardiomyopathy: A 10-year follow-up study. *Heart* **2010**, *96*, 352–356. [CrossRef] [PubMed]
42. Fananapazir, L.; Epstein, N.D.; Curiel, R.V.; Panza, J.A.; Tripodi, D.; McAreavey, D. Long-term results of dual-chamber (DDD) pacing in obstructive hypertrophic cardiomyopathy. Evidence for progressive symptomatic and hemodynamic improvement and reduction of left ventricular hypertrophy. *Circulation* **1994**, *90*, 2731–2742. [CrossRef] [PubMed]
43. Dimitrow, P.P.; Podolec, P.; Grodecki, J.; Plazak, W.; Dudek, D.; Pieniazek, P.; Bacior, B.; Legutko, J.; Olszowska, M.; Kostkiewicz, M.; et al. Comparison of dual-chamber pacing with nonsurgical septal reduction effect in patients with hypertrophic obstructive cardiomyopathy. *Int. J. Cardiol.* **2004**, *94*, 31–34. [CrossRef]
44. Krejci, J.; Gregor, P.; Zemanek, D.; Vyskocilova, K.; Curila, K.; Stepanova, R.; Novak, M.; Groch, L.; Veselka, J. Comparison of long-term effect of dual-chamber pacing and alcohol septal ablation in patients with hypertrophic obstructive cardiomyopathy. *Sci. World J.* **2013**, *2013*, 629650. [CrossRef] [PubMed]
45. Pavin, D.; de Place, C.; Le Breton, H.; Leclercq, C.; Gras, D.; Victor, F.; Mabo, P.; Daubert, J.C. Effects of permanent dual-chamber pacing on mitral regurgitation in hypertrophic obstructive cardiomyopathy. *Eur. Heart J.* **1999**, *20*, 203–210. [CrossRef] [PubMed]
46. Ommen, S.R.; Nishimura, R.A.; Squires, R.W.; Schaff, H.V.; Danielson, G.K.; Tajik, A.J. Comparison of dual-chamber pacing versus septal myectomy for the treatment of patients with hypertrophic obstructive cardiomyopathy: A comparison of objective hemodynamic and exercise end points. *J. Am. Coll. Cardiol.* **1999**, *34*, 191–196. [CrossRef]
47. Liu, L.; Li, J.; Zuo, L.; Zhang, J.; Zhou, M.; Xu, B.; Hahn, R.T.; Leon, M.B.; Hsi, D.H.; Ge, J.; et al. Percutaneous Intramyocardial Septal Radiofrequency Ablation for Hypertrophic Obstructive Cardiomyopathy. *J. Am. Coll. Cardiol.* **2018**, *72*, 1898–1909. [CrossRef]
48. Shelke, A.B.; Menon, R.; Kapadiya, A.; Yalagudri, S.; Saggu, D.; Nair, S.; Narasimhan, C. A novel approach in the use of radiofrequency catheter ablation of septal hypertrophy in hypertrophic obstructive cardiomyopathy. *Indian Heart J.* **2016**, *68*, 618–623. [CrossRef]
49. Lawrenz, T.; Borchert, B.; Leuner, C.; Bartelsmeier, M.; Reinhardt, J.; Strunk-Mueller, C.; Meyer Zu Vilsendorf, D.; Schloesser, M.; Beer, G.; Lieder, F.; et al. Endocardial radiofrequency ablation for hypertrophic obstructive cardiomyopathy: Acute results and 6 months' follow-up in 19 patients. *J. Am. Coll. Cardiol.* **2011**, *57*, 572–576. [CrossRef]
50. Liu, L.W.; Zuo, L.; Zhou, M.Y.; Li, J.; Zhou, X.D.; He, G.B.; Zhang, J.; Zhang, J.Z.; Liu, B.; Yang, J.; et al. Efficacy and safety of transthoracic echocardiography-guided percutaneous intramyocardial septal radiofrequency ablation for the treatment of patients with obstructive hypertrophic cardiomyopathy. *Zhonghua Xin Xue Guan Bing Za Zhi* **2019**, *47*, 284–290.
51. Crossen, K.; Jones, M.; Erikson, C. Radiofrequency septal reduction in symptomatic hypertrophic obstructive cardiomyopathy. *Heart Rhythm* **2016**, *13*, 1885–1890. [CrossRef] [PubMed]
52. Maron, B.J.; Harding, A.M.; Spirito, P.; Roberts, W.C.; Waller, B.F. Systolic anterior motion of the posterior mitral leaflet: A previously unrecognized cause of dynamic subaortic obstruction in patients with hypertrophic cardiomyopathy. *Circulation* **1983**, *68*, 282–293. [CrossRef] [PubMed]
53. Wang, R.; Chen, X.; Xu, M.; Shi, K.H.; Wang, L.M.; Xiao, L.Q.; Liu, P.S. Surgical treatment of obstructive hypertrophic cardiomyopathy with ventricular septal myectomy concomitant mitral valve replacement. *Zhonghua Wai Ke Za Zhi* **2008**, *46*, 1572–1574. [PubMed]

54. McIntosh, C.L.; Maron, B.J.; Cannon, R.O., 3rd; Klues, H.G. Initial results of combined anterior mitral leaflet plication and ventricular septal myotomy-myectomy for relief of left ventricular outflow tract obstruction in patients with hypertrophic cardiomyopathy. *Circulation* **1992**, *86* (Suppl. S5), II60–II67. [PubMed]
55. Collis, R.; Watkinson, O.; Pantazis, A.; Tome-Esteban, M.; Elliott, P.M.; McGregor, C.G.A. Early and medium-term outcomes of Alfieri mitral valve repair in the management of systolic anterior motion during septal myectomy. *J. Card. Surg.* **2017**, *32*, 686–690. [CrossRef] [PubMed]
56. Fritzsche, D.; Krakor, R.; Goos, H.; Lindenau, K.F.; Will-Shahab, L. Comparison of myectomy alone or in combination with mitral valve repair for hypertrophic obstructive cardiomyopathy. *Thorac. Cardiovasc. Surg.* **1992**, *40*, 65–69. [CrossRef] [PubMed]
57. Nasseri, B.A.; Stamm, C.; Siniawski, H.; Kukucka, M.; Komoda, T.; Delmo Walter, E.M.; Hetzer, R. Combined anterior mitral valve leaflet retention plasty and septal myectomy in patients with hypertrophic obstructive cardiomyopathy. *Eur. J. Cardiothorac. Surg.* **2011**, *40*, 1515–1520. [CrossRef]
58. van der Lee, C.; Kofflard, M.J.; van Herwerden, L.A.; Vletter, W.B.; ten Cate, F.J. Sustained improvement after combined anterior mitral leaflet extension and myectomy in hypertrophic obstructive cardiomyopathy. *Circulation* **2003**, *108*, 2088–2092. [CrossRef]
59. Shimahara, Y.; Fujita, T.; Kobayashi, J.; Fukushima, S.; Kume, Y.; Yamashita, K.; Matsumoto, Y.; Kawamoto, N.; Tadokoro, N.; Kakuta, T.; et al. Combined mechanical mitral valve replacement and transmitral myectomy for hypertrophic obstructive cardiomyopathy treatment: An experience of over 20 years. *J. Cardiol.* **2019**, *73*, 318–325. [CrossRef]
60. Song, B.R.; Ren, Y.; Zhang, H.J. Surgical Treatment for Hypertrophic Obstructive Cardiomyopathy with Concomitant Mitral Valve Abnormalities: A Cohort of 26 Cases. *Heart Surg. Forum.* **2018**, *21*, E443–E447. [CrossRef]
61. Wehman, B.; Ghoreishi, M.; Foster, N.; Wang, L.; D'Ambra, M.N.; Maassel, N.; Maghami, S.; Quinn, R.; Dawood, M.; Fisher, S.; et al. Transmitral Septal Myectomy for Hypertrophic Obstructive Cardiomyopathy. *Ann. Thorac. Surg.* **2018**, *105*, 1102–1108. [CrossRef] [PubMed]
62. Bogachev-Prokophiev, A.; Afanasyev, A.; Zheleznev, S.; Fomenko, M.; Sharifulin, R.; Kretov, E.; Karaskov, A. Mitral valve repair or replacement in hypertrophic obstructive cardiomyopathy: A prospective randomized study. *Interact. Cardiovasc. Thorac. Surg.* **2017**, *25*, 356–362. [CrossRef] [PubMed]
63. Afanasyev, A.; Bogachev-Prokophiev, A.; Lenko, E.; Sharifulin, R.; Ovcharov, M.; Kozmin, D.; Karaskov, A. Myectomy with mitral valve repair versus replacement in adult patients with hypertrophic obstructive cardiomyopathy: A systematic review and meta-analysis. *Interact. Cardiovasc. Thorac. Surg.* **2019**, *28*, 465–472. [CrossRef] [PubMed]
64. Kaple, R.K.; Murphy, R.T.; DiPaola, L.M.; Houghtaling, P.L.; Lever, H.M.; Lytle, B.W.; Blackstone, E.H.; Smedira, N.G. Mitral valve abnormalities in hypertrophic cardiomyopathy: Echocardiographic features and surgical outcomes. *Ann. Thorac. Surg.* **2008**, *85*, 1527–1535.e1–2. [CrossRef]
65. Nguyen, A.; Schaff, H.V.; Nishimura, R.A.; Dearani, J.A.; Geske, J.B.; Lahr, B.D.; Ommen, S.R. Does septal thickness influence outcome of myectomy for hypertrophic obstructive cardiomyopathy? *Eur. J. Cardiothorac. Surg.* **2018**, *53*, 582–589. [CrossRef]
66. Shingu, Y.; Sugiki, H.; Ooka, T.; Kato, H.; Wakasa, S.; Tachibana, T.; Matsui, Y. Surgery for Left Ventricular Outflow Tract Obstruction with a Relatively Thin Interventricular Septum. *Thorac. Cardiovasc. Surg.* **2018**, *66*, 307–312. [CrossRef]
67. van der Lee, C.; ten Cate, F.J.; Geleijnse, M.L.; Kofflard, M.J.; Pedone, C.; van Herwerden, L.A.; Biagini, E.; Vletter, W.B.; Serruys, P.W. Percutaneous versus surgical treatment for patients with hypertrophic obstructive cardiomyopathy and enlarged anterior mitral valve leaflets. *Circulation* **2005**, *112*, 482–488. [CrossRef]
68. Delling, F.N.; Sanborn, D.Y.; Levine, R.A.; Picard, M.H.; Fifer, M.A.; Palacios, I.F.; Lowry, P.A.; Vlahakes, G.J.; Vaturi, M.; Hung, J. Frequency and mechanism of persistent systolic anterior motion and mitral regurgitation after septal ablation in obstructive hypertrophic cardiomyopathy. *Am. J. Cardiol.* **2007**, *100*, 1691–1695. [CrossRef]
69. Sakaguchi, T.; Totsugawa, T.; Tamura, K.; Hiraoka, A.; Chikazawa, G.; Yoshitaka, H. Minimally invasive trans-mitral septal myectomy for diffuse-type hypertrophic obstructive cardiomyopathy. *Gen. Thorac. Cardiovasc. Surg.* **2018**, *66*, 321–326. [CrossRef]
70. Gilmanov, D.; Bevilacqua, S.; Solinas, M.; Ferrarini, M.; Kallushi, E.; Santarelli, P.; Farneti, P.A.; Glauber, M. Minimally invasive septal myectomy for the treatment of hypertrophic obstructive cardiomyopathy and intrinsic mitral valve disease. *Innovations* **2015**, *10*, 106–113. [CrossRef]
71. Raffa, G.M.; Pilato, M. Hypertrophic Obstructive Cardiomyopathy and Subvalvular Mitral Apparatus Remodeling. *Ann. Thorac. Surg.* **2019**, *108*, 964. [CrossRef] [PubMed]
72. Silbiger, J.J. Abnormalities of the Mitral Apparatus in Hypertrophic Cardiomyopathy: Echocardiographic, Pathophysiologic, and Surgical Insights. *J. Am. Soc. Echocardiogr.* **2016**, *29*, 622–639. [CrossRef] [PubMed]
73. Klues, H.G.; Roberts, W.C.; Maron, B.J. Anomalous insertion of papillary muscle directly into anterior mitral leaflet in hypertrophic cardiomyopathy. Significance in producing left ventricular outflow obstruction. *Circulation* **1991**, *84*, 1188–1197. [CrossRef] [PubMed]
74. Ferrazzi, P.; Spirito, P.; Iacovoni, A.; Calabrese, A.; Migliorati, K.; Simon, C.; Pentiricci, S.; Poggio, D.; Grillo, M.; Amigoni, P.; et al. Transaortic Chordal Cutting: Mitral Valve Repair for Obstructive Hypertrophic Cardiomyopathy with Mild Septal Hypertrophy. *J. Am. Coll. Cardiol.* **2015**, *66*, 1687–1696. [CrossRef]
75. Wang, S.; Cui, H.; Yu, Q.; Chen, H.; Zhu, C.; Wang, J.; Xiao, M.; Zhang, Y.; Wu, R.; Hu, S. Excision of anomalous muscle bundles as an important addition to extended septal myectomy for treatment of left ventricular outflow tract obstruction. *J. Thorac. Cardiovasc. Surg.* **2016**, *152*, 461–468. [CrossRef]

76. Song, H.K.; Turner, J.; Macfie, R.; Kumar, S.; Mannello, M.J.; Smith, D.; Bhamidipati, C.; Raman, J.; Tibayan, F.; Heitner, S.B. Routine Papillary Muscle Realignment and Septal Myectomy for Obstructive Hypertrophic Cardiomyopathy. *Ann. Thorac. Surg.* **2018**, *106*, 670–675. [CrossRef]
77. Minakata, K.; Dearani, J.A.; Nishimura, R.A.; Maron, B.J.; Danielson, G.K. Extended septal myectomy for hypertrophic obstructive cardiomyopathy with anomalous mitral papillary muscles or chordae. *J. Thorac. Cardiovasc. Surg.* **2004**, *127*, 481–489. [CrossRef]
78. Schoendube, F.A.; Klues, H.G.; Reith, S.; Flachskampf, F.A.; Hanrath, P.; Messmer, B.J. Long-term clinical and echocardiographic follow-up after surgical correction of hypertrophic obstructive cardiomyopathy with extended myectomy and reconstruction of the subvalvular mitral apparatus. *Circulation* **1995**, *92* (Suppl. S9), II122–II127. [CrossRef]
79. Kwon, D.H.; Smedira, N.G.; Thamilarasan, M.; Lytle, B.W.; Lever, H.; Desai, M.Y. Characteristics and surgical outcomes of symptomatic patients with hypertrophic cardiomyopathy with abnormal papillary muscle morphology undergoing papillary muscle reorientation. *J. Thorac. Cardiovasc. Surg.* **2010**, *140*, 317–324. [CrossRef]
80. Bogachev-Prokophiev, A.; Afanasyev, A.V.; Zheleznev, S.; Pivkin, A.; Sharifulin, R.; Kozmin, D.; Karaskov, A. Septal Myectomy with Vs without Subvalvular Apparatus Intervention in Patients with Hypertrophic Obstructive Cardiomyopathy: A Prospective Randomized Study. *Semin. Thorac. Cardiovasc. Surg.* **2019**, *31*, 424–431. [CrossRef]
81. Said, S.M.; Schaff, H.V.; Abel, M.D.; Dearani, J.A. Transapical approach for apical myectomy and relief of midventricular obstruction in hypertrophic cardiomyopathy. *J. Card. Surg.* **2012**, *27*, 443–448. [CrossRef]
82. Minami, Y.; Kajimoto, K.; Terajima, Y.; Yashiro, B.; Okayama, D.; Haruki, S.; Nakajima, T.; Kawashiro, N.; Kawana, M.; Hagiwara, N. Clinical implications of midventricular obstruction in patients with hypertrophic cardiomyopathy. *J. Am. Coll. Cardiol.* **2011**, *57*, 2346–2355. [CrossRef]
83. Nguyen, A.; Schaff, H.V.; Nishimura, R.A.; Geske, J.B.; Dearani, J.A.; King, K.S.; Ommen, S.R. Apical myectomy for patients with hypertrophic cardiomyopathy and advanced heart failure. *J. Thorac. Cardiovasc. Surg.* **2019**, *159*, 145–152. [CrossRef]
84. Kunkala, M.R.; Schaff, H.V.; Nishimura, R.A.; Abel, M.D.; Sorajja, P.; Dearani, J.A.; Ommen, S.R. Transapical approach to myectomy for midventricular obstruction in hypertrophic cardiomyopathy. *Ann. Thorac. Surg.* **2013**, *96*, 564–570. [CrossRef]
85. Hang, D.; Schaff, H.V.; Ommen, S.R.; Dearani, J.A.; Nishimura, R.A. Combined transaortic and transapical approach to septal myectomy in patients with complex hypertrophic cardiomyopathy. *J. Thorac. Cardiovasc. Surg.* **2018**, *155*, 2096–2102. [CrossRef]
86. Tang, Y.; Song, Y.; Duan, F.; Deng, L.; Ran, J.; Gao, G.; Liu, S.; Liu, Y.; Wang, H.; Zhao, S.; et al. Extended myectomy for hypertrophic obstructive cardiomyopathy patients with midventricular obstruction. *Eur. J. Cardiothorac. Surg.* **2018**, *54*, 875–883. [CrossRef]
87. Husaini, M.; Baker, J.N.; Cresci, S.; Bach, R.; LaRue, S.J. Recurrent Takotsubo Cardiomyopathy in a Patient with Hypertrophic Cardiomyopathy Leading to Cardiogenic Shock Requiring VA-ECMO. *JACC Case Rep.* **2020**, *2*, 1014–1018. [CrossRef]
88. Basic, D.; Mollmann, H.; Haas, M.A.; Rolf, A.; Jovanovic, A.; Liebetrau, C.; Szardien, S.; Leick, J.; Dorr, O.; Skwara, A.; et al. A TASH experience: Post-infarction myocardial oedema necessitating the support of ECMO and occurrence of significant mitral regurgitation. *Clin. Res. Cardiol.* **2012**, *101*, 149–153. [CrossRef]
89. Williams, L.; Kermeen, F.; Mullany, D.; Thomson, B. Successful use of pre and post-operative ECMO for pulmonary endarterectomy, mitral valve replacement and myomectomy in a patient with chronic thromboembolic pulmonary hypertension and hypertrophic cardiomyopathy. *Heart Lung Circ.* **2015**, *24*, e153–e156. [CrossRef]
90. Gordon, J.S.; Blazoski, C.M.; Wood, C.T.; Zuber, C.; Massey, H.T.; Throckmorton, A.; Tchantchaleishvili, V. Mechanical and interventional support for heart failure with preserved ejection fraction: A review. *Artif. Organs.* **2022**. Epub ahead of print. [CrossRef]
91. Miyagi, C.; Miyamoto, T.; Karimov, J.H.; Starling, R.C.; Fukamachi, K. Device-based treatment options for heart failure with preserved ejection fraction. *Heart Fail. Rev.* **2021**, *26*, 749–762, Epub ahead of print. [CrossRef]
92. Lanmueller, P.; Eulert-Grehn, J.J.; Schoenrath, F.; Pieske, B.; Mulzer, J.; Mueller, M.; Falk, V.; Potapov, E. Durable mechanical circulatory support in patients with heart failure with preserved ejection fraction. *Interact. Cardiovasc. Thorac. Surg.* **2021**, *33*, 628–630. [CrossRef]
93. Epstein, A.E.; DiMarco, J.P.; Ellenbogen, K.A.; Estes, N.A., 3rd; Freedman, R.A.; Gettes, L.S.; Gillinov, A.M.; Gregoratos, G.; Hammill, S.C.; Hayes, D.L.; et al. ACC/AHA/HRS 2008 Guidelines for Device-Based Therapy of Cardiac Rhythm Abnormalities: A report of the American College of Cardiology/American Heart Association Task Force on Practice Guidelines (Writing Committee to Revise the ACC/AHA/NASPE 2002 Guideline Update for Implantation of Cardiac Pacemakers and Antiarrhythmia Devices): Developed in collaboration with the American Association for Thoracic Surgery and Society of Thoracic Surgeons. *Circulation* **2008**, *117*, e350–e408.
94. European Society of Cardiology (ESC); European Heart Rhythm Association (EHRA); Brignole, M.; Auricchio, A.; Baron-Esquivias, G.; Bordachar, P.; Boriani, G.; Breithardt, O.A.; Cleland, J.; Deharo, J.C.; et al. 2013 ESC guidelines on cardiac pacing and cardiac resynchronization therapy: The task force on cardiac pacing and resynchronization therapy of the European Society of Cardiology (ESC). Developed in collaboration with the European Heart Rhythm Association (EHRA). *Europace* **2013**, *15*, 1070–1118.

95. Gersh, B.J.; Maron, B.J.; Bonow, R.O.; Dearani, J.A.; Fifer, M.A.; Link, M.S.; Naidu, S.S.; Nishimura, R.A.; Ommen, S.R.; Rakowski, H.; et al. 2011 ACCF/AHA Guideline for the Diagnosis and Treatment of Hypertrophic Cardiomyopathy: A report of the American College of Cardiology Foundation/American Heart Association Task Force on Practice Guidelines. Developed in collaboration with the American Association for Thoracic Surgery, American Society of Echocardiography, American Society of Nuclear Cardiology, Heart Failure Society of America, Heart Rhythm Society, Society for Cardiovascular Angiography and Interventions, and Society of Thoracic Surgeons. *J. Am. Coll. Cardiol.* **2011**, *58*, e212–e260.
96. Glikson, M.; Nielsen, J.C.; Kronborg, M.B.; Michowitz, Y.; Auricchio, A.; Barbash, I.M.; Barrabés, J.A.; Boriani, G.; Braunschweig, F.; Brignole, M.; et al. 2021 ESC Guidelines on cardiac pacing and cardiac resynchronization therapy. *Eur. Heart J.* **2021**, *42*, 3427–3520, Erratum in *Eur. Heart J.* **2022**, *43*, 1651. [CrossRef]
97. van Velzen, H.G.; Vriesendorp, P.A.; Oldenburg, R.A.; van Slegtenhorst, M.A.; van der Velden, J.; Schinkel, A.F.L.; Michels, M. Value of Genetic Testing for the Prediction of Long-Term Outcome in Patients with Hypertrophic Cardiomyopathy. *Am. J. Cardiol.* **2016**, *118*, 881–887. [CrossRef]
98. Pasipoularides, A. Challenges and Controversies in Hypertrophic Cardiomyopathy: Clinical, Genomic and Basic Science Perspectives. *Rev. Esp. Cardiol.* **2018**, *71*, 132–138. [CrossRef]
99. Prondzynski, M.; Mearini, G.; Carrier, L. Gene therapy strategies in the treatment of hypertrophic cardiomyopathy. *Pflug. Arch.* **2019**, *471*, 807–815. [CrossRef]
100. Bos, J.M.; Hebl, V.B.; Oberg, A.L.; Sun, Z.; Herman, D.S.; Teekakirikul, P.; Seidman, J.G.; Seidman, C.E.; Dos Remedios, C.G.; Maleszewski, J.J.; et al. Marked Up-Regulation of ACE2 in Hearts of Patients with Obstructive Hypertrophic Cardiomyopathy: Implications for SARS-CoV-2-Mediated COVID-19. *Mayo Clin. Proc.* **2020**, *95*, 1354–1368. [CrossRef]
101. Ammirati, E.; Contri, R.; Coppini, R.; Cecchi, F.; Frigerio, M.; Olivotto, I. Pharmacological treatment of hypertrophic cardiomyopathy: Current practice and novel perspectives. *Eur. J. Heart Fail.* **2016**, *18*, 1106–1118. [CrossRef] [PubMed]
102. Cohen, L.S.; Braunwald, E. Amelioration of angina pectoris in idiopathic hypertrophic subaortic stenosis with beta-adrenergic blockade. *Circulation* **1967**, *35*, 847–851. [CrossRef] [PubMed]
103. Dybro, A.M.; Rasmussen, T.B.; Nielsen, R.R.; Andersen, M.J.; Jensen, M.K.; Poulsen, S.H. Randomized Trial of Metoprolol in Patients with Obstructive Hypertrophic Cardiomyopathy. *J. Am. Coll. Cardiol.* **2021**, *78*, 2505–2517. [CrossRef] [PubMed]
104. Dybro, A.M.; Rasmussen, T.B.; Nielsen, R.R.; Ladefoged, B.T.; Andersen, M.J.; Jensen, M.K.; Poulsen, S.H. Effects of Metoprolol on Exercise Hemodynamics in Patients with Obstructive Hypertrophic Cardiomyopathy. *J. Am. Coll. Cardiol.* **2022**, *79*, 1565–1575. [CrossRef]
105. Monda, E.; Lioncino, M.; Palmiero, G.; Franco, F.; Rubino, M.; Cirillo, A.; Verrillo, F.; Fusco, A.; Caiazza, M.; Mazzella, M.; et al. Bisoprolol for treatment of symptomatic patients with obstructive hypertrophic cardiomyopathy. The BASIC (bisoprolol AS therapy in hypertrophic cardiomyopathy) study. *Int. J. Cardiol.* **2022**, *354*, 22–28. [CrossRef]
106. Sherrid, M.V.; Barac, I.; McKenna, W.J.; Elliott, P.M.; Dickie, S.; Chojnowska, L.; Casey, S.; Maron, B.J. Multicenter study of the efficacy and safety of disopyramide in obstructive hypertrophic cardiomyopathy. *J. Am. Coll. Cardiol.* **2005**, *45*, 1251–1258. [CrossRef]
107. Ananthakrishna, R.; Lee, S.L.; Foote, J.; Sallustio, B.C.; Binda, G.; Mangoni, A.A.; Woodman, R.; Semsarian, C.; Horowitz, J.D.; Selvanayagam, J.B. Randomized controlled trial of perhexiline on regression of left ventricular hypertrophy in patients with symptomatic hypertrophic cardiomyopathy (RESOLVE-HCM trial). *Am. Heart J.* **2021**, *240*, 101–113. [CrossRef]
108. Olivotto, I.; Camici, P.G.; Merlini, P.A.; Rapezzi, C.; Patten, M.; Climent, V.; Sinagra, G.; Tomberli, B.; Marin, F.; Ehlermann, P.; et al. Efficacy of Ranolazine in Patients with Symptomatic Hypertrophic Cardiomyopathy: The RESTYLE-HCM Randomized, Double-Blind, Placebo-Controlled Study. *Circ. Heart Fail.* **2018**, *11*, e004124. [CrossRef]
109. Olivotto, I.; Oreziak, A.; Barriales-Villa, R.; Abraham, T.P.; Masri, A.; Garcia-Pavia, P.; Saberi, S.; Lakdawala, N.K.; Wheeler, M.T.; Owens, A.; et al. Mavacamten for treatment of symptomatic obstructive hypertrophic cardiomyopathy (EXPLORER-HCM): A randomised, double-blind, placebo-controlled, phase 3 trial. *Lancet* **2020**, *396*, 759–769. [CrossRef]
110. Desai, M.Y.; Wolski, K.; Owens, A.; Naidu, S.S.; Geske, J.B.; Smedira, N.G.; Schaff, H.; Lampl, K.; McErlean, E.; Sewell, C.; et al. Study design and rationale of VALOR-HCM: Evaluation of mavacamten in adults with symptomatic obstructive hypertrophic cardiomyopathy who are eligible for septal reduction therapy. *Am. Heart J.* **2021**, *239*, 80–89. [CrossRef]
111. Desai, M.Y. Mavacamten in Adults with Symptomatic Obstructive HCM Who Are Eligible for Septal Reduction Therapy—VALOR-HCM. In Proceedings of the American College of Cardiology Annual Scientific Session (ACC 2022), Washington, DC, USA, 2 April 2022.
112. Totsugawa, T.; Suzuki, K.; Hiraoka, A.; Tamura, K.; Yoshitaka, H.; Sakaguchi, T. Concomitant septal myectomy during minimally invasive aortic valve replacement through a right mini-thoracotomy for the treatment of aortic stenosis with systolic anterior motion of the mitral valve. *Gen. Thorac. Cardiovasc. Surg.* **2017**, *65*, 657–660. [CrossRef] [PubMed]
113. Bayburt, S.; Senay, S.; Gullu, A.U.; Kocyigit, M.; Karakus, G.; Batur, M.K.; Alhan, C. Robotic Septal Myectomy and Mitral Valve Repair for Idiopathic Hypertrophic Subaortic Stenosis with Systolic Anterior Motion. *Innovations* **2016**, *11*, 146–149. [CrossRef] [PubMed]
114. Mazine, A.; Ghoneim, A.; Bouhout, I.; Fortin, W.; Berania, I.; L'Allier, P.L.; Garceau, P.; Bouchard, D. A Novel Minimally Invasive Approach for Surgical Septal Myectomy. *Can. J. Cardiol.* **2016**, *32*, 1340–1347. [CrossRef] [PubMed]
115. Musharbash, F.N.; Schill, M.R.; Hansalia, V.H.; Schuessler, R.B.; Leidenfrost, J.E.; Melby, S.J.; Damiano, R.J., Jr. Minimally Invasive versus Full-Sternotomy Septal Myectomy for Hypertrophic Cardiomyopathy. *Innovations* **2018**, *13*, 261–266. [CrossRef] [PubMed]

116. Jiang, Z.; Tang, M.; Liu, H.; Ma, N.; Ding, F.; Bao, C.; Mei, J. Minimally invasive surgery for hypertrophic obstructive cardiomyopathy with mitral regurgitation. *Ann. Thorac. Surg.* **2020**, *111*, 1345–1350. [CrossRef]
117. Philipson, D.J.; DePasquale, E.C.; Yang, E.H.; Baas, A.S. Emerging pharmacologic and structural therapies for hypertrophic cardiomyopathy. *Heart Fail. Rev.* **2017**, *22*, 879–888. [CrossRef]
118. Schafer, U.; Frerker, C.; Thielsen, T.; Schewel, D.; Bader, R.; Kuck, K.H.; Kreidel, F. Targeting systolic anterior motion and left ventricular outflow tract obstruction in hypertrophic obstructed cardiomyopathy with a MitraClip. *EuroIntervention* **2015**, *11*, 942–947. [CrossRef]
119. Sorajja, P.; Pedersen, W.A.; Bae, R.; Lesser, J.R.; Jay, D.; Lin, D.; Harris, K.; Maron, B.J. First Experience with Percutaneous Mitral Valve Plication as Primary Therapy for Symptomatic Obstructive Hypertrophic Cardiomyopathy. *J. Am. Coll. Cardiol.* **2016**, *67*, 2811–2818. [CrossRef]

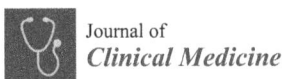

Review

Molecular Diagnosis of Hypertrophic Cardiomyopathy (HCM): In the Heart of Cardiac Disease

Marilena Melas [1,*], Eleftherios T. Beltsios [2], Antonis Adamou [3], Konstantinos Koumarelas [4] and Kim L. McBride [5,6]

1. New York Genome Center, New York, NY 10013, USA
2. West Germany Heart Center, Department of Thoracic and Cardiovascular Surgery, University Hospital Essen, 45147 Essen, Germany
3. Department of Radiology—Medical Imaging, University Hospital Larissa, 41110 Larissa, Greece
4. Faculty of Medicine, School of Health Sciences, University of Thessaly, 41110 Larissa, Greece
5. Center for Cardiovascular Research, Nationwide Children's Hospital, and Department of Pediatrics, Ohio State University, Columbus, OH 43205, USA
6. Department of Pediatrics, Nationwide Children's Hospital, Ohio State University, Columbus, OH 43205, USA
* Correspondence: mmelas@nygenome.org

Abstract: Hypertrophic cardiomyopathy (HCM) is an inherited myocardial disease with the presence of left ventricular hypertrophy (LVH). The disease is characterized by high locus, allelic and phenotypic heterogeneity, even among members of the same family. The list of confirmed and potentially relevant genes implicating the disease is constantly increasing, with novel genes frequently reported. Heterozygous alterations in the five main sarcomeric genes (*MYBPC3*, *MYH7*, *TNNT2*, *TNNI3*, and *MYL2*) are estimated to account for more than half of confirmed cases. The genetic discoveries of recent years have shed more light on the molecular pathogenic mechanisms of HCM, contributing to substantial advances in the diagnosis of the disease. Genetic testing applying next-generation sequencing (NGS) technologies and early diagnosis prior to the clinical manifestation of the disease among family members demonstrate an important improvement in the field.

Keywords: hypertrophic cardiomyopathy (HCM); next generation sequencing; genetic testing

1. Background and Medical Diagnosis of HCM

Hypertrophic cardiomyopathy (HCM) is an inherited cardiomyopathy defined as the presence of left ventricular hypertrophy (LVH) in the absence of any other disease that might result in secondary LVH. Individuals diagnosed with HCM are at higher risk of developing atrial fibrillation, which can lead to blood clots, stroke, and other heart-related complications. HCM may also lead to heart failure and sudden cardiac arrest. The disease is caused by transcriptomic defects in certain proteins of the sarcomere as a result of specific genomic alterations on thick and thin filaments and Z-disks (Figure 1). These mutations initiate a series of events leading to histological or morphological changes to the myocardial cell, which eventually becomes hypertrophic and/or fibrotic [1].

HCM remains a clinical diagnosis, and despite the molecular identification of the previously mentioned genetic loci, molecular findings cannot be used solely for the diagnosis of HCM. Clinical practice guidelines for the evaluation of HCM in children and adults have been developed [2,3]. Evaluation of an individual includes a detailed pedigree with attention to heart disease and early death in the family. Signs that can indicate the diagnosis of HCM are usually detected clinically by a physician cardiologist, depending on the skills of the examiner. A rapid rise in the carotid pulse rate with a forceful presystolic hump of the apex beat followed by a prolonged upstroke is indicative of disease. In case of severe obstruction in the absence of severe mitral regurgitation and significant septal defect, a bisferiens contour might be observed. The presence of a triple impulse of the apex beat in case of severe obstruction without significant mitral regurgitation is pathognomonic. Electrocardiography and imaging modalities such as echocardiography, magnetic resonance imaging (MRI), and computed tomography are used to confirm a diagnosis, preferably modalities with non-ionizing radiation. In adults, a maximal end-diastolic wall thickness ≥15 mm anywhere in the left ventricle measured through echocardiography or MRI is sufficient for the diagnosis of HCM in the absence of another cause of hypertrophy [2]. Hypertrophy of 13–14 mm may be diagnostic in the presence of a positive family history of HCM or a positive genetic test.

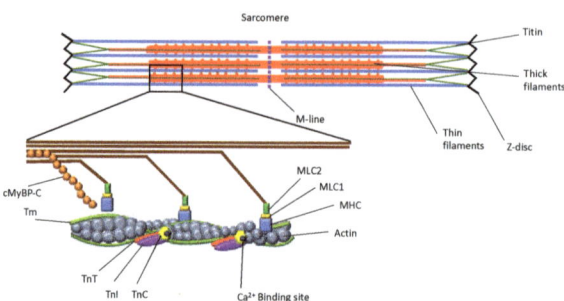

Figure 1. Hypertrophic cardiomyopathy (HCM) is caused by transcriptomic defects in certain proteins of the sarcomere as a result of specific genomic alterations on thick and thin filaments and Z-disks. Abbreviations: cMyBP-C, cardiac myosin binding protein C; Tm, tropomyosin; TnT, troponin T; TnI, troponin I; TnC, troponin C; MHC, myosin heavy chain; MLC1-2, myosin light chain 1-2.

2. Epidemiology of HCM

The prevalence of HCM has been previously reported to reach as high as 0.2% [4]. However, more recent studies suggested a prevalence between 0.03% and 0.07% [5,6]. The prevalence of the condition has presented an increasing trend in recent years, as reported in a recent study conducted in Germany including five million patients [5]. The same study suggests that HCM is more frequent in male patients in all studied age groups, and the prevalence increases successively with age, reported as 298.7/100,000 in individuals > 80 years of age. It is worth mentioning that the reported prevalence in the literature may substantially vary based on the investigated population and the diagnostic tools. The disease is present in all races, and defining differences among them would be controversial, as the degree of prevalence, the severity of the disease, and consequences are closely associated with access to genetic testing or possible inequities in care, with potentially lower use of invasive septal reduction therapy [7]. Therefore, some population groups tend to have higher rates of functionally limited heart failure. Furthermore, diagnosis of HCM based on morphological criteria (left ventricular wall thickness ≥ 15 mm present in any left ventricular segment measured by echocardiography) suggests a 10 times higher prevalence of the disease compared to studies based on the presence of symptoms and approximately a 50% lower prevalence compared to studies based on echocardiographic screening [6].

3. Molecular Diagnosis of HCM and Genetic Testing

HCM is inherited with an autosomal dominant pattern and a variable degree of penetrance and expression between affected individuals [1]. It is an entity characterized by high locus, allelic and phenotypic heterogeneity. Approximately 50–65% of individuals with a known or suspected diagnosis of familial HCM harbor a variant in one of several genes encoding components of the sarcomere and cytoskeleton [8]. Carriers of double heterozygous, compound heterozygous, and homozygous mutations often exhibit more severe forms of cardiomyopathies, ultimately leading to premature death. Inconsistencies within the same family (intrafamiliar) not explained by mutational heterogeneity could be attributed to environmental factors.

The molecular genetic basis of HCM was initially investigated by the innovative studies of Christine and Jonathan Seidman. Pare et al. [9] shed more light on the field with the discovery of the p.Arg403Glu variant in the MYH7 gene, which encodes the β-myosin heavy-chain sarcomere protein. The identification of multiple further variants in principal genes encoding sarcomere proteins elucidated the genetic heterogeneity of HCM [1]. Among the most common causal genes, *MYBPC3* (myosin-binding protein C) and *MYH7* (Myosin Heavy Chain 7) have been reported as being responsible for almost half of familiar HCM cases. However, the disease is genetically heterogeneous, and sequencing additional genes should be considered if familial HCM is suspected or the underlying etiology remains unknown. Compound heterozygous mutations have been reported in *MYBPC3* and other genes associated with HCM [10]. Notably, alterations in the *MYBPC3* gene have been primarily associated with HCM but can also be associated with other types of heart muscle disease, including dilated cardiomyopathy, restrictive cardiomyopathy, and left-ventricular non-compaction [11].

Other common associated genes include *ACTC1* (cardiac α-actin), *MYL2*, (myosin light chain 2) *MYL3* (myosin light chain 3), and SCRP3 (cysteine- and glycine-rich protein 3). The most common type of the reported causal mutations in HCM are missense variants, which often change the encoded protein structure and function by altering the protein's amino acid composition. Less commonly reported variants include deletions in *MYH7* and *TNNT2* genes. In addition, *LMNA* C591F and *LMNA* R644C alterations are reported to lead to phenotypes consistent with HCM [12,13]. How *LMNA* mutations can influence HCM-related mechanisms is not entirely clear. The loss of lamins A/C in isolated cardiomyocytes does not impact Ca^{2+} transients, but the shortening of cardiomyocytes is reduced [14]. This implies that whereas the function of SERCA appears to be normal, the activation of myofilaments is hindered and may point to a mechanism involving reduced availability of ATP to the myofilaments.

Although important causal genes have been reported for HCM, there is a great discussion in the literature regarding the HCM-associated genes in sporadic cases and small families. This is largely due to the difficulty in evaluating the causality of the genetic variants in an unambiguous manner. The gradient of effect sizes that genetic variants present results in a wide spectrum of causality, which varies from clearly causal to clinically unimportant. Frequently, members of the same family present with a disease of varying severity. The list of confirmed and potentially relevant genes associated with the disease is ever-increasing, with novel genes constantly being reported. Heterozygous alterations in the five main sarcomeric genes (*MYBPC3*, *MYH7*, *TNNT2*, *TNNI3*, and *MYL2*) are estimated to account for about 50% to 70% of HCM cases and are therefore routinely screened for diagnosis, predictive testing, genetic counseling, and surveillance [15]. Furthermore, next-generation sequencing methods contributed to the discovery of modifiers in specific regions of the genome. Particularly, polymorphisms of genomic regions encoding major components of the renin–angiotensin–aldosterone system have been reported in several meta-analyses as potential risk factors for HCM [16,17]. Additionally, four single-nucleotide polymorphisms (SNPs) (three of which are novel) were reported in a recent article as potential modifier loci in sarcomere-positive cases [18].

Despite alterations in the sarcomeric genes representing the most frequent cause of HCM in adults, the diagnosis of the disease in up to 35% of affected children is due to non-sarcomeric causes. Causal factors can be neuromuscular or mitochondrial diseases and inherited errors of metabolism (glycogen storage diseases, lysosomal storage diseases, and fatty acid oxidation disorders) [19,20]. Several diagnostic markers, such as family history, physical examination, electrocardiography, echocardiography, and genetic analysis have been recommended to guide diagnostic testing and early detection of non-sarcomeric HCM. Should a diagnosis of a non-sarcomeric cause of HCM be established, etiological therapy is vital (e.g., Fabry disease and Pompe disease) [21]. Interestingly, the age of presentation plays a prognostic role. For instance, HCM presenting before one year of age is associated with a worse prognosis and is mainly caused by inherited errors of metabolism or malformation syndrome such as RASopathies [22].

Genetic testing for HCM is a class 1 (strong) recommended action by the American College of Cardiology and the American Heart Association [2]. The diagnostic yield of genetic testing in children and adults with HCM is about 30% for sporadic cases and 60% for familial cases [23,24]. HCM in children may require a more specialized evaluation and diagnostic testing because of the rate of syndromic conditions and inborn errors of metabolism associated with HCM at these ages [25]. Following a well-established principle that generates the most informative outcome in clinical genetics, diagnostic genetic testing should be initiated on an affected individual within a family with a confirmed diagnosis of cardiomyopathy; usually, the individual with the most severe phenotype and/or the earliest disease onset. This approach increases the possibility of finding a genetic etiology of the disease. If a specimen from this individual is unavailable, comprehensive genomic testing should be performed on another affected family member. Nonetheless, the greatest utility of testing is for asymptomatic family members. Identification of a pathogenic variant can guide appropriate targeted sequencing in other family members, with that information used to guide the need for ongoing genetic counseling and surveillance [26].

In recent years, the molecular diagnosis of HCM has been facilitated by the advancement of next-generation sequencing (NGS) technology. NGS has arisen from DNA sequencing methodologies. Most notably massively parallel signature sequencing [27] NGS enables high-throughput sequencing of large and complex DNA specimens such as whole human exomes and genomes [28]. Geneticists first applied NGS to accurately and rapidly sequence the human germline genome [29], allowing for insights into the cause of inherited disease [30]. New applications have allowed for the assessment of not only single-nucleotide variation and nucleotide insertions and deletions but also the transcriptome to assess gene expression [31], copy number variation [32], and complex genomic structural variation [33].

NGS can be applied to the diagnosis of HCM in three ways: targeted sequencing for a number of genes (multigene panels), whole-exome sequencing (WES), and whole-genome sequencing (WGS) [34]. It has been recommended that the most cost-effective first line of testing is gene panels or exome-sequencing-based analysis of genes, which have been established to cause HCM or other diseases that could be misdiagnosed as HCM. If this initial genetic test does not detect a causal variant, no further testing is recommended for individuals with late-onset HCM and a mild phenotype. However, if there is no family history of the disease but a severe clinical phenotype, a search for de novo variants with WGS of a family trio may be considered. For gene-elusive patients with a family history of HCM, WGS-based analysis of intronic regions and the mitochondrial genome may reveal a pathogenic variant in an additional 9% of this HCM cohort.

4. Gene Panels

The advantage of targeted sequencing using gene panels is that the region of sequencing can be highly specific and can be covered in great depth with many samples analyzed at the same time. For diseases in which only a small number of genes are involved, the cost of targeted sequencing is considerably less than WES and WGS. For HCM, panels including many genes relevant to the phenotype have become the standard of practice, as they are usually feasible and cost-effective [35]. Genetic testing using multigene panels is recommended over Sanger-sequencing-based single-gene testing due to the genetic heterogeneity of cardiomyopathies [23].

Large gene panels for cardiomyopathy may include genes that cause genetic syndromes associated with cardiomyopathy (such as Noonan syndrome, Fabry disease, Danon disease, and Alström syndrome), neuromuscular conditions associated with cardiomyopathy (such as limb girdle muscular dystrophies), or metabolic conditions. These large gene panels increase the likelihood of identifying a molecular etiology, especially for patients with complex phenotypes [36]. Panels also increase the likelihood of identifying individuals who harbor disease-causing alterations in multiple genes, which are estimated to occur in 5% of HCM cases, with a typically more severe phenotype [37]. Larger panels are not necessarily better than smaller panels. Many large panels include genes that are likely not causative of HCM; thus, variant detection in those genes can make clinical interpretation rather challenging [38].

5. Whole-Exome Sequencing (WES) and Whole-Genome Sequencing (WGS)

WES is an approach that works through attempts to capture and sequence protein-coding regions in the human genome. These capture regions are predesigned through commercially marketed kits. This approach has the advantage of covering the entire exome; however, the coverage of the exome is typically not complete, owing to difficulties in the design of probes. The use of WES in HCM is somewhat controversial, as the gain in yield may be limited, whereas the possibility of identifying variants of unknown significance (VUS) increases. Genes related to cardiovascular phenotypes have always been included on the list of secondary findings [39] due to the morbidity and mortality of sudden cardiac death (SCD) and heart failure (HF), which can both be prevented or treated with well-established interventions [3,40]. These secondary findings can pose challenges in the clinical setting of an individual without a personal or family history of HCM [41].

In a recent study [42], the authors examined the coverage and diagnostic yield of WES on HCM-related genes variants compared to four different commercial gene panels studying a cohort of forty HCM patients. With a diagnostic yield of 43%, the coverage was found to be similar to that of four existing commercial gene panels due to the clustering of alterations within *MYH7, MYBPC3, TPM1, TNT2,* and *TTN* genes. In addition, the coverage of WES appeared suboptimal for TNNI3 and *PLN* genes. It has been debated that most of the pathogenic variants for HCM can be adequately detected via gene panels and that the application of WES did not improve the diagnostic yield. Most recently, WES has gained momentum for the genetic diagnosis of HCM, revealing potential digenic inheritance of familial HCM. In particular, a genomic deletion in chromosome 19 encompassing the troponin I3 gene (*TNNI3*) and the p.Ile736Thr variant in the myosin heavy chain 7 gene (*MYH7*) were detected in two patients with familial HCM [43]. The *MYH7* variant was confirmed by Sanger sequencing and was predicted as a pathogenic variant by in silico tools.

Whole-genome sequencing (WGS) is valuable in detecting variants in intronic regions, and new in silico tools can predict which variants located in introns, exons, or splice regions are more likely to alter splicing. According to Cirino et al. [44], WGS in 41 patients with HCM was able to reveal almost all variants identified by panel testing, providing one new diagnostic finding. Several variants of uncertain significance (VUS) and a number of secondary genetic findings were also detected. Whereas gene panel testing and WGS provided similar diagnostic yield, the WGS approach can enable reanalysis, allowing for the incorporation of new knowledge; however, certain expertise in variant interpretation is required to appropriately incorporate WGS into the clinical setting.

WGS has also identified additional genetic causes of HCM over targeted gene sequencing approaches [45]. In this study, it was demonstrated how WGS can detect genetic variants not identified with sequencing of protein-coding exons only, therefore improving the yield of genetic testing for HCM. In particular, they found that an additional 9% of gene-elusive HCM patients have pathogenic variants in deep intronic regions of *MYBPC3*, which result in a splice gain. It was also demonstrated that WGS, as a first-line genetic test, can detect pathogenic variants in 42% of patients tested. These outcomes enable a more accurate diagnosis of HCM and diseases that can be misdiagnosed as HCM, therefore facilitating more targeted therapies with the ultimate goal of improving clinical management [45].

6. RNA Sequencing (RNA-Seq)

RNA-seq is emerging as the major transcriptome profiling system, with considerable advantages in many aspects, such as novel transcript identification through de novo assembly, splice junction identification, and allele-specific expression analysis. Developments in RNA analysis have improved diagnosis by identifying new variants that interfere with splicing [46]. Non-coding RNAs, particularly microRNAs (miRNAs), are also attracting considerable attention as biomarkers of cardiac disease and potential therapeutic targets. Altered expression levels of circulating miRNAs have been reported in association with HCM, and the forced overexpression of stress-inducible miRNAs was shown to induce cardiomyocyte hypertrophy. However, it remains to be established whether the modulation of miRNA levels is sufficient to revert the HCM phenotype [46].

Recent studies using single-cell approaches have comprehensively characterized the transcriptional landscape at the cellular level in patients with HCM. These findings extend the understanding of the molecular basis of cardiomyopathies both on the genomic and transcriptomic level, therefore providing insights into the pathways involved and potential therapeutic targets for these morbid cardiac conditions [47]. Compared with the standard RNA-seq protocol, strand-specific RNA-seq retains strand-of-origin information; therefore, it can provide a greater resolution for sense/antisense profiling, which is important for antisense lncRNA identification. A strand-specific RNA-seq dataset for coding and lncRNA profiling in myocardial tissues from 28 HCM patients and 9 healthy donors was recently developed [48]. This dataset was systemically reanalyzed by another group, which focused on the identification of functional variants, differentially expressed coding and noncoding genes, and the interpretation of their potential functional roles associated with HCM [49].

RNA analysis is essential to demonstrate the consequences of potential splice-disrupting alterations. Recent studies have succeeded in reclassifying variants from uncertain significance to likely pathogenic through an analysis of RNA isolated from fresh venous blood, from myectomy samples, or induced pluripotent stem-cell-derived cardiomyocytes from patients [46]. In addition to improving the precision of molecular diagnostics, the discovery of disease-causing aberrantly spliced mRNA in HCM patients opens new venues for the development of RNA-targeted therapies. Splice-switching antisense oligonucleotides and short interfering RNAs are promising strategies. Although further developments are needed to overcome major challenges related to safety and delivery, RNA-targeting drugs hold great potential for the treatment of HCM [50,51].

7. Gene Therapy Strategies in the Treatment of HCM

Current therapies for HCM are mainly focused on symptomatic relief and improving clinical outcomes such as myosin modulators [52] rather than the genetic etiology of HCM. Several strategies have been developed in the last decades to remove genetic defects, including genome editing, allele-specific silencing, exon skipping, gene replacement, and spliceosome-mediated RNA trans-splicing. These approaches have already been tested for their efficacy and efficiency, with promising results, most of them in animal- or human-induced pluripotent stem cell models of HCM.

Gene therapy targeting the cause of HCM is particularly attractive for rare, severe forms with biallelic truncating mutations in *MYBPC3* leading to heart failure and premature death in infants [53,54]. Among the different gene therapy options tested, gene replacement with AAV9-mediated delivery of functional *MYBPC3* cDNA has already proven to be the most successful in mice [55] and in human pluripotent stem-cell-derived cardiomyocytes [56,57].

High-fidelity gene repair in human embryos harboring HCM alterations has demonstrated promising results. Using sperm from a heterozygous *MYBPC3* mutation male carrier, oocytes from healthy women were inseminated. Simultaneous injection of a mutation-specific CRISPR/Cas9 system during the early metaphase resulted in the successful editing of the mutation [58].

Allele-specific gene silencing is another gene-based therapeutic technology that holds promise for monogenic diseases. This involves the transduction of an adenovirus vector containing short-interfering ribonucleic acid segments designed to inhibit the expression of a specific pathogenic allele—a method more broadly known as ribonucleic acid interference (RNAi). In preclinical models, RNAi was demonstrated to attenuate the phenotype of specific alterations causing HCM [59]. This approach is more tailored to conditions caused by gain-of-function alterations (e.g., *MYH7*) and likely not the full spectrum of HCM (e.g.,

MYBPC3). Additional limitations include off-target effects (e.g., knockdown of non-target mRNAs) and the current need for adenovirus delivery.

8. Challenges of Molecular Diagnosis and Future Perspectives

Genetic testing in HCM plays an important role in the management of affected individuals and their families, allowing for cascade testing. It can provide a molecular diagnosis and differentiate HCM from other diseases causing LV wall thickening, guiding the clinical management of patients and their families. Genetic testing results are based on the strength of evidence of specific variants to be disease-causing (pathogenic or likely pathogenic). If a pathogenic variant is detected, discovery testing strategies can definitively identify relatives at risk and guide longitudinal family screening. However, understanding the clinical relevance of genetic testing is complicated, and classifying variants may be complex. As such, pretest and post-test genetic counseling is fundamental to help establish appropriate expectations and assist the patient and their family to better understand the results. If results are difficult to interpret, further expertise and consultation should be sought.

Recent standards and guidelines are routinely used in order to standardize and increase the clarity of variant classification [60]. Nevertheless, the interpretations provided for a given variant may differ between molecular diagnostics laboratories [61]. In addition, frequent revisions of variant interpretation may occur as more information is obtained from larger patient and healthy control cohorts, sometimes leading to the amendment of a clinical report with a modified diagnostic interpretation. Because genetic testing results are probabilistic rather than determinative, they must always be interpreted in the context of the patient's medical and family history [62]. For example, family history and the segregation of a putative causal variant within the family may be important information for clinical interpretation, especially when a novel genetic variant is identified.

The inability to identify a causative alteration in 50%–60% of HCM patients is a significant limiting factor of genetic testing [63]. Factors enabling the development of HCM in patients with a negative genetic test and asymptomatic carriers of a pathogenic alteration have not been fully described yet. Initially, the theory that patients with a negative genetic test could harbor mutations in genes not yet associated to the pathogenesis of HCM was universally accepted. Patients without a pathogenic variant are now suspected to have HCM through a non-Mendelian mechanism, with a more favorable prognosis compared to patients with sarcomeric pathogenic alterations [64]. As comprehensive whole-exome and whole-genome sequencing approaches become more widely accessible, ongoing research efforts are key to expanding our knowledge of the full spectrum of HCM-related genes and facilitating variant interpretation and classification. However, although such comprehensive molecular testing can identify new genes associated with HCM, a large number of variants of uncertain significance (VUS) are also expected to be detected, potentially increasing overall uncertainty as a result of inconclusive results and causing psychological stress to the patients and their families.

A more sophisticated understanding of genetic variation and novel strategies for the assessment of the pathogenicity of variants are decisive to precisely translate the massive amount of data obtained from comprehensive NGS-based genetic testing. Due to the enormous heterogeneity of HCM and the diverse clinical manifestations of the disease, larger patient cohorts including longitudinal clinical phenotypes and genotyping are needed to provide further insights into the genetic etiology and pathogenesis of HCM. In addition, multicenter collaborations and interdisciplinary cooperation of cardiologists, molecular biologists, clinical geneticists, bioinformaticians, and genetic counselors are required to efficiently interpret and communicate NGS-based genetic testing results to patients and their families.

Author Contributions: Conceptualization, E.T.B. and M.M.; methodology, E.T.B., M.M. and A.A.; writing—original draft preparation, M.M., E.T.B., A.A. and K.K. writing—review and editing, M.M., E.T.B., A.A. and K.L.M.; visualization, E.T.B.; supervision, K.L.M.; project administration K.L.M. All authors have read and agreed to the published version of the manuscript.

Funding: This research received no external funding.

Conflicts of Interest: The authors declare no conflict of interest.

References

1. Marian, A.J.; Braunwald, E. Hypertrophic Cardiomyopathy: Genetics, Pathogenesis, Clinical Manifestations, Diagnosis, and Therapy. *Circ. Res.* **2017**, *121*, 749–770. [CrossRef] [PubMed]
2. Writing Committee Members; Ommen, S.R.; Mital, S.; Burke, M.A.; Day, S.M.; Deswal, A.; Elliott, P.; Evanovich, L.L.; Hung, J.; Joglar, J.A.; et al. 2020 AHA/ACC Guideline for the Diagnosis and Treatment of Patients With Hypertrophic Cardiomyopathy. *Circulation* **2020**, *142*, e558–e631. [CrossRef]
3. Hershberger, R.E.; Givertz, M.M.; Ho, C.Y.; Judge, D.P.; Kantor, P.F.; McBride, K.L.; Morales, A.; Taylor, M.R.G.; Vatta, M.; Ware, S.M. Genetic Evaluation of Cardiomyopathy—A Heart Failure Society of America Practice Guideline. *J. Card. Fail.* **2018**, *24*, 281–302. [CrossRef] [PubMed]
4. Maron, B.J.; Gardin, J.M.; Flack, J.M.; Gidding, S.S.; Kurosaki, T.T.; Bild, D.E. Prevalence of Hypertrophic Cardiomyopathy in a General Population of Young Adults. Echocardiographic Analysis of 4111 Subjects in the CARDIA Study. Coronary Artery Risk Development in (Young) Adults. *Circulation* **1995**, *92*, 785–789. [CrossRef]
5. Husser, D.; Ueberham, L.; Jacob, J.; Heuer, D.; Riedel-Heller, S.; Walker, J.; Hindricks, G.; Bollmann, A. Prevalence of Clinically Apparent Hypertrophic Cardiomyopathy in Germany—An Analysis of over 5 Million Patients. *PLoS ONE* **2018**, *13*, e0196612. [CrossRef]
6. Maron, M.S.; Hellawell, J.L.; Lucove, J.C.; Farzaneh-Far, R.; Olivotto, I. Occurrence of Clinically Diagnosed Hypertrophic Cardiomyopathy in the United States. *Am. J. Cardiol.* **2016**, *117*, 1651–1654. [CrossRef]
7. Eberly, L.A.; Day, S.M.; Ashley, E.A.; Jacoby, D.L.; Jefferies, J.L.; Colan, S.D.; Rossano, J.W.; Semsarian, C.; Pereira, A.C.; Olivotto, I.; et al. Association of Race With Disease Expression and Clinical Outcomes Among Patients With Hypertrophic Cardiomyopathy. *JAMA Cardiol.* **2020**, *5*, 83–91. [CrossRef]
8. Morita, H.; Rehm, H.L.; Menesses, A.; McDonough, B.; Roberts, A.E.; Kucherlapati, R.; Towbin, J.A.; Seidman, J.G.; Seidman, C.E. Shared Genetic Causes of Cardiac Hypertrophy in Children and Adults. *N. Engl. J. Med.* **2008**, *358*, 1899–1908. [CrossRef]
9. Pare, J.A.; Fraser, R.G.; Pirozynski, W.J.; Shanks, J.A.; Stubington, D. Hereditary Cardiovascular Dysplasia. A Form of Familial Cardiomyopathy. *Am. J. Med.* **1961**, *31*, 37–62. [CrossRef]
10. Van Driest, S.L.; Vasile, V.C.; Ommen, S.R.; Will, M.L.; Tajik, A.J.; Gersh, B.J.; Ackerman, M.J. Myosin Binding Protein C Mutations and Compound Heterozygosity in Hypertrophic Cardiomyopathy. *J. Am. Coll. Cardiol.* **2004**, *44*, 1903–1910. [CrossRef]
11. Hershberger, R.E.; Norton, N.; Morales, A.; Li, D.; Siegfried, J.D.; Gonzalez-Quintana, J. Coding Sequence Rare Variants Identified in MYBPC3, MYH6, TPM1, TNNC1, and TNNI3 from 312 Patients with Familial or Idiopathic Dilated Cardiomyopathy. *Circ. Cardiovasc. Genet.* **2010**, *3*, 155–161. [CrossRef] [PubMed]
12. Mercuri, E.; Brown, S.C.; Nihoyannopoulos, P.; Poulton, J.; Kinali, M.; Richard, P.; Piercy, R.J.; Messina, S.; Sewry, C.; Burke, M.M.; et al. Extreme Variability of Skeletal and Cardiac Muscle Involvement in Patients with Mutations in Exon 11 of the Lamin A/C Gene. *Muscle Nerve* **2005**, *31*, 602–609. [CrossRef] [PubMed]
13. Araújo-Vilar, D.; Lado-Abeal, J.; Palos-Paz, F.; Lattanzi, G.; Bandín, M.A.; Bellido, D.; Domínguez-Gerpe, L.; Calvo, C.; Pérez, O.; Ramazanova, A.; et al. A Novel Phenotypic Expression Associated with a New Mutation in LMNA Gene, Characterized by Partial Lipodystrophy, Insulin Resistance, Aortic Stenosis and Hypertrophic Cardiomyopathy. *Clin. Endocrinol.* **2008**, *69*, 61–68. [CrossRef] [PubMed]
14. Nikolova, V.; Leimena, C.; McMahon, A.C.; Tan, J.C.; Chandar, S.; Jogia, D.; Kesteven, S.H.; Michalicek, J.; Otway, R.; Verheyen, F.; et al. Defects in Nuclear Structure and Function Promote Dilated Cardiomyopathy in Lamin A/C-Deficient Mice. *J. Clin. Investig.* **2004**, *113*, 357–369. [CrossRef] [PubMed]
15. Bos, J.M.; Ackerman, M.J. Chapter 7—Hypertrophic Cardiomyopathy in the Era of Genomic Medicine. In *Genomic and Precision Medicine*, 3rd ed.; Ginsburg, G.S., Willard, H.F., Eds.; Academic Press: Boston, MA, USA, 2018; pp. 103–126, ISBN 978-0-12-801812-5.
16. Yuan, Y.; Meng, L.; Zhou, Y.; Lu, N. Genetic Polymorphism of Angiotensin-Converting Enzyme and Hypertrophic Cardiomyopathy Risk: A Systematic Review and Meta-Analysis. *Medicine* **2017**, *96*, e8639. [CrossRef]
17. Zhen, Z.; Gao, L.; Wang, Q.; Chen, X.; Na, J.; Xu, X.; Yuan, Y. Angiotensinogen M235T Polymorphism and Susceptibility to Hypertrophic Cardiomyopathy in Asian Population: A Meta Analysis. *J. Renin. Angiotensin. Aldosterone. Syst.* **2020**, *21*, 1470320320978100. [CrossRef] [PubMed]
18. Harper, A.R.; Goel, A.; Grace, C.; Thomson, K.L.; Petersen, S.E.; Xu, X.; Waring, A.; Ormondroyd, E.; Kramer, C.M.; Ho, C.Y.; et al. Common Genetic Variants and Modifiable Risk Factors Underpin Hypertrophic Cardiomyopathy Susceptibility and Expressivity. *Nat. Genet.* **2021**, *53*, 135–142. [CrossRef]

19. Monda, E.; Rubino, M.; Lioncino, M.; Di Fraia, F.; Pacileo, R.; Verrillo, F.; Cirillo, A.; Caiazza, M.; Fusco, A.; Esposito, A.; et al. Hypertrophic Cardiomyopathy in Children: Pathophysiology, Diagnosis, and Treatment of Non-Sarcomeric Causes. *Front. Pediatr.* 2021, *9*, 632293. [CrossRef]
20. Limongelli, G.; Adorisio, R.; Baggio, C.; Bauce, B.; Biagini, E.; Castelletti, S.; Favilli, S.; Imazio, M.; Lioncino, M.; Merlo, M.; et al. Diagnosis and Management of Rare Cardiomyopathies in Adult and Paediatric Patients. A Position Paper of the Italian Society of Cardiology (SIC) and Italian Society of Paediatric Cardiology (SICP). *Int. J. Cardiol.* 2022, *357*, 55–71. [CrossRef]
21. Rubino, M.; Monda, E.; Lioncino, M.; Caiazza, M.; Palmiero, G.; Dongiglio, F.; Fusco, A.; Cirillo, A.; Cesaro, A.; Capodicasa, L.; et al. Diagnosis and Management of Cardiovascular Involvement in Fabry Disease. *Heart Fail. Clin.* 2022, *18*, 39–49. [CrossRef]
22. Colan, S.D.; Lipshultz, S.E.; Lowe, A.M.; Sleeper, L.A.; Messere, J.; Cox, G.F.; Lurie, P.R.; Orav, E.J.; Towbin, J.A. Epidemiology and Cause-Specific Outcome of Hypertrophic Cardiomyopathy in Children: Findings from the Pediatric Cardiomyopathy Registry. *Circulation* 2007, *115*, 773–781. [CrossRef]
23. Alfares, A.A.; Kelly, M.A.; McDermott, G.; Funke, B.H.; Lebo, M.S.; Baxter, S.B.; Shen, J.; McLaughlin, H.M.; Clark, E.H.; Babb, L.J.; et al. Results of Clinical Genetic Testing of 2912 Probands with Hypertrophic Cardiomyopathy: Expanded Panels Offer Limited Additional Sensitivity. *Genet. Med.* 2015, *17*, 880–888. [CrossRef] [PubMed]
24. Ingles, J.; Sarina, T.; Yeates, L.; Hunt, L.; Macciocca, I.; McCormack, L.; Winship, I.; McGaughran, J.; Atherton, J.; Semsarian, C. Clinical Predictors of Genetic Testing Outcomes in Hypertrophic Cardiomyopathy. *Genet. Med.* 2013, *15*, 972–977. [CrossRef] [PubMed]
25. Ware, S.M. Genetics of Pediatric Cardiomyopathies. *Curr. Opin. Pediatr.* 2017, *29*, 534–540. [CrossRef]
26. Teekakirikul, P.; Zhu, W.; Huang, H.C.; Fung, E. Hypertrophic Cardiomyopathy: An Overview of Genetics and Management. *Biomolecules* 2019, *9*, 878. [CrossRef]
27. Mardis, E.R. Next-Generation DNA Sequencing Methods. *Annu. Rev. Genom. Hum. Genet.* 2008, *9*, 387–402. [CrossRef] [PubMed]
28. Hu, T.; Chitnis, N.; Monos, D.; Dinh, A. Next-Generation Sequencing Technologies: An Overview. *Hum. Immunol.* 2021, *82*, 801–811. [CrossRef]
29. Bentley, D.R.; Balasubramanian, S.; Swerdlow, H.P.; Smith, G.P.; Milton, J.; Brown, C.G.; Hall, K.P.; Evers, D.J.; Barnes, C.L.; Bignell, H.R.; et al. Accurate Whole Human Genome Sequencing Using Reversible Terminator Chemistry. *Nature* 2008, *456*, 53–59. [CrossRef]
30. Mardis, E.R. The Impact of Next-Generation Sequencing Technology on Genetics. *Trends Genet.* 2008, *24*, 133–141. [CrossRef]
31. Reinartz, J.; Bruyns, E.; Lin, J.-Z.; Burcham, T.; Brenner, S.; Bowen, B.; Kramer, M.; Woychik, R. Massively Parallel Signature Sequencing (MPSS) as a Tool for in-Depth Quantitative Gene Expression Profiling in All Organisms. *Brief. Funct. Genom. Proteomic* 2002, *1*, 95–104. [CrossRef]
32. Wang, H.; Nettleton, D.; Ying, K. Copy Number Variation Detection Using next Generation Sequencing Read Counts. *BMC Bioinform.* 2014, *15*, 109. [CrossRef]
33. Medvedev, P.; Stanciu, M.; Brudno, M. Computational Methods for Discovering Structural Variation with Next-Generation Sequencing. *Nat. Methods* 2009, *6*, S13–S20. [CrossRef]
34. Sun, Y.; Ruivenkamp, C.A.L.; Hoffer, M.J.V.; Vrijenhoek, T.; Kriek, M.; van Asperen, C.J.; den Dunnen, J.T.; Santen, G.W.E. Next-Generation Diagnostics: Gene Panel, Exome, or Whole Genome? *Hum. Mutat.* 2015, *36*, 648–655. [CrossRef]
35. Wilson, K.D.; Shen, P.; Fung, E.; Karakikes, I.; Zhang, A.; InanlooRahatloo, K.; Odegaard, J.; Sallam, K.; Davis, R.W.; Lui, G.K.; et al. A Rapid, High-Quality, Cost-Effective, Comprehensive and Expandable Targeted Next-Generation Sequencing Assay for Inherited Heart Diseases. *Circ. Res.* 2015, *117*, 603–611. [CrossRef] [PubMed]
36. Long, P.A.; Evans, J.M.; Olson, T.M. Exome Sequencing Establishes Diagnosis of Alström Syndrome in an Infant Presenting with Non-Syndromic Dilated Cardiomyopathy. *Am. J. Med. Genet. A* 2015, *167A*, 886–890. [CrossRef] [PubMed]
37. Maron, B.J.; Maron, M.S.; Semsarian, C. Double or Compound Sarcomere Mutations in Hypertrophic Cardiomyopathy: A Potential Link to Sudden Death in the Absence of Conventional Risk Factors. *Heart Rhythm* 2012, *9*, 57–63. [CrossRef] [PubMed]
38. Ingles, J.; Goldstein, J.; Thaxton, C.; Caleshu, C.; Corty, E.W.; Crowley, S.B.; Dougherty, K.; Harrison, S.M.; McGlaughon, J.; Milko, L.V.; et al. Evaluating the Clinical Validity of Hypertrophic Cardiomyopathy Genes. *Circ. Genom. Precis. Med.* 2019, *12*, e002460. [CrossRef]
39. Miller, D.T.; Lee, K.; Chung, W.K.; Gordon, A.S.; Herman, G.E.; Klein, T.E.; Stewart, D.R.; Amendola, L.M.; Adelman, K.; Bale, S.J.; et al. ACMG SF v3.0 List for Reporting of Secondary Findings in Clinical Exome and Genome Sequencing: A Policy Statement of the American College of Medical Genetics and Genomics (ACMG). *Genet. Med.* 2021, *23*, 1381–1390. [CrossRef]
40. Al-Khatib, S.M.; Stevenson, W.G.; Ackerman, M.J.; Bryant, W.J.; Callans, D.J.; Curtis, A.B.; Deal, B.J.; Dickfeld, T.; Field, M.E.; Fonarow, G.C.; et al. 2017 AHA/ACC/HRS Guideline for Management of Patients With Ventricular Arrhythmias and the Prevention of Sudden Cardiac Death. *J. Am. Coll. Cardiol.* 2018, *72*, e91–e220. [CrossRef]
41. Lacaze, P.; Sebra, R.; Riaz, M.; Ingles, J.; Tiller, J.; Thompson, B.A.; James, P.A.; Fatkin, D.; Semsarian, C.; Reid, C.M.; et al. Genetic Variants Associated with Inherited Cardiovascular Disorders among 13,131 Asymptomatic Older Adults of European Descent. *NPJ Genom. Med.* 2021, *6*, 51. [CrossRef]
42. Mak, T.S.H.; Lee, Y.-K.; Tang, C.S.; Hai, J.S.H.; Ran, X.; Sham, P.-C.; Tse, H.-F. Coverage and Diagnostic Yield of Whole Exome Sequencing for the Evaluation of Cases with Dilated and Hypertrophic Cardiomyopathy. *Sci. Rep.* 2018, *8*, 10846. [CrossRef]
43. Ren, M.-B.; Chai, X.-R.; Li, L.; Wang, X.; Yin, C. Potential Digenic Inheritance of Familial Hypertrophic Cardiomyopathy Identified by Whole-Exome Sequencing. *Mol. Genet. Genom. Med.* 2020, *8*, e1150. [CrossRef] [PubMed]

44. Cirino, A.L.; Lakdawala, N.K.; McDonough, B.; Conner, L.; Adler, D.; Weinfeld, M.; O'Gara, P.; Rehm, H.L.; Machini, K.; Lebo, M.; et al. A Comparison of Whole Genome Sequencing to Multigene Panel Testing in Hypertrophic Cardiomyopathy Patients. *Circ. Cardiovasc. Genet.* **2017**, *10*, e001768. [CrossRef] [PubMed]
45. Bagnall, R.D.; Ingles, J.; Dinger, M.E.; Cowley, M.J.; Ross, S.B.; Minoche, A.E.; Lal, S.; Turner, C.; Colley, A.; Rajagopalan, S.; et al. Whole Genome Sequencing Improves Outcomes of Genetic Testing in Patients With Hypertrophic Cardiomyopathy. *J. Am. Coll. Cardiol.* **2018**, *72*, 419–429. [CrossRef] [PubMed]
46. Ribeiro, M.; Furtado, M.; Martins, S.; Carvalho, T.; Carmo-Fonseca, M. RNA Splicing Defects in Hypertrophic Cardiomyopathy: Implications for Diagnosis and Therapy. *Int. J. Mol. Sci.* **2020**, *21*, 1329. [CrossRef]
47. Chaffin, M.; Papangeli, I.; Simonson, B.; Akkad, A.-D.; Hill, M.C.; Arduini, A.; Fleming, S.J.; Melanson, M.; Hayat, S.; Kost-Alimova, M.; et al. Single-Nucleus Profiling of Human Dilated and Hypertrophic Cardiomyopathy. *Nature* **2022**, *608*, 174–180. [CrossRef] [PubMed]
48. Liu, X.; Ma, Y.; Yin, K.; Li, W.; Chen, W.; Zhang, Y.; Zhu, C.; Li, T.; Han, B.; Liu, X.; et al. Long Non-Coding and Coding RNA Profiling Using Strand-Specific RNA-Seq in Human Hypertrophic Cardiomyopathy. *Sci Data* **2019**, *6*, 90. [CrossRef]
49. Gao, J.; Collyer, J.; Wang, M.; Sun, F.; Xu, F. Genetic Dissection of Hypertrophic Cardiomyopathy with Myocardial RNA-Seq. *Int. J. Mol. Sci.* **2020**, *21*, 3040. [CrossRef]
50. Roma-Rodrigues, C.; Raposo, L.R.; Fernandes, A.R. MicroRNAs Based Therapy of Hypertrophic Cardiomyopathy: The Road Traveled So Far. *Biomed. Res. Int.* **2015**, *2015*, 983290. [CrossRef]
51. Robinson, E.L.; Port, J.D. Utilization and Potential of RNA-Based Therapies in Cardiovascular Disease. *JACC Basic Transl. Sci.* **2022**, *7*, 956–969. [CrossRef]
52. Lekaditi, D.; Sakellaropoulos, S. Myosin Modulators: The New Era of Medical Therapy for Systolic Heart Failure and Hypertrophic Cardiomyopathy. *Cardiol. Res.* **2021**, *12*, 146–148. [CrossRef]
53. Wessels, M.W.; Herkert, J.C.; Frohn-Mulder, I.M.; Dalinghaus, M.; van den Wijngaard, A.; de Krijger, R.R.; Michels, M.; de Coo, I.F.; Hoedemaekers, Y.M.; Dooijes, D. Compound Heterozygous or Homozygous Truncating MYBPC3 Mutations Cause Lethal Cardiomyopathy with Features of Noncompaction and Septal Defects. *Eur. J. Hum. Genet.* **2015**, *23*, 922–928. [CrossRef] [PubMed]
54. Carrier, L. Targeting the Population for Gene Therapy with MYBPC3. *J. Mol. Cell. Cardiol.* **2021**, *150*, 101–108. [CrossRef]
55. Mearini, G.; Stimpel, D.; Geertz, B.; Weinberger, F.; Krämer, E.; Schlossarek, S.; Mourot-Filiatre, J.; Stoehr, A.; Dutsch, A.; Wijnker, P.J.M.; et al. Mybpc3 Gene Therapy for Neonatal Cardiomyopathy Enables Long-Term Disease Prevention in Mice. *Nat. Commun.* **2014**, *5*, 5515. [CrossRef]
56. Monteiro da Rocha, A.; Guerrero-Serna, G.; Helms, A.; Luzod, C.; Mironov, S.; Russell, M.; Jalife, J.; Day, S.M.; Smith, G.D.; Herron, T.J. Deficient CMyBP-C Protein Expression during Cardiomyocyte Differentiation Underlies Human Hypertrophic Cardiomyopathy Cellular Phenotypes in Disease Specific Human ES Cell Derived Cardiomyocytes. *J. Mol. Cell. Cardiol.* **2016**, *99*, 197–206. [CrossRef]
57. Prondzynski, M.; Krämer, E.; Laufer, S.D.; Shibamiya, A.; Pless, O.; Flenner, F.; Müller, O.J.; Münch, J.; Redwood, C.; Hansen, A.; et al. Evaluation of MYBPC3 Trans-Splicing and Gene Replacement as Therapeutic Options in Human IPSC-Derived Cardiomyocytes. *Mol. Ther. Nucleic Acids* **2017**, *7*, 475–486. [CrossRef] [PubMed]
58. Ma, H.; Marti-Gutierrez, N.; Park, S.-W.; Wu, J.; Lee, Y.; Suzuki, K.; Koski, A.; Ji, D.; Hayama, T.; Ahmed, R.; et al. Correction of a Pathogenic Gene Mutation in Human Embryos. *Nature* **2017**, *548*, 413–419. [CrossRef] [PubMed]
59. Jiang, J.; Wakimoto, H.; Seidman, J.G.; Seidman, C.E. Allele-Specific Silencing of Mutant Myh6 Transcripts in Mice Suppresses Hypertrophic Cardiomyopathy. *Science* **2013**, *342*, 111–114. [CrossRef] [PubMed]
60. Richards, S.; Aziz, N.; Bale, S.; Bick, D.; Das, S.; Gastier-Foster, J.; Grody, W.W.; Hegde, M.; Lyon, E.; Spector, E.; et al. Standards and Guidelines for the Interpretation of Sequence Variants: A Joint Consensus Recommendation of the American College of Medical Genetics and Genomics and the Association for Molecular Pathology. *Genet. Med.* **2015**, *17*, 405–423. [CrossRef]
61. Van Driest, S.L.; Wells, Q.S.; Stallings, S.; Bush, W.S.; Gordon, A.; Nickerson, D.A.; Kim, J.H.; Crosslin, D.R.; Jarvik, G.P.; Carrell, D.S.; et al. Association of Arrhythmia-Related Genetic Variants With Phenotypes Documented in Electronic Medical Records. *JAMA* **2016**, *315*, 47–57. [CrossRef]
62. Ingles, J.; Semsarian, C. Conveying a Probabilistic Genetic Test Result to Families with an Inherited Heart Disease. *Heart Rhythm.* **2014**, *11*, 1073–1078. [CrossRef] [PubMed]
63. Thomson, K.L.; Ormondroyd, E.; Harper, A.R.; Dent, T.; McGuire, K.; Baksi, J.; Blair, E.; Brennan, P.; Buchan, R.; Bueser, T.; et al. Analysis of 51 Proposed Hypertrophic Cardiomyopathy Genes from Genome Sequencing Data in Sarcomere Negative Cases Has Negligible Diagnostic Yield. *Genet. Med.* **2019**, *21*, 1576–1584. [CrossRef] [PubMed]
64. Bonaventura, J.; Polakova, E.; Vejtasova, V.; Veselka, J. Genetic Testing in Patients with Hypertrophic Cardiomyopathy. *Int. J. Mol. Sci.* **2021**, *22*, 10401. [CrossRef] [PubMed]

Disclaimer/Publisher's Note: The statements, opinions and data contained in all publications are solely those of the individual author(s) and contributor(s) and not of MDPI and/or the editor(s). MDPI and/or the editor(s) disclaim responsibility for any injury to people or property resulting from any ideas, methods, instructions or products referred to in the content.

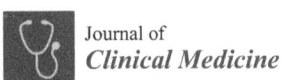

Article

Association of Types of Sleep Apnea and Nocturnal Hypoxemia with Atrial Fibrillation in Patients with Hypertrophic Cardiomyopathy

Haobo Xu, Juan Wang *, Shubin Qiao, Jiansong Yuan, Fenghuan Hu, Weixian Yang, Chao Guo, Xiaoliang Luo, Xin Duan, Shengwen Liu, Rong Liu and Jingang Cui *

Department of Cardiology, Fuwai Hospital, National Center for Cardiovascular Diseases, Chinese Academy of Medical Sciences, Beijing 100037, China
* Correspondence: dr_juan@163.com (J.W.); doctorcjg@163.com (J.C.); Fax: +86-10-8832-2415 (J.W.)

Abstract: Background: Data regarding the association between sleep apnea (SA) and atrial fibrillation (AF) in hypertrophic cardiomyopathy (HCM) are still limited. We aim to investigate the association of both types of SA, obstructive sleep apnea (OSA) and central sleep apnea (CSA), and nocturnal hypoxemia with AF in HCM. Methods: A total of 606 patients with HCM who underwent sleep evaluations were included. Logistic regression was used to assess the association between sleep disorder and AF. Results: SA was presented in 363 (59.9%) patients, of whom 337 (55.6%) had OSA and 26 (4.3%) had CSA. Patients with SA were older, more often male, had a higher body mass index, and more clinical comorbidities. Prevalence of AF was higher in patients with CSA than patients with OSA and without SA (50.0% versus 24.9% and 12.8%, $p < 0.001$). After adjustment for age, sex, body mass index, hypertension, diabetes mellitus, cigarette use, New York Heart Association class and severity of mitral regurgitation, SA (OR, 1.79; 95% CI, 1.09–2.94) and nocturnal hypoxemia (higher tertile of percentage of total sleep time with oxygen saturation < 90% [OR, 1.81; 95% CI, 1.05–3.12] compared with lower tertile) were significantly associated with AF. The association was much stronger in the CSA group (OR, 3.98; 95% CI, 1.56–10.13) than in OSA group (OR, 1.66; 95% CI, 1.01–2.76). Similar associations were observed when analyses were restricted to persistent/permanent AF. Conclusion: Both types of SA and nocturnal hypoxemia were independently associated with AF. Attention should be paid to the screening of both types of SA in the management of AF in HCM.

Keywords: hypertrophic cardiomyopathy; obstructive sleep apnea; central sleep apnea; nocturnal hypoxemia; atrial fibrillation

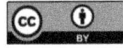

1. Introduction

Hypertrophic cardiomyopathy (HCM) is the most common hereditary cardiomyopathy characterized by left ventricular hypertrophy and a spectrum of clinical manifestations [1]. Atrial fibrillation (AF) is the most common cardiac arrhythmia and is associated with significant morbidity and mortality in patients with HCM [2]. Nowadays, considerable evidence supports sleep apnea (SA) as a risk factor for AF [3]. Previous studies including our works showed a high prevalence of SA in HCM and the most common type of SA, obstructive sleep apnea (OSA), is independently associated with AF in HCM [4–6]. Unlike OSA, central sleep apnea (CSA) is characterized by a lack of drive to breathe during sleep and is less common [7]. Recently, an increasing number of investigations have linked CSA to AF [8,9]. Whether CSA also has a relationship with AF in HCM is still unknown. In addition, few studies have analyzed the respective relations of OSA and CSA to AF in HCM and there is also a paucity of evidence on the association between nocturnal hypoxemia, an essential pathophysiological feature in SA, and AF. To address the above limitations, the overall aim of the current study was designed to examine the association of both types of SA and nocturnal hypoxemia with AF in a large HCM cohort.

2. Materials and Methods

2.1. Study population

This retrospective cross-sectional study included consecutive patients who were diagnosed with HCM and underwent overnight diagnostic sleep examination at the inpatient department of Fuwai Hospital between February 2010 and January 2019. The study cohort has been described in detail previously [10]. Diagnostic criteria of HCM were consistent with the 2020 American Heart Association/American College of Cardiology which mainly include unexplained septal hypertrophy with a thickness of at least 15 mm [11]. Patients with rest left ventricular outflow tract (LVOT) peak gradient $\geq$ 30 mmHg or rest LVOT peak gradient < 30 mmHg with provoked LVOT peak gradient $\geq$ 30 mmHg were considered as obstructive. Otherwise, patients were considered as nonobstructive. Patients were excluded if they had New York Heart Association (NYHA) class IV, incomplete sleep data, were younger than 18 years old, had septal reduction therapy before (septal myectomy or alcohol septal ablation), or had a history of heart transplantation. Patients were also excluded if they were receiving treatment with continuous positive airway pressure or oxygen therapy. According to the exclusion criteria, a total of 606 patients were finally enrolled. All patients provided informed consent before enrollment. The study was approved by the ethics committee of Fuwai Hospital (2020-ZX25). All studies were conducted in accordance with the ethical principles stated in the Declaration of Helsinki.

2.2. Definition of AF

Prevalence of AF was documented. Data including medical histories, 12-lead electrocardiograms and 24-h Holter electrocardiography were collected to help with diagnosis during inpatient stays. Type of AF was defined according to the 2017 HRS/EHRA/ECAS/APHRS/SOLAECE expert consensus statement on catheter and surgical ablation of atrial fibrillation [12]. Briefly, paroxysmal AF was defined as AF that terminated without intervention within 7 days of onset. Persistent AF was defined as continuous AF that is sustained over 7 days. Long-standing persistent AF that lasted at least 1 year when deciding to adopt a rhythm control strategy was classified into persistent AF in our study. Permanent AF was defined when AF was accepted by the patients and physicians and stop further attempts to restore or maintain sinus rhythm.

2.3. Diagnosis of Sleep Apnea

Portable polysomnography monitoring was performed before the time of septal reduction therapy by using the system Embletta (Medcare Flaga, Reykjavik, Iceland) in all included patients. All patients underwent testing on room air. This device records nasal airflow by an airflow pressure transducer, finger pulse oximetry, thoracic and abdominal movement, body position, snoring, heart rate, and ECG, and has been validated against full polysomnography [13]. All polysomnograms were scored blindly. Apnea was defined when cessation of airflow or airflow reduction to $\leq$10% of the baseline value lasted for 10 s or more. An apnea was scored as obstructive if a respiratory effort was present during the event or central in the absence of effort during the event. Hypopnea was defined as a 50% or discernible decrement in airflow lasting 10 s or longer associated with oxygen desaturation of 3%. Hypopneas were scored as obstructive if snoring, and/or flow limitation was noted on the nasal pressure signal or if paradoxical movement was noted on respiratory inductance plethysmography during the event. In the absence of snoring, flow limitation, and paradoxical movement, the hypopnea was scored as a central event. It should be noted that the precise scoring of obstructive or central hypopnea is difficult without the measurement of esophageal pressure. The apnea–hypopnea index (AHI) was the number of apneas and hypopneas per hour of total sleep time. Diagnosis of SA was made solely when the AHI was 5 events/h or more, irrespective of daytime symptoms, which allowed objective evaluation of the disease severity [14]. Patients with SA were grouped into CSA when at least 50% of the disordered breathing events were central (apnea or hypopnea); whereas, if greater than 50% of disordered breathing events were obstructive (apnea or hypopnea), patients were grouped into OSA. The oxygen desaturation index, mean oxygen saturation (SaO_2), minimal SaO_2, average pulse frequency and snoring proportion were also recorded. The severity of nocturnal hypoxemia was measured based on percentage of total sleep time (TST) spent with $SaO_2 < 90\%$. It was assessed as a categorical variable (tertiles with T1 [<0.3%], T2 [$\geq$0.3 to <5.1%] and T3 [$\geq$5.2%]) or as a continuous variable in regression models.

2.4. Statistical Analysis

The numeric variables were expressed as mean and standard deviation, and the categorical variables were expressed as number (percentage). Continuous variables were tested for normal distribution with the Kolmogorov–Smirnov test. Comparison of categorical variables was performed using the χ^2 or Fisher's exact test, as appropriate. Differences of continuous variables between groups were compared using the Student's unpaired *t*-test or Mann–Whitney U test, as appropriate. Univariate and multivariate logistic regression analyses were used to determine the association between the presence of both types of SA or severity of nocturnal hypoxemia and prevalence of AF. The results are expressed as odds ratio (OR) and 95% confidence interval (CI). Covariates including age, sex, body mass index (BMI), hypertension, diabetes mellitus, cigarette use, NYHA class, and severity of mitral regurgitation were adjusted. Tests of interaction were performed to assess whether the association of SA and nocturnal hypoxemia with AF was affected by obstruction of LVOT, sex, or obesity using the abovementioned multivariate model. All reported probability values were 2-tailed, and a *p*-value of <0.05 was considered statistically significant. SPSS version 24.0 (IBM Corp., Armonk, NY, USA) was used for calculations and illustrations.

3. Results

3.1. Baseline Characteristics

A total of 606 patients were enrolled. The study flowchart is shown in Figure 1. SA was diagnosed in 363 (59.9%), of whom 337 (55.6%) had OSA and 26 (4.3%) had CSA. Patients with SA were older, more likely to be male and smokers and had more clinical comorbidities such as hypertension, hyperlipidemia, diabetes mellitus, and coronary heart disease (Table 1). Compared with patients without SA, the prevalence of AF was higher in patients with SA (26.7% versus 12.8%, $p < 0.001$) (Table 1) and the prevalence was even higher in the CSA group when compared with the OSA group (Table 1 and Figure 2A). In addition, patients with CSA had higher NYHA class and N-terminal brain natriuretic peptide (NT-pro BNP) level. Prevalence of AF increased with tertiles of percentage of TST spent with $SaO_2 < 90\%$ (14.9% in T1, 16.8% in T2 and 31.7% in T3, $p < 0.001$) (Figure 2B).

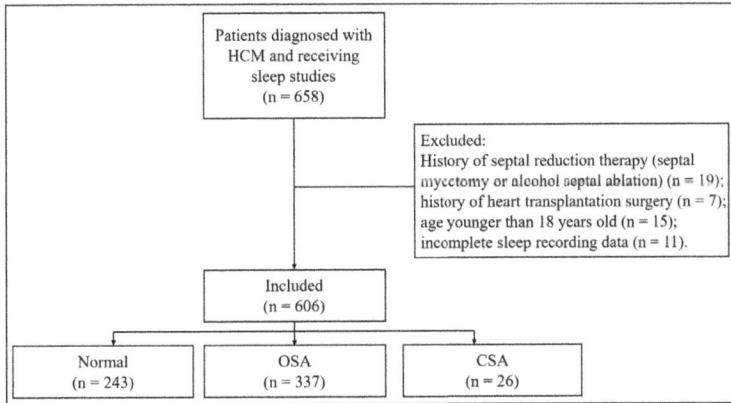

Figure 1. The study flowchart. HCM: hypertrophic cardiomyopathy; OSA: obstructive sleep apnea; CSA: central sleep apnea.

Table 1. Clinical characteristics of patients with HCM grouped according to types of sleep apnea.

Variables	None (n = 243)	SA (n = 363)	* p-Value	Pooled Patients with SA		# p-Value
				OSA (n = 337)	CSA (n = 26)	
Male	157 (64.6)	278 (76.6)	0.001	258 (76.6)	20 (76.9)	0.966
Age (y)	45.7 ± 13.7	54.0 ± 10.9	<0.001	53.7 ± 11.1	57.2 ± 7.1	0.120
BMI (kg/m2)	24.7 ± 3.3	27.2 ± 3.6	<0.001	27.2 ± 3.6	26.7 ± 3.5	0.501
Cigarette use	92 (37.9)	198 (54,5)	<0.001	181 (53.7)	17 (65.4)	0.249
Hypertension	72 (29.6)	215 (59.2)	<0.001	202 (59.9)	13 (50.0)	0.320
Hyperlipidemia	49 (20.2)	171 (47.1)	<0.001	156 (46.3)	15 (57.7)	0.262
Diabetes	21 (8.6)	63 (17.4)	0.002	56 (16.6)	7 (28.0)	0.148
Coronary heart disease	22 (9.1)	67 (18.5)	0.001	59 (17.5)	8 (32.0)	0.072
History of stroke	9 (3.7)	35 (9.7)	0.006	32 (9.5)	3 (12.0)	0.683
AF	31 (12.8)	97 (26.7)	<0.001	84 (24.9)	13 (50.0)	0.005
Paroxysmal AF	23 (9.5)	55 (15.2)	0.040	50 (14.8)	5 (19.2)	0.547
Persistent or permanent AF	8 (3.3)	42 (11.6)	<0.001	34 (10.1)	8 (30.8)	0.001
NYHA class II–III	154 (63.4)	257 (71.0)	0.049	234 (69.4)	23 (92.0)	0.016
Fasting glucose (mmol/L)	4.8 ± 1.2	5.3 ± 1.5	<0.001	5.3 ± 1.5	5.4 ± 1.3	0.761
TC (mmol/L)	4.4 ± 0.9	4.4 ± 1.0	0.891	4.4 ± 1.0	3.9 ± 1.2	0.009
LDL-C (mmol/L)	2.7 ± 0.8	2.7 ± 0.9	0.810	2.7 ± 0.8	2.4 ± 1.0	0.032
Creatinine (mmol/L)	82.4 ± 15.8	87.4 ± 19.0	0.001	87.2 ± 19.2	90.1 ± 15.4	0.470
NT-pro BNP (pg/mL)	1585.3 ± 2313.9	1276.2 ± 1851.1	0.074	1208.4 ± 1832.8	2188.8 ± 1892.4	0.012

Values are presented as mean ± standard deviation, or as n (%). * p-value represented comparison between patients with and without sleep apnea. # p-value represented comparison between patients with OSA and CSA. HCM: hypertrophic cardiomyopathy; OSA: obstructive sleep apnea; CSA: central sleep apnea; BMI: body mass index; AF: atrial fibrillation; NYHA: New York Heart Association; AF: atrial fibrillation; TC: total cholesterol; LDL-C: low-density lipoprotein cholesterol; NT-pro BNP: N-terminal brain natriuretic peptide.

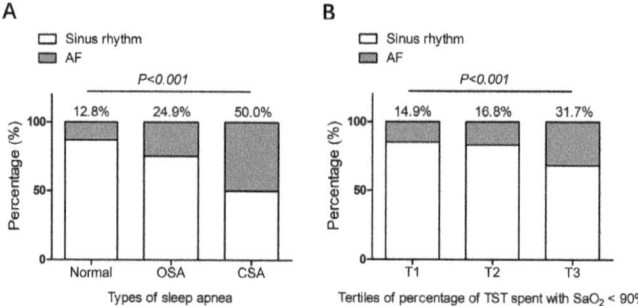

Figure 2. Prevalence of atrial fibrillation in patients with hypertrophic cardiomyopathy grouped by types of sleep apnea (**A**) or severity of nocturnal hypoxemia (**B**). Severity of nocturnal hypoxemia was measured based on percentage of TST spent with SaO_2 < 90%. Tertiles of percentage of TST spent with SaO_2 < 90% were classified as following: T1 (<0.3%), T2 ($\geq$0.3 to <5.1%) and T3 ($\geq$5.2%). AF: atrial fibrillation; OSA: obstructive sleep apnea; CSA: central sleep apnea; TST: total sleep time; SaO_2: oxygen saturation.

3.2. Echocardiographic Data

Echocardiographic data are shown in Table 2. Obstruction of LVOT was more common in patients without SA, while the LVOT gradient in obstructive HCM was not different between groups. Patients with SA were associated with enlarged left atrial diameter (LAD), left ventricular end-diastolic diameter, and ascending aorta diameter compared with patients without SA. LAD was even larger in the CSA group than the OSA group. The mean LVEF was lower and the ratio of patients with LFEV < 50% was higher in the CSA group than the OSA group.

Table 2. Echocardiographic data of HCM patients grouped according to types of sleep apnea.

Variables	None (n = 243)	SA (n = 363)	* p-Value	Pooled Patients with SA		# p-Value
				OSA (n = 337)	CSA (n = 26)	
Obstructive HCM	166 (68.3)	187 (51.5)	<0.001	179 (53.1)	8 (30.8)	0.028
LVOTG at rest in obstructive HCM (mm Hg)	67.3 ± 34.0	63.3 ± 32.4	0.261	62.8 ± 32.5	73.6 ± 31.0	0.358
LAD (mm)	42.1 ± 6.5	43.6 ± 7.7	0.013	43.2 ± 7.5	48.4 ± 7.6	0.001
LVEDD (mm)	43.8 ± 6.3	46.5 ± 5.9	<0.001	46.5 ± 5.9	46.2 ± 6.1	0.825
AAD (mm)	30.2 ± 4.9	32.9 ± 4.3	<0.001	32.9 ± 4.3	33.1 ± 3.8	0.857
IVST (mm)	18.6 ± 5.0	17.2 ± 4.6	0.001	17.1 ± 4.6	18.2 ± 4.2	0.268
PWT (mm)	11.5 ± 3.2	11.6 ± 2.6	0.496	11.6 ± 2.6	11.5 ± 2.1	0.719
Moderate to severe MR	94 (38.7)	104 (28.7)	0.010	96 (28.5)	8 (30.8)	0.804
LVEF (%)	66.6 ± 8.6	65.1 ± 9.4	0.049	65.4 ± 8.9	60.9 ± 13.2	0.016
LVEF < 50%	12 (4.9)	18 (5.0)	0.991	13 (3.9)	5 (19.2)	0.001

Values are presented as mean ± standard deviation, or as n (%). The representation of * p-value and # p-value are shown in Table 1. HCM: hypertrophic cardiomyopathy; OSA: obstructive sleep apnea; CSA: central sleep apnea; LVOTG: left ventricular outflow tract gradient; LAD: left atrial diameter; LVEDD: left ventricular end-diastolic dimension; AAD: ascending aorta diameter; IVST: Interventricular septum thickness; PWT: Posterior wall thickness; MR: mitral regurgitation; LVEF: left ventricular ejection fraction.

3.3. Sleep Parameters

Data from sleep study are summarized in Table 3. Patients with SA had a significantly higher value of AHI and oxygen desaturation index compared with patients without SA. The value was even higher in the CSA group than OSA group. The longest apnea/hypopnea time, percentage of TST spent with $SaO_2 < 90\%$, and snoring time ratio were higher, and the lowest SaO_2 and mean SaO_2 were lower in patients with SA than those without.

Table 3. Sleep data of patients with HCM grouped according to types of sleep apnea.

Variables	None (n = 243)	SA (n = 363)	* p-Value	Pooled Patients with SA		# p-Value
				OSA (n = 337)	CSA (n = 26)	
AHI (events/h)	1.8 ± 1.4	22.5 ± 16.7	<0.001	21.8 ± 16.6	31.5 ± 15.0	0.004
OAI (events/h)	0.6 ± 0.7	9.1 ± 10.9	<0.001	9.6 ± 11.2	3.1 ± 2.8	0.003
CAI (events/h)	0.1 ± 0.2	2.2 ± 5.5	<0.001	1.0 ± 2.0	17.1 ± 11.4	<0.001
OHI (events/h)	1.1 ± 1.1	9.9 ± 7.9	<0.001	10.4 ± 7.9	3.4 ± 3.3	<0.001
CHI (events/h)	0.0 ± 0.0	1.3 ± 3.3	<0.001	0.7 ± 2.1	8.1 ± 6.7	<0.001
ODI (events/h)	2.8 ± 2.7	21.1 ± 16.1	<0.001	20.6 ± 15.9	27.4 ± 17.4	0.040
Longest apnea/hypopnea time (s)	41.0 ± 25.1	72.2 ± 25.3	<0.001	72.1 ± 25.6	73.2 ± 7.9	0.839
Lowest SaO_2 (%)	88.0 ± 4.0	80.2 ± 7.9	<0.001	80.3 ± 7.7	78.6 ± 9.9	0.294
Mean SaO_2 (%)	94.5 ± 1.7	93.1 ± 2.2	<0.001	93.2 ± 2.1	92.4 ± 2.5	0.080
Percentage of TST spent with SaO_2 <90% (%)	1.7 ± 6.6	11.6 ± 17.2	<0.001	11.1 ± 16.9	17.6 ± 20.1	0.063
Snoring time ratio (%)	5.1 ± 6.6	11.8 ± 13.6	<0.001	12.0 ± 13.5	9.1 ± 14.8	0.292
Mean HR during sleep (rpm)	59.9 ± 7.3	61.4 ± 7.8	0.019	61.2 ± 7.6	64.4 ± 10.2	0.040
TST (min)	486.7 ± 94.2	456.2 ± 78.7	<0.001	456.4 ± 80.2	453.1 ± 58.3	0.838

Values are presented as mean ± standard deviation. The representation of * p-value and # p-value are shown in Table 1. HCM: hypertrophic cardiomyopathy; OSA: obstructive sleep apnea; CSA: central sleep apnea; AHI: apnea hypopnea index; OAI: obstructive apnea index; CAI: central apnea index; OHI: obstructive hypopnea index; CHI: central hypopnea index; ODI: oxygen desaturation index; SaO_2: oxygen saturation; TST: total sleep time; HR: heart rate.

3.4. Association of Sleep Apnea and Nocturnal Hypoxemia with AF

In the univariate analyses, SA as well as both types of SA, OSA and CSA, were significantly associated with AF (Table 4). OSA was associated with an OR of 3.24 (95% CI, 1.63–6.44), meanwhile, CSA was associated with a higher OR of 6.84 (95% CI, 2.91–16.10). Significant associations were also observed between measures of nocturnal hypoxemia and

AF. After controlling for age, sex, BMI, hypertension, diabetes mellitus, cigarette use, NYHA class, and severity of mitral regurgitation, the association of SA (OR, 1.79; 95% CI, 1.09–2.94) and nocturnal hypoxemia (higher tertile of percentage of TST spent with $SaO_2 < 90$% with OR, 1.81; 95% CI, 1.05–3.12) with AF remained statistically significant. Adjusted risk of AF was also stronger in the CSA group (OR, 3.98; 95% CI, 1.56–10.13) than the OSA group (OR, 1.66; 95% CI, 1.01–2.76). Similar associations were observed when analyses were restricted to persistent/permanent AF.

Table 4. Association of types of sleep apnea and nocturnal hypoxemia with AF in patients with HCM.

Terms	Univariate	p-Value	Multivariate	p-Value
Atrial fibrillation				
Sleep apnea	2.49 (1.60–3.88)	<0.001	1.79 (1.09–2.94)	0.022
Types of sleep apnea		<0.001		0.010
None	Reference		Reference	
OSA	2.27 (1.45–3.56)	<0.001	1.66 (1.01–2.76)	0.048
CSA	6.84 (2.91–16.10)	<0.001	3.98 (1.56–10.13)	0.004
Percentage of TST spent with $SaO_2 <90$%				
Continuous variable	1.02 (1.01–1.03)	0.001	1.01 (0.99–1.02)	0.257
Tertiles		<0.001		0.012
T1	Reference		Reference	
T2	1.16 (0.68–1.98)	0.586	0.88 (0.50–1.55)	0.652
T3	2.66 (1.63–4.33)	<0.001	1.81 (1.05–3.12)	0.034
ODI	1.01 (1.00–1.03)	0.019	1.00 (0.99–1.02)	0.557
Persistent/permanent atrial fibrillation				
Sleep apnea	3.84 (1.77–8.34)	0.001	2.79 (1.19–6.53)	0.018
Types of sleep apnea		<0.001		0.007
None	Reference		Reference	
OSA	3.30 (1.50–7.25)	0.003	2.47 (1.04–5.88)	0.040
CSA	13.06 (4.39–38.87)	<0.001	7.09 (2.10–23.89)	0.002
Percentage of TST spent with $SaO_2 <90$%				
Continuous variable	1.02 (1.01–1.03)	0.009	1.00 (0.99–1.02)	0.642
Tertiles		0.007		0.197
T1	Reference		Reference	
T2	1.10 (0.47–2.55)	0.830	0.86 (0.36–2.08)	0.738
T3	2.68 (1.29–5.56)	0.008	1.65 (0.73–3.69)	0.226
ODI	1.02 (1.01–1.04)	0.006	1.01 (0.99–1.03)	0.221

Data are presented as odds ratio (95% confidence interval). Multivariate analysis was adjusted for age, sex, body mass index, hypertension, diabetes mellitus, cigarette use, NYHA class, and moderate to severe mitral regurgitation. AF: atrial fibrillation; HCM: hypertrophic cardiomyopathy; OSA: obstructive sleep apnea; CSA: central sleep apnea; TST: total sleep time; SaO_2: oxygen saturation; ODI: oxygen desaturation index; NYHA: New York Heart Association.

The interaction analysis is shown in Table 5. The association of SA or nocturnal hypoxemia with AF was stronger in obstructive HCM compared with non-obstructive HCM (p for interaction = 0.025 and 0.074, respectively). Additionally, associations between SA and AF were greater in obese (BMI $\geq$ 25 kg/m^2) patients compared with non-obese (BMI < 25 kg/m^2) patients (p for interaction = 0.024). No significant interaction was present between nocturnal hypoxemia and obesity for AF (p for interaction = 0.396). There was no significant interaction between SA or nocturnal hypoxemia and sex for AF (p for interaction = 0.534 and 0.793, respectively).

Table 5. Association of sleep apnea and nocturnal hypoxemia with AF in different subgroups of HCM patients.

Terms	Non-Obstructive	Obstructive	p for Interaction	Non-Obese (BMI < 25 kg/m^2)	Obese (BMI ≥ 25 kg/m^2)	p for Interaction	Male	Female	p for Interaction
Sleep apnea	1.10 (0.53–2.28)	2.45 (1.15–5.19)	0.025	1.28 (0.57–2.86)	2.29 (1.17–4.47)	0.024	1.92 (1.03–3.56)	1.82 (0.73–4.55)	0.534
Tertiles of percentage of TST spent with SaO$_2$ <90%			0.074			0.396			0.793
T1	Reference	Reference		Reference	Reference		Reference	Reference	
T2	0.57 (0.21–1.29)	1.41 (0.56–3.53)		0.90 (0.36–2.28)	0.78 (0.37–1.66)		0.74 (0.37–1.50)	1.09 (0.39–3.03)	
T3	0.95 (0.44–2.07)	3.45 (1.43–8.33)		1.81 (0.70–4.71)	1.63 (0.81–3.31)		1.62 (0.85–3.10)	2.27 (0.77–6.71)	

Data are presented as odds ratio (95% confidence interval). Tertiles of percentage of TST spent with SaO$_2$ <90% were classified as following: T1 (<0.3%), T2 (≥0.3 to <5.1%) and T3 (≥5.2%). Mul-tivariate analysis was adjusted for age, sex, BMI, hypertension, diabetes mellitus, cigarette use, NYHA class, and moderate to severe mitral regurgitation. AF: atrial fibrillation; HCM: hypertrophic cardiomyopathy; TST: total sleep time; SaO$_2$: oxygen saturation; BMI: body mass index.

4. Discussion

The current investigation demonstrated that SA was common and was independently associated with AF in patients with HCM. Even though CSA was less common compared with OSA, CSA was more strongly associated with AF than OSA after adjusting for confounders. Nocturnal hypoxemia, an important pathophysiological feature in SA, was also independently associated with AF.

Previous studies have reported a prevalence of SA ranging from 40% to 83% in HCM [15]. Findings from the current study showed that nearly 60% of patients with HCM had SA which was congruent with previous reports, demonstrating that SA was a much more common condition in HCM. The independent association of SA with AF in HCM had been demonstrated in studies with small sample sizes [5,6]. In our study, a significant association between SA and AF was found in a larger HCM cohort. Clinical comorbidities such as obesity, hypertension, and coronary heart disease as well as heart remodeling such as enlarged LAD, which were contributors to AF, were found more common in patients with SA. Several physiologic stressors involved in SA could enhance arrhythmogenicity in HCM including intermittent hypoxemia, hypercapnia, autonomic nervous system fluctuations, and intrathoracic pressure swings.

However, much of previous data are focused on analyzing the association between OSA and AF, while, the link between CSA and AF is not as well studied. In our study, we first found that both types of SA were independently associated with AF in HCM. Interestingly, CSA was more strongly associated with AF than OSA. These results were in alignment with previous investigations. Sin et al. found AF to be associated with CSA, but not OSA, in a sample of 450 individuals with heart failure [16]. Mehra et al. also documented a stronger cross-sectional relationship of CSA than OSA to AF in an unselected community cohort of 2911 men [17]. Additionally, Tung et al. showed a similar finding that CSA, but not OSA, was a predictor of incident AF in a community-based cohort [9]. CSA may be linked with increased risk for AF beyond OSA through the following mechanisms. Intermittent fluctuations in PaCO2 levels and periodic arousals, occurs to be greater in CSA than OSA, and may predispose to arrhythmia by enhancing sympathetic activation and then resulting in electrical and structural remodeling [18]. CSA is often concomitantly found in patients with systolic heart failure which usually occurred frequently with AF and would exacerbate each other [19]. In our study, the CSA group had higher NYHA class and NT-pro BNP level, enlarged LAD, and decreased LVEF com-pared with the OSA group. These results indicated that the above mechanisms contribute to the stronger association between CSA and AF. Interestingly, only a small proportion of patients with CSA had systolic heart failure. We propose that these patients are more likely to have diastolic dysfunction which is a prominent clinical feature in HCM [20].

Nocturnal hypoxemia is an important pathophysiological feature in SA. Previous works had proved the relationship between nocturnal hypoxemia and AF [21]. However, studies have failed to find out the association between nocturnal hypoxemia and AF in HCM, which was possibly due to a relatively small study population [5,6]. In our works, patients in highest tertiles of percentage of TST spent with $SaO_2 < 90\%$ were associated with AF prevalence. We proposed that patients with HCM were associated with AF only with more severe hypoxemia which were consistent with results of previous studies performed in the general population [22]. It is well established that obesity and male sex are risk factors for SA. Our interaction analysis showed that the association between SA and AF was more prominent in patients with obesity but not in the male sex. Meanwhile, the association between nocturnal hypoxemia and AF was irrespective of obesity and sex. Therefore, the association between SA and AF in HCM was not different between males and females. It is still unknown whether LVOT obstruction, a special hemodynamic feature in HCM, plays a role between SA and AF. Our interaction results showed that the association of SA and nocturnal hypoxemia with AF was stronger in HCM patients with LVOT obstruction than those without. These results indicated that obesity and LVOT obstruction might exert synergistic effects on AF together with SA.

To date, SA remains underestimated in HCM. Therefore, a high degree of suspicion for SA is warranted and clinicians should have a low threshold to refer for diagnostic sleep evaluation. Importantly, treatment of OSA was shown to be associated with reduced AF burden as well as cardiovascular benefits in the general population [23,24]. We expect that identification and treatment of both types of SA may serve to further improve outcomes in HCM.

Several limitations in the current study merit discussion. First, this study is a cross-sectional study. Although our results suggested an independent association be-tween SA and AF in HCM, the retrospective nature of this study limited our ability to determine a causal relationship. Second, the sample size of the present study was relatively low, especially in the CSA group, which should be increased in the future to confirm the findings. Third, prevalence of SA and AF in this HCM cohort may represent an overestimation of the prevalence in a general HCM population because of selection bias as patients presented to a tertiary medical center for their care and many were symptomatic. Finally, it is not possible to ensure that all confounding variables were fully adjusted in multivariate analysis. These facts limit the generalizability of our findings.

5. Conclusions

Both types of SA and nocturnal hypoxemia were independently associated with AF. Even though CSA was not as popular as OSA in HCM, the association of CSA with AF was stronger than OSA. These results suggest that attention should be paid to the screening of both types of SA in the management of AF in HCM.

Author Contributions: Conceptualization, H.X. and J.W.; methodology, H.X. and J.W.; validation, S.Q. and J.C.; formal analysis, J.Y., F.H. and W.Y.; investigation, C.G., X.L. and X.D.; data curation, R.L. and S.L.; writing—original draft preparation, H.X. and J.W.; writing—review and editing, J.C.; supervision, J.C.; funding acquisition, J.W. All authors have read and agreed to the published version of the manuscript.

Funding: This research was funded by Chinese Clinical and Scientific Funds for High Level Hospitals (2022-1752).

Institutional Review Board Statement: The study was conducted in accordance with the Declaration of Helsinki, and approved by the Ethics Committee of Fuwai Hospital (2020-ZX25).

Informed Consent Statement: Informed consent was obtained from all subjects involved in the study. Written informed consent has been obtained from the patients to publish this paper.

Data Availability Statement: The data underlying this article will be shared on reasonable request to the corresponding author.

Conflicts of Interest: The authors declare no conflict of interest.

References

1. Maron, B.J. Clinical Course and Management of Hypertrophic Cardiomyopathy. *N. Engl. J. Med.* **2018**, *379*, 655–668. [CrossRef] [PubMed]
2. Garg, L.; Gupta, M.; Sabzwari, S.R.A.; Agrawal, S.; Agarwal, M.; Nazir, T.; Gordon, J.; Bozorgnia, B.; Martinez, M.W. Atrial fibrillation in hypertrophic cardiomyopathy: Prevalence, clinical impact, and management. *Heart Fail. Rev.* **2019**, *24*, 189–197. [CrossRef] [PubMed]
3. Javaheri, S.; Barbe, F.; Campos-Rodriguez, F.; Dempsey, J.A.; Khayat, R.; Javaheri, S.; Malhotra, A.; Martinez-Garcia, M.A.; Mehra, R.; Pack, A.I.; et al. Sleep Apnea: Types, Mechanisms, and Clinical Cardiovascular Consequences. *J. Am. Coll. Cardiol.* **2017**, *69*, 841–858. [CrossRef] [PubMed]
4. Xu, H.; Wang, J.; Yuan, J.; Hu, F.; Yang, W.; Guo, C.; Luo, X.; Liu, R.; Cui, J.; Gao, X.; et al. Implication of Apnea-Hypopnea Index, a Measure of Obstructive Sleep Apnea Severity, for Atrial Fibrillation in Patients with Hypertrophic Cardiomyopathy. *J. Am. Heart Assoc.* **2020**, *9*, e015013. [CrossRef]
5. Pedrosa, R.P.; Drager, L.F.; Genta, P.R.; Amaro, A.C.; Antunes, M.O.; Matsumoto, A.Y.; Arteaga, E.; Mady, C.; Lorenzi-Filho, G. Obstructive sleep apnea is common and independently associated with atrial fibrillation in patients with hypertrophic cardiomyopathy. *Chest* **2010**, *137*, 1078–1084. [CrossRef]
6. Konecny, T.; Brady, P.A.; Orban, M.; Lin, G.; Pressman, G.S.; Lehar, F.; Tomas, K.; Gersh, B.J.; Tajik, A.J.; Ommen, S.R.; et al. Interactions between sleep disordered breathing and atrial fibrillation in patients with hypertrophic cardiomyopathy. *Am. J. Cardiol.* **2010**, *105*, 1597–1602. [CrossRef]
7. Randerath, W.; Verbraecken, J.; Andreas, S.; Arzt, M.; Bloch, K.E.; Brack, T.; Buyse, B.; De Backer, W.; Eckert, D.J.; Grote, L.; et al. Definition, discrimination, diagnosis and treatment of central breathing disturbances during sleep. *Eur. Respir. J.* **2017**, *49*, 1600959. [CrossRef]
8. May, A.M.; Blackwell, T.; Stone, P.H.; Stone, K.L.; Cawthon, P.M.; Sauer, W.H.; Varosy, P.D.; Redline, S.; Mehra, R. Central Sleep-disordered Breathing Predicts Incident Atrial Fibrillation in Older Men. *Am. J. Respir. Crit. Care Med.* **2016**, *193*, 783–791. [CrossRef]
9. Tung, P.; Levitzky, Y.S.; Wang, R.; Weng, J.; Quan, S.F.; Gottlieb, D.J.; Rueschman, M.; Punjabi, N.M.; Mehra, R.; Bertisch, S.; et al. Obstructive and Central Sleep Apnea and the Risk of Incident Atrial Fibrillation in a Community Cohort of Men and Women. *J. Am. Heart Assoc.* **2017**, *6*, e004500. [CrossRef]
10. Wang, J.; Xu, H.; Yuan, J.; Guo, C.; Hu, F.; Yang, W.; Song, L.; Luo, X.; Liu, R.; Cui, J.; et al. Association between Obstructive Sleep Apnea and Metabolic Abnormalities in Patients with Hypertrophic Cardiomyopathy. *J. Clin. Endocrinol. Metab.* **2021**, *106*, e2309–e2321. [CrossRef]
11. Ommen, S.R.; Mital, S.; Burke, M.A.; Day, S.M.; Deswal, A.; Elliott, P.; Evanovich, L.L.; Hung, J.; Joglar, J.A.; Kantor, P.; et al. 2020 AHA/ACC Guideline for the Diagnosis and Treatment of Patients with Hypertrophic Cardiomyopathy: Executive Summary: A Report of the American College of Cardiology/American Heart Association Joint Committee on Clinical Practice Guidelines. *Circulation* **2020**, *142*, e533–e557. [CrossRef]
12. Calkins, H.; Hindricks, G.; Cappato, R.; Kim, Y.H.; Saad, E.B.; Aguinaga, L.; Akar, J.G.; Badhwar, V.; Brugada, J.; Camm, J.; et al. 2017 HRS/EHRA/ECAS/APHRS/SOLAECE expert consensus statement on catheter and surgical ablation of atrial fibrillation. *Europace* **2018**, *20*, e1–e160. [CrossRef]
13. Santos-Silva, R.; Sartori, D.E.; Truksinas, V.; Truksinas, E.; Alonso, F.F.; Tufik, S.; Bittencourt, L.R. Validation of a portable monitoring system for the diagnosis of obstructive sleep apnea syndrome. *Sleep* **2009**, *32*, 629–636. [CrossRef]
14. American Academy of Sleep Medicine Task Force. Sleep-related breathing disorders in adults: Recommendations for syndrome definition and measurement techniques in clinical research. The Report of an American Academy of Sleep Medicine Task Force. *Sleep* **1999**, *22*, 667–689. [CrossRef]
15. Konecny, T.; Somers, V.K. Sleep-disordered breathing in hypertrophic cardiomyopathy: Challenges and opportunities. *Chest* **2014**, *146*, 228–234. [CrossRef]
16. Sin, D.D.; Fitzgerald, F.; Parker, J.D.; Newton, G.; Floras, J.S.; Bradley, T.D. Risk factors for central and obstructive sleep apnea in 450 men and women with congestive heart failure. *Am. J. Respir. Crit. Care Med.* **1999**, *160*, 1101–1106. [CrossRef]
17. Mehra, R.; Stone, K.L.; Varosy, P.D.; Hoffman, A.R.; Marcus, G.M.; Blackwell, T.; Ibrahim, O.A.; Salem, R.; Redline, S. Nocturnal Arrhythmias across a spectrum of obstructive and central sleep-disordered breathing in older men: Outcomes of sleep disorders in older men (MrOS sleep) study. *Arch. Intern. Med.* **2009**, *169*, 1147–1155. [CrossRef]
18. Sanchez, A.M.; Germany, R.; Lozier, M.R.; Schweitzer, M.D.; Kosseifi, S.; Anand, R. Central sleep apnea and atrial fibrillation: A review on pathophysiological mechanisms and therapeutic implications. *Int. J. Cardiology. Heart Vasc.* **2020**, *30*, 100527. [CrossRef]
19. Ling, L.H.; Kistler, P.M.; Kalman, J.M.; Schilling, R.J.; Hunter, R.J. Comorbidity of atrial fibrillation and heart failure. *Nat. Rev. Cardiol.* **2016**, *13*, 131–147. [CrossRef]
20. Kato, T.; Noda, A.; Izawa, H.; Nishizawa, T.; Somura, F.; Yamada, A.; Nagata, K.; Iwase, M.; Nakao, A.; Yokota, M. Myocardial velocity gradient as a noninvasively determined index of left ventricular diastolic dysfunction in patients with hypertrophic cardiomyopathy. *J. Am. Coll. Cardiol.* **2003**, *42*, 278–285. [CrossRef]

21. Chen, C.Y.; Ho, C.H.; Chen, C.L.; Yu, C.C. Nocturnal Desaturation is Associated with Atrial Fibrillation in Patients with Ischemic Stroke and Obstructive Sleep Apnea. *J. Clin. Sleep Med.* **2017**, *13*, 729–735. [CrossRef] [PubMed]
22. Patel, S.K.; Hanly, P.J.; Smith, E.E.; Chan, W.; Coutts, S.B. Nocturnal Hypoxemia Is Associated with White Matter Hyperintensities in Patients with a Minor Stroke or Transient Ischemic Attack. *J. Clin. Sleep Med.* **2015**, *11*, 1417–1424. [CrossRef] [PubMed]
23. Bradley, T.D.; Logan, A.G.; Kimoff, R.J.; Sériès, F.; Morrison, D.; Ferguson, K.; Belenkie, I.; Pfeifer, M.; Fleetham, J.; Hanly, P.; et al. Continuous positive airway pressure for central sleep apnea and heart failure. *N. Engl. J. Med.* **2005**, *353*, 2025–2033. [CrossRef] [PubMed]
24. Shukla, A.; Aizer, A.; Holmes, D.; Fowler, S.; Park, D.S.; Bernstein, S.; Bernstein, N.; Chinitz, L. Effect of Obstructive Sleep Apnea Treatment on Atrial Fibrillation Recurrence: A Meta-Analysis. *JACC. Clin. Electrophysiol.* **2015**, *1*, 41–51. [CrossRef]

Disclaimer/Publisher's Note: The statements, opinions and data contained in all publications are solely those of the individual author(s) and contributor(s) and not of MDPI and/or the editor(s). MDPI and/or the editor(s) disclaim responsibility for any injury to people or property resulting from any ideas, methods, instructions or products referred to in the content.

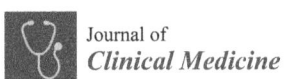

Opinion

Genetic Testing and Counselling in Hypertrophic Cardiomyopathy: Frequently Asked Questions

Francesca Girolami [1,*], Alessia Gozzini [1], Eszter Dalma Pálinkás [2,3], Adelaide Ballerini [1], Alessia Tomberli [1], Katia Baldini [3], Alberto Marchi [1], Mattia Zampieri [1], Silvia Passantino [1], Giulio Porcedda [1], Giovanni Battista Calabri [1], Elena Bennati [1], Gaia Spaziani [1], Lia Crotti [4,5], Franco Cecchi [4], Silvia Favilli [1] and Iacopo Olivotto [1,6]

1. Pediatric Cardiology Unit, Meyer Children's Hospital IRCCS, 50139 Florence, Italy
2. Doctoral School of Clinical Medicine, University of Szeged, 6720 Szeged, Hungary
3. Cardiomyopathy Unit, Careggi University Hospital, 50134 Florence, Italy
4. Department of Cardiovascular, Neural and Metabolic Sciences, San Luca Hospital, Istituto Auxologico Italiano, IRCCS, 20100 Milan, Italy
5. Department of Medicine and Surgery, University Milano Bicocca, 20126 Milan, Italy
6. Department of Experimental and Clinical Medicine, University of Florence, 50121 Florence, Italy
* Correspondence: francesca.girolami@meyer.it

Abstract: Genetic counselling and genetic testing in hypertrophic cardiomyopathy (HCM) represent an integral part of the diagnostic algorithm to confirm the diagnosis, distinguish it from phenocopies, and suggest tailored therapeutic intervention strategies. Additionally, they enable cascade genetic testing in the family. With the implementation of Next Generation Sequencing technologies (NGS), the interpretation of genetic data has become more complex. In this regard, cardiologists play a central role, aiding geneticists to correctly evaluate the pathogenicity of the identified genetic alterations. In the ideal setting, geneticists and cardiologists must work side by side to diagnose HCM as well as convey the correct information to patients in response to their many questions and concerns. After a brief overview of the role of genetics in the diagnosis of HCM, we present and discuss the frequently asked questions by HCM patients throughout our 20-year genetic counselling experience. Appropriate communication between the team and the families is key to the goal of delivering the full potential of genetic testing to our patients.

Keywords: hypertrophic cardiomyopathy; genetic testing; genetic counselling; cascade testing; multidisciplinary team; next-generation sequencing

1. Introduction

Hypertrophic Cardiomyopathy (HCM) is a genetic heart condition characterized by the presence of asymmetric hypertrophy of the left ventricle (LVH) that is not solely explained by abnormal loading conditions [1–5]. However, in the latest AHA/ACC HCM guidelines, the term is applied only to patients that have a sarcomeric gene variant or a negative gene test in the absence of another cardiac, systemic, or metabolic disease [5]. In the 1990s, an *MYH7* (β myosin heavy chain) variant was identified in a large Canadian family with four generations of HCM-affected subjects [6,7]. Over the past 30 years, the complexity of the genetic basis of HCM has been increasingly elucidated. Today HCM is considered the most common genetic cardiac disease, transmitted in an autosomal dominant manner. HCM has a prevalence of roughly 1:500 in adults, thus affecting an estimated 1 million individuals in Europe [8]. Mutation penetrance varies widely and may be significantly delayed [9]. HCM is known to be associated with over ~1500 mutations, described in about 40 genes, especially in genes encoding for cardiac sarcomeric proteins. HCM has been designed as the "disease of the sarcomere" [10]. *MYH7* and *MYBPC3* (cardiac myosin-binding protein C) are the two most commonly mutated sarcomeric genes, and they account for about 40% of diagnoses. In addition, *MYL2* (regulatory myosin light chain), *MYL3* (essential myosin light chain), *TPM1* (α tropomyosin), *TNNT2* (cardiac troponin T), *TNNI3* (cardiac troponin I), and *ACTC1* (cardiac actin) represent the "core disease" genes which are considered essential for establishing a reliable and accurate molecular diagnosis. Rare mutations have been found in additional sarcomere genes or genes coding for proteins from the nearby Z-disc, such as *MYH6* (α myosin heavy chain), *CSRP3* (muscle LIM protein), *TCAP* (telethonin), and genes implicated in calcium homeostasis pathways, such as *VCL* (vinculin) and *JPH2* (junctophilin 2) [11–14]. A small number of hypertrophic patients exhibit Fabry syndrome (*GLA* gene), Danon disease (*LAMP2* gene), cardiac amyloidosis (*TTR* gene), Wolff—Parkinson—White syndrome (*PRKAG2* gene), and mitochondrial cardiomyopathies [15–18]. These phenocopies are different disease entities with distinct heredity, pathogenesis, natural history, extra-cardiac characteristics, and therapy. Moreover, HCM phenotype may be associated with malformation syndromes, mainly RASophaties, a heterogeneous group of diseases caused by mutations in genes of RAS-MAPK cascade, including *PTPN11, BRAF, RAF1, SOS1, HRAS*, and *KRAS* [14]. For these diseases, the genetic test, in conjunction with a detailed diagnostic examination of the patient and their family, is a critical tool for the diagnosis and proper treatment [19].

Currently, with Next Generation Sequencing (NGS) technologies, it is possible to identify a responsible mutation in 30–60% of HCM patients. However, it is true that the yield of positive genetic testing is higher in the case of positive family history of HCM and is lower in sporadic cases [5,20]. The genetic cause remains unknown and may be polygenic in the rest of the cases, together with some environmental factors, such as obesity, arterial hypertension, and intense sports activity [14,20]. About 5–10% of patients have been reported to have complex genotypes carrying multiple (two or more rarely three) mutations in sarcomere genes; this condition is usually associated with a poorer prognosis [21]. Since 2005, NGS technologies have enabled a breakthrough rise in high-throughput sequencing capabilities by analyzing multigene panels, whole-exome (WES), and whole-genome sequencing (WGS). The latter is mostly aimed at discovering novel disease-causing genes and is mostly used for research purposes. In selected cases, for example, in children with HCM, the WES analysis in a trio (together with the parent's DNA sequencing) should be performed [22]. The NGS strategy is to sequence millions of short-DNA fragments in massively parallel arrays, then realign and map the short reads back to the reference genome [23]. The accurate interpretation of data sequencing is the weakness of the NGS strategy. It may be very difficult to predict if a DNA variant identified in a patient is truly disease-causing (pathogenic or likely pathogenic), a benign polymorphism (negative test) or a rare variant with unclear clinical significance and not predicted to cause HCM (variant of uncertain significance, VUS) [24]. In this last case, the genetic test's result is not clinically actionable and may be considered one limitation of the genetic study. Private and public cardiogenetic laboratories often use commercial panels for genetic tests. The panels are typically designed to contain genes having a definitive or moderate association with the disorders; the panels must be assessed on a regular basis and may potentially be expanded if new genes are identified [10,20,25].

2. Genetic Counselling

Genetic counselling represents an essential part of genetic testing and is recommended for all patients with HCM who choose to undergo genetic testing [5]. The main objective of counselling is informing patients and families about the genetic aspects of their disease, the advantages and the limitations of the test and the possibility of transmitting the disease to their relatives [26–29]. It is also critical to help ensure that patients and families have realistic expectations about the benefits of genetic testing. Counselling can be divided into pre-test and post-test counselling (Figure 1). According to the latest guidelines on HCM, pre-and post-test genetic counselling should be performed by a trained genetic counsellor or by other experts in the genetics of cardiovascular diseases (Class 1, level of evidence B) [5]. Due to technological advances and new recommendations, the number of genetic testing requests is increasing rapidly, which may expose cardiologists to more often facing similar questions about the implication of genetic testing results. Therefore, in this article, we collected and discussed the frequently asked questions by our HCM patients to help cardiologists manage genetic testing-related scenarios more easily and confidently.

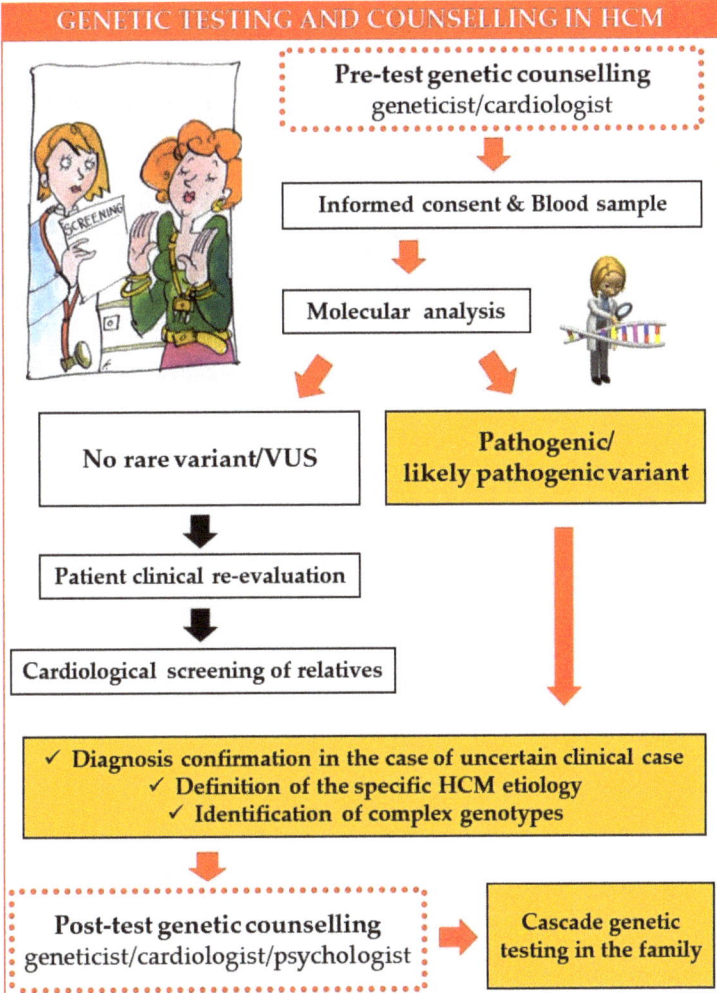

Figure 1. Genetic testing strategy in HCM. Abbreviations: HCM: hypertrophic cardiomyopathy; VUS: variant of uncertain significance.

Pre-test counselling. During pre-test counselling, the patient should be informed about the specific type of test that will be performed on the DNA sample (for example, which are the genes studied and by which technologies), the possible test results, the potential clinical benefit, and the test turn-around time. Pre-test counselling is of paramount importance to identify other clinically affected family members, patterns of disease transmission, consanguinity within the family, and history of sudden cardiac death in a relative. Moreover, it helps to assist decision-making by fully informing patients [5,23]. A three generations pedigree of the family, written informed consent and a blood sample are collected during this interview.

Post-test counselling. Test results should be communicated during post-test genetic counselling. Post-test genetic counselling should involve skilled healthcare professionals working in multidisciplinary teams to assist patients in understanding and handling the psychological, social, professional, ethical, and legal consequences of test results. During post-test genetic counselling, the patient becomes aware of the impact of test results on himself/herself and his/her relatives. Importantly, the patient is informed about the clinical implications and the possibility of performing cascade testing screening on other family members (predictive genetic testing in relatives). In young patients, the risk of transmission when planning future pregnancies should be discussed [5].

3. Patients' Questions, Real-World Answers

Interpreting the clinical significance of genetic variants is a complex process in which the role of clinicians is key by providing evidence that supports the variants' classification, both in the proband and in family members [23]. Cardiologists need to be able to answer questions from patients with genetic heart diseases, collaborating closely with the geneticist. In this article, we present and discuss the frequently asked questions by HCM patients over our 20-year genetic counselling experience.

Why is it useful to undergo a genetic test for me? Genetic testing in HCM adult patients remains critical for the identification of at-risk asymptomatic relatives. In addition, it provides a definitive molecular diagnosis and allows the identification of phenocopies (for example Anderson-Fabry disease, *TTR* amyloidosis, Danon disease, or *PRKAG2* cardiac glycogenosis). Conversely, the impact on risk stratification and the prognosis is limited as genotype status alone cannot predict patient-specific outcomes. However, it is important to note that patients with pathogenic or likely pathogenic sarcomere mutations had a greater risk for adverse outcomes compared with patients without mutations [5,10,11,21].

Will the identified DNA mutation predict the course and outcome of my disease? Because HCM is a genetic disease with incomplete penetrance and variable expressivity, the possibility of associating mutations with a specific disease course is limited. Some genes or specific mutations have been linked to a high rate of sudden mortality and adverse remodeling (e.g., *TNNT2* mutations; *MYH7* p.Arg403Gln), a low rate of LVH (*TNNT2*), or delayed cardiac expression (*MYBPC3*). Additionally, patients with complex genotypes are more likely to have severe phenotypes or early disease manifestations [21]. Yet, no clear and consistent associations have been discovered for the majority of mutations to date [20,22,23,30–32].

Is it possible that I will never develop the disease, even if I have inherited the familial mutation? HCM is known to be a disease with incomplete penetrance and an intra-family variability of phenotype expression. Hence, the identification of a sarcomeric mutation (genotype positive) in an otherwise healthy individual (phenotype negative) does not necessarily mean that the subject will develop the disease but does indicate an increased risk of developing it. Although HCM may rarely be present in neonates and children, usually, the mean age of onset in HCM ranges from the third to the fifth decade of life. However, it has been reported that in a proportion of cases, it may remain latent or be identified even after age 60 [33].

If my genetic mutation gets identified, will I have targeted therapies? Although experimental studies hold hope for the future, no etiological/preventive therapies are available today. Nonetheless, the identification of a pathogenic mutation may help the cardiologist make tailored therapeutic choices and distinguish rare mimics such as Fabry disease, Danon disease, amyloidosis caused by *TTR* mutation, or atypical glycogenosis due to mutations in the *PRKAG2* gene. Emerging, targeted therapies, including gene therapy for HCM patients, are now opening new perspectives [24,34–38].

In the case of an uncertain clinical diagnosis, can the identification of a genetic mutation definitively help to clarify it? In the case of inconclusive clinical findings, the identification of a pathogenic/likely pathogenic HCM rare variant can confirm the diagnosis [39].

My echocardiography is normal, but my genetic test is positive. Should I stop the physical activity? In general, for most patients with HCM, mild- to moderate-intensity recreational exercise is beneficial and is recommended to improve cardiorespiratory fitness, quality of life, and overall health. For phenotype-negative individuals, due to their low risk of sudden cardiac death (SCD), there is no restriction from competitive sports unless the family history indicates a high risk for SCD. However, serial echocardiography is recommended to assess for any phenotype development at periodic intervals depending on age [1,5,40].

Can a positive genetic test influence my insurance policies? Genetic data are strictly personal and protected by different regulations from country to country. In the USA, The Genetic Information Non-discrimination Act (GINA) protects individuals against discrimination based on their genetic information in health coverage and employment. Italy also has these types of laws (Authorization No. 8/2016—Garante Privacy). For this reason, it is not required to declare to have carried out the genetic test, either in the working environment or during the stipulation of life insurance [41].

How likely is it that my children will inherit the mutation? Sarcomeric HCM is inherited in an autosomal dominant manner, which means that both female and male children have a 50% probability of carrying the disease-causing variant, although variable penetrance can result in differences in the onset and severity of clinical manifestations [5].

I know genetic test needs a long time to be performed. However, once a mutation has been identified, is it going to take that much time to test my family? Once the mutation is identified in the first patient of the family, we can easily look for it in the other family members. We already know which "word" is misspelled and on which "page" it is located. Therefore, the predictive test takes only a few days [42].

Since I have HCM and a causative mutation has been found, is it possible to perform the genetic test on my five-year-old son/daughter, even if he/she does not show any sign of the disease? Performing a genetic test on an unaffected child is generally not recommended [43]. The fundamental justification behind this is the lack of knowledge on the severity, age of onset, and phenotypic manifestations associated with HCM, as well as the inability to stop its progression. For these reasons, the medical benefit of a pre-symptomatic diagnosis of HCM is questionable, and since the request is made by the parents, the child is often not mature enough to understand the consequences of the test and make any decision. In our opinion, it is of utmost importance to balance benefits and harms, case by case, and keep in mind that he/she should be free to choose by himself to know whether he/she has inherited the mutation. Therefore, in the case of an unaffected child, a genetic test should be carried out after 10–12 years of age. However, in certain situations, such as a possible competitive sports career or a family history of malignant early-onset disease, it may be performed earlier [22,44].

After the identification of the mutation in my husband, is it possible to perform a prenatal test on our child? The decision to pursue a prenatal diagnosis is a personal one. Through invasive prenatal diagnosis (by amniocentesis or chorionic villus sample), it is possible to obtain the fetus's DNA and proceed with searching for the known mutation [5,23,26]. Nonetheless, in our opinion, it is not appropriate to carry out this type of test due to the above-mentioned reasons: the uncertain age of onset of symptoms, the severity of symptoms, the risk of complications, etc. Clinicians cannot precisely anticipate the clinical course of an individual with a mutation since extremely different manifestations of HCM can occur in family members carrying the same mutation. Both incomplete penetrance and variable expressivity are probably due to a combination of genetic, environmental, and lifestyle factors. In our experience, none of the couples persisted to request prenatal testing after the first steps of the multidisciplinary shared decision-making process.

If the mutation is not identified, does it mean that my cardiomyopathy does not have a genetic base? The available genetic test in the cardiogenetic laboratories involves the analysis of a panel of genes known to be associated with HCM. The probability of identifying a disease-causing mutation in these genes is about 40–60% (test sensitivity). It is believed that both familial and isolated HCM forms are genetically determined. Therefore, even if no causative variant gets identified, a genetic basis cannot be excluded [5]. In this scenario, the causative variant could lie in modulator or unknown genes or in DNA regions that we are not able to analyze yet. For these reasons, both the HCM patients with negative genetic tests and their relatives should undergo regular cardiological follow-ups [5].

What does "Inconclusive genetic test result" mean? It means that a rare variant was identified in the patient's DNA, called a variant of uncertain significance (VUS). It is unclear whether this variant is associated with the health condition or not. Due to their rarity in the population, only a limited amount of information is available on VUS. Thus, when a VUS gets identified, the test result is ambiguous and inconclusive at a clinical level. For this reason, a VUS should not be used to establish a genetic diagnosis and guide cascade family screening. Future knowledge or scientific reports may ameliorate our understanding of the VUS and help to re-evaluate them. The identification of a VUS, even if it represents one of the three possible results of a genetic test (1, positive: pathogenic/likely pathogenic causative variant; 2, rare VUS; 3, no identified rare variant) can be considered a limitation of genetic testing [24,45,46].

In Table 1, we have collected some pieces of information for cardiologists who deem it appropriate to have the patient undergo genetic testing. We consider these recommendations necessary to avoid setting unrealistic expectations and to ensure that it is consistent with the information provided during genetic counselling.

Table 1. Recommendations for the cardiologist on genetic testing in HCM.

Genetic Testing in HCM: Tips for the Cardiologist
It is important to inform the patient that genetic testing:
Usually needs a long time (up to three months) before results are ready.
Has a chance of finding a causative mutation ranging from 30 to 60%, depending on the cardiomyopathy and its presence in other family members.
Can be extended to other family members **ONLY** in the presence of a pathogenic/likely pathogenic variant in the proband.
It is undesirable to suggest:
Performing the test as a matter of urgency.
Waiting for the test result to start treatment.
Submitting the entire family to genetic testing before determining the proband's mutation.
Advising a prenatal diagnosis before genetic counselling.
Waiting for test results to decide on physical and sport activity.
Performing genetic testing for individuals in the family without phenotypic evidence of HCM, including relatives of sudden cardiac death victims.

4. Conclusions

For cardiologists to achieve confidence in ordering genetic testing for HCM and counselling, they must be able to answer the major questions of their patients. Continuing close collaboration with geneticists is the key to success.

Funding: This research received no external funding. E.D.P. was a recipient of the Erasmus+ grant for medical and doctorate students in Florence from September to December 2021 and January to December 2022.

Institutional Review Board Statement: The study was conducted following the Declaration of Helsinki.

Informed Consent Statement: Informed consent was obtained from all subjects involved in the study.

Data Availability Statement: No new data were created or analyzed in this study. Data sharing is not applicable to this article.

Acknowledgments: We are thankful to all patients.

Conflicts of Interest: The authors declare no conflict of interest.

References

1. Elliott, P.M.; Anastasakis, A.; Borger, M.A.; Borggrefe, M.; Cecchi, F.; Charron, P.; Hagege, A.A.; Lafont, A.; Limongelli, G.; Mahrholdt, H.; et al. 2014 ESC Guidelines on diagnosis and management of hypertrophic cardiomyopathy: The Task Force for the Diagnosis and Management of Hypertrophic Cardiomyopathy of the European Society of Cardiology (ESC). *Eur. Heart J.* **2014**, *35*, 2733–2779.
2. Maron, B.J.; Desai, M.Y.; Nishimura, R.A.; Spirito, P.; Rakowski, H.; Towbin, J.A.; Dearani, J.A.; Rowin, E.J.; Maron, M.S.; Sherrid, M.V. Management of Hypertrophic Cardiomyopathy: JACC State-of-the-Art Review. *J. Am. Coll. Cardiol.* **2022**, *79*, 390–414. [CrossRef] [PubMed]
3. Maron, B.J.; Maron, M.S. Hypertrophic cardiomyopathy. *Lancet* **2013**, *381*, 242–255. [CrossRef]
4. Braunwald, E.; Lambrew, C.T.; Rockoff, S.D.; Ross, J., Jr.; Morrow, A.G. Idiopathic Hypertrophic Subaortic Stenosis. I. A Description of the Disease Based Upon an Analysis of 64 Patients. *Circulation* **1964**, *30* (Suppl. S4), 3–119. [CrossRef]
5. Ommen, S.R.; Mital, S.; Burke, M.A.; Day, S.M.; Deswal, A.; Elliott, P.; Evanovich, L.L.; Hung, J.; Joglar, J.A.; Kantor, P.; et al. 2020 AHA/ACC Guideline for the Diagnosis and Treatment of Patients with Hypertrophic Cardiomyopathy: Executive Summary: A Report of the American College of Cardiology/American Heart Association Joint Committee on Clinical Practice Guidelines. *J. Am. Coll. Cardiol.* **2020**, *76*, 3022–3055. [CrossRef]
6. Jarcho, J.A.; McKenna, W.; Pare, J.A.; Solomon, S.D.; Holcombe, R.F.; Dickie, S.; Levi, T.; Donis-Keller, H.; Seidman, J.G.; Seidman, C.E. Mapping a gene for familial hypertrophic cardiomyopathy to chromosome 14q1. *N. Engl. J. Med.* **1989**, *321*, 1372–1378. [CrossRef]
7. Seidman, C.E.; Seidman, J.G. Identifying sarcomere gene mutations in hypertrophic cardiomyopathy: A personal history. *Circ. Res.* **2011**, *108*, 743–750. [CrossRef] [PubMed]
8. Maron, B.J.; Maron, M.S.; Semsarian, C. Genetics of hypertrophic cardiomyopathy after 20 years: Clinical perspectives. *JACC* **2012**, *60*, 705–715. [CrossRef]
9. Semsarian, C.; Semsarian, C.R. Variable Penetrance in Hypertrophic Cardiomyopathy: In Search of the Holy Grail. *JACC* **2020**, *76*, 560–562. [CrossRef]
10. Ho, C.Y.; Charron, P.; Richard, P.; Girolami, F.; Van Spaendonck-Zwarts, K.Y.; Pinto, Y. Genetic advances in sarcomeric cardiomyopathies: State of the art. *Cardiovasc. Res.* **2015**, *105*, 397–408. [CrossRef] [PubMed]
11. Olivotto, I.; Girolami, F.; Ackerman, M.J.; Nistri, S.; Bos, J.M.; Zachara, E.; Ommen, S.R.; Theis, J.L.; Vaubel, R.A.; Re, F.; et al. Myofilament protein gene mutation screening and outcome of patients with hypertrophic cardiomyopathy. *Mayo. Clin. Proc.* **2008**, *83*, 630–638. [CrossRef] [PubMed]
12. Ingles, J.; Goldstein, J.; Thaxton, C.; Caleshu, C.; Corty, E.W.; Crowley, S.B.; Dougherty, K.; Harrison, S.M.; McGlaughon, J.; Milko, L.V.; et al. Evaluating the Clinical Validity of Hypertrophic Cardiomyopathy Genes. *Circ. Genom. Precis. Med.* **2019**, *12*, e002460. [CrossRef]
13. Walsh, R.; Thomson, K.L.; Ware, J.S.; Funke, B.H.; Woodley, J.; McGuire, K.J.; Mazzarotto, F.; Blair, E.; Seller, A.; Taylor, J.C.; et al. Reassessment of Mendelian gene pathogenicity using 7855 cardiomyopathy cases and 60,706 reference samples. *Genet. Med.* **2017**, *19*, 192–203. [CrossRef]
14. Hershberger, R.E.; Givertz, M.M.; Ho, C.Y.; Judge, D.P.; Kantor, P.F.; McBride, K.L.; Morales, A.; Taylor, M.R.G.; Vatta, M.; Ware, S.M.; et al. Genetic evaluation of cardiomyopathy: A clinical practice resource of the American College of Medical Genetics and Genomics (ACMG). *Genet. Med.* **2018**, *20*, 899–909. [CrossRef] [PubMed]
15. Maron, B.J.; Roberts, W.C.; Arad, M.; Haas, T.S.; Spirito, P.; Wright, G.B.; Almquist, A.K.; Baffa, J.M.; Saul, J.P.; Ho, C.Y.; et al. Clinical outcome and phenotypic expression in LAMP2 cardiomyopathy. *JAMA* **2009**, *301*, 1253–1259. [CrossRef] [PubMed]
16. Banankhah, P.; Fishbein, G.A.; Dota, A.; Ardehali, R. Cardiac manifestations of PRKAG2 mutation. *BMC Med. Genet.* **2018**, *19*, 1. [CrossRef]
17. Arends, M.; Wijburg, F.A.; Wanner, C.; Vaz, F.M.; van Kuilenburg, A.B.P.; Hughes, D.A.; Biegstraaten, M.; Mehta, A.; Hollak, C.E.M.; Langeveld, M. Favourable effect of early versus late start of enzyme replacement therapy on plasma globotriaosylsphingosine levels in men with classical Fabry disease. *Mol. Genet. Metab.* **2017**, *121*, 157–161. [CrossRef]
18. Gagliardi, C.; Perfetto, F.; Lorenzini, M.; Ferlini, A.; Salvi, F.; Milandri, A.; Quarta, C.C.; Taborchi, G.; Bartolini, S.; Frusconi, S.; et al. Phenotypic profile of Ile68Leu transthyretin amyloidosis: An underdiagnosed cause of heart failure. *Eur. J. Heart Fail.* **2018**, *20*, 1417–1425. [CrossRef]
19. Girolami, F.; Vergaro, G.; Pieroni, M.; Passantino, S.; Giannotti, G.; Grippo, G.; Canale, M.L.; Favilli, S.; Cappelli, F.; Olivotto, I.; et al. Clinical pathway for cardiomyopathies: A genetic testing strategy proposed by ANMCO in Tuscany. *G. Ital. Cardiol.* **2020**, *21*, 926–934.
20. Mazzarotto, F.; Girolami, F.; Boschi, B.; Barlocco, F.; Tomberli, A.; Baldini, K.; Coppini, R.; Tanini, I.; Bardi, S.; Contini, E.; et al. Defining the diagnostic effectiveness of genes for inclusion in panels: The experience of two decades of genetic testing for hypertrophic cardiomyopathy at a single center. *Genet. Med.* **2019**, *21*, 284–292. [CrossRef] [PubMed]
21. Ho, C.Y.; Day, S.M.; Ashley, E.A.; Michels, M.; Pereira, A.C.; Jacoby, D.; Cirino, A.L.; Fox, J.C.; Lakdawala, N.K.; Ware, J.S.; et al. Genotype and Lifetime Burden of Disease in Hypertrophic Cardiomyopathy: Insights from the Sarcomeric Human Cardiomyopathy Registry (SHaRe). *Circulation* **2018**, *138*, 1387–1398. [CrossRef]

22. Girolami, F.; Iascone, M.; Pezzoli, L.; Passantino, S.; Limongelli, G.; Monda, E.; Rubino, M.; Adorisio, R.; Lombardi, M.; Ragni, L.; et al. Clinical pathway on pediatric cardiomyopathies: A genetic testing strategy proposed by the Italian Society of Pediatric Cardiology. *G. Ital. Cardiol.* **2022**, *23*, 505–515.
23. Girolami, F.; Frisso, G.; Benelli, M.; Crotti, L.; Iascone, M.; Mango, R.; Mazzaccara, C.; Pilichou, K.; Arbustini, E.; Tomberli, B.; et al. Contemporary genetic testing in inherited cardiac disease: Tools, ethical issues, and clinical applications. *J. Cardiovasc. Med.* **2018**, *19*, 1. [CrossRef] [PubMed]
24. Arbustini, E.; Behr, E.R.; Carrier, L.; van Duijn, C.; Evans, P.; Favalli, V.; van der Harst, P.; Haugaa, K.H.; Jondeau, G.; Kääb, S.; et al. Interpretation and actionability of genetic variants in cardiomyopathies: A position statement from the European Society of Cardiology Council on cardiovascular genomics. *Eur. Heart J.* **2022**, *43*, 1901–1916. [CrossRef] [PubMed]
25. Alfares, A.A.; Kelly, M.A.; McDermott, G.; Funke, B.H.; Lebo, M.S.; Baxter, S.B.; Shen, J.; McLaughlin, H.M.; Clark, E.H.; Babb, L.J.; et al. Results of clinical genetic testing of 2,912 probands with hypertrophic cardiomyopathy: Expanded panels offer limited additional sensitivity. *Genet. Med.* **2015**, *17*, 880–888. [CrossRef]
26. Charron, P.; Héron, D.; Gargiulo, M.; Richard, P.; Dubourg, O.; Desnos, M.; Bouhour, J.B.; Feingold, J.; Carrier, L.; Hainque, B.; et al. Genetic testing and genetic counselling in hypertrophic cardiomyopathy: The French experience. *J. Med. Genet.* **2002**, *39*, 741–746. [CrossRef]
27. Cirino, A.L.; Seidman, C.E.; Ho, C.Y. Genetic Testing and Counselling for Hypertrophic Cardiomyopathy. *Cardiol. Clin.* **2019**, *37*, 35–43. [CrossRef]
28. Skrzynia, C.; Demo, E.M.; Baxter, S.M. Genetic counselling and testing for hypertrophic cardiomyopathy: An adult perspective. *J. Cardiovasc. Transl. Res.* **2009**, *2*, 493–499. [CrossRef]
29. Cirino, A.L.; Harris, S.L.; Murad, A.M.; Hansen, B.; Malinowski, J.; Natoli, J.L.; Kelly, M.A.; Christian, S. The uptake and utility of genetic testing and genetic counselling for hypertrophic cardiomyopathy—A systematic review and meta-analysis. *J. Genet. Couns.* **2022**, *31*, 1290–1305. [CrossRef]
30. Chen, Y.; Xu, F.; Munkhsaikhan, U.; Boyle, C.; Borcky, T.; Zhao, W.; Purevjav, E.; Towbin, J.A.; Liao, F.; Williams, R.W.; et al. Identifying modifier genes for hypertrophic cardiomyopathy. *J. Mol. Cell. Cardiol.* **2020**, *144*, 119–126. [CrossRef]
31. Torricelli, F.; Girolami, F.; Olivotto, I.; Passerini, I.; Frusconi, S.; Vargiu, D.; Richard, P.; Cecchi, F. Prevalence and clinical profile of troponin T mutations among patients with hypertrophic cardiomyopathy in Tuscany. *Am. J. Cardiol.* **2003**, *92*, 1358–1362. [CrossRef]
32. Girolami, F.; Ho, C.Y.; Semsarian, C.; Baldi, M.; Will, M.L.; Baldini, K.; Torricelli, F.; Yeates, L.; Cecchi, F.; Ackerman, M.J.; et al. Clinical features and outcome of hypertrophic cardiomyopathy associated with triple sarcomere protein gene mutations. *J. Am. Coll. Cardiol.* **2010**, *55*, 1444–1453. [CrossRef] [PubMed]
33. Maurizi, N.; Michels, M.; Rowin, E.J.; Semsarian, C.; Girolami, F.; Tomberli, B.; Cecchi, F.; Maron, M.S.; Olivotto, I.; Maron, B.J. Clinical Course and Significance of Hypertrophic Cardiomyopathy Without Left Ventricular Hypertrophy. *Circulation* **2019**, *139*, 830–833. [CrossRef] [PubMed]
34. Iavarone, M.; Monda, E.; Vritz, O.; Albert, D.C.; Rubino, M.; Verrillo, F.; Caiazza, M.; Lioncino, M.; Amodio, F.; Guarnaccia, N.; et al. Medical treatment of patients with hypertrophic cardiomyopathy: An overview of current and emerging therapy. *Arch. Cardiovasc. Dis.* **2022**, *115*, 529–537. [CrossRef] [PubMed]
35. Helms, A.S.; Thompson, A.D.; Day, S.M. Translation of New and Emerging Therapies for Genetic Cardiomyopathies. *JACC* **2021**, *7*, 70–83. [CrossRef]
36. Investor Portal. Tenaya Therapeutics Receives Orphan Drug Designation and Presents Pre-Clinical Data for Its Most Advanced Gene Therapy Product Candidate for Genetic Hypertrophic Cardiomyopathy. Available online: https://investors.tenayatherapeutics.com/news-releases/news-release-details/tenaya-therapeutics-receives-orphan-drug-designation-and (accessed on 11 February 2023).
37. Globe Newswire. LEXEO Therapeutics Expands Cardiac Gene Therapy Pipeline with Acquisition of Stelios Therapeutics and its Gene Therapy Programs for Rare Cardiovascular Diseases. Available online: https://www.globenewswire.com/news-release/2021/07/21/2266478/0/en/LEXEO-Therapeutics-Expands-Cardiac-Gene-Therapy-Pipeline-with-Acquisition-of-Stelios-Therapeutics-and-its-Gene-Therapy-Programs-for-Rare-Cardiovascular-Diseases.html (accessed on 11 February 2023).
38. Olivotto, I.; Oreziak, A.; Barriales-Villa, R.; Abraham, T.P.; Masri, A.; Garcia-Pavia, P.; Saberi, S.; Lakdawala, N.K.; Wheeler, M.T.; Owens, A.; et al. Mavacamten for treatment of symptomatic obstructive hypertrophic cardiomyopathy (EXPLORER-HCM): A randomised, double-blind, placebo-controlled, phase 3 trial. *Lancet* **2020**, *396*, 759–769. [CrossRef]
39. Baldi, M.; Girolami, F. A new type of "tracing" for cardiologists? *G. Ital. Cardiol.* **2009**, *10*, 266.
40. Semsarian, C.; Gray, B.; Haugaa, K.H.; Lampert, R.; Sharma, S.; Kovacic, J.C. Athletic Activity for Patients with Hypertrophic Cardiomyopathy and Other Inherited Cardiovascular Diseases: JACC Focus Seminar 3/4. *JACC* **2022**, *80*, 1268–1283. [CrossRef]
41. GPDP. Autorizzazione Generale al Trattamento Dei Dati Genetici. Autorizzazione n. 8/2016, 15 Dicembre 2016. Available online: https://www.garanteprivacy.it/home/docweb/-/docweb-display/docweb/5803688 (accessed on 11 February 2023).
42. Kassem, H.S.; Girolami, F.; Sanoudou, D. Molecular genetics made simple. *Glob. Cardiol. Sci. Pract.* **2012**, *2012*, 6. [CrossRef]
43. Semsarian, C.; Ho, C.Y. Screening children at risk for hypertrophic cardiomyopathy: Balancing benefits and harms. *Eur. Heart J.* **2019**, *40*, 3682–3684. [CrossRef]
44. Mital, S.; Ommen, S. To Screen or Not to Screen, That Is the Question. *Circulation* **2019**, *140*, 193–195. [CrossRef] [PubMed]

45. Richards, S.; Aziz, D.; Bale, S.; Bick, J.; Das, W.W.; Gastier-Foster, M.; Grody, E.; Hegde, E.; Lyon, K.; Spector, H.L.; et al. Standards and guidelines for the interpretation of sequence variants: A joint consensus recommendation of the American College of Medical Genetics and Genomics and the Association for Molecular Pathology. *Genet. Med.* **2015**, *17*, 405–424. [CrossRef] [PubMed]
46. Wilde, A.A.M.; Semsarian, C.; Márquez, M.F.; Shamloo, A.S.; Ackerman, M.J.; Barajas-Martinez, H.S.; Behr, E.R.; Breckpot, B.J.; Charron, P.; Chockalingam, P.; et al. N EHRA/HRS/APHRS/LAHRS. Expert Consensus Statement on the state of genetic testing for cardiac diseases. *Europace* **2022**, *24*, 1307–1367. [CrossRef] [PubMed]

Disclaimer/Publisher's Note: The statements, opinions and data contained in all publications are solely those of the individual author(s) and contributor(s) and not of MDPI and/or the editor(s). MDPI and/or the editor(s) disclaim responsibility for any injury to people or property resulting from any ideas, methods, instructions or products referred to in the content.

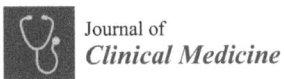

Article

Real-World Use and Predictors of Response to Disopyramide in Patients with Obstructive Hypertrophic Cardiomyopathy

Niccolò Maurizi [1,2,*], Chiara Chiriatti [3], Carlo Fumagalli [3], Mattia Targetti [3], Silvia Passantino [3], Panagiotis Antiochos [2], Ioannis Skalidis [2], Chiara Chiti [3], Giulia Biagioni [3], Alessia Tomberli [3], Sara Giovani [3], Raffaele Coppini [4], Franco Cecchi [5] and Iacopo Olivotto [1,6]

1. Department of Clinical and Experimental Medicine, University of Florence, 50121 Florence, Italy
2. Service of Cardiology, University Hospital of Lausanne, 1009 Lausanne, Switzerland
3. Cardiomyopathy Unit, Careggi University Hospital, 50134 Florence, Italy
4. Department NeuroFarBa, University of Florence, 50121 Florence, Italy
5. Fondazione AICARM, 50100 Florence, Italy
6. Service of Cardiology, Meyer Children's Hospital IRCCS, 50139 Florence, Italy
* Correspondence: niccolo.maurizi@gmail.com; Tel.: +41-076-5568-981

Abstract: Background: Although disopyramide has been widely used to reduce left ventricular outflow obstruction (LVOTO) and to improve symptoms in patients with obstructive hypertrophic cardiomyopathy (oHCM), its use in real world as well as patient characteristics associated with a positive treatment response are still unclear. **Methods:** From 1980 to 2021, 1527 patients with HCM were evaluated and 372 (23%) had a LVOTO with active follow-up. The efficacy and safety of disopyramide were assessed systematically during 12 months (2-, 6-, and 12-month visits). Responders were patients with a final NYHA = I and a LVOTO < 30 mmHg; incomplete responders were those patients with NYHA > I and a LVOTO < 30 mmHg; and non-responders were symptomatic patients with no change in functional class NYHA and a LVOT gradient > 30 mmHg. **Results:** Two-hundred-fifty-four (66%) patients were in functional class NYHA I/II and 118 (34%) in NYHA III/IV. A total of 118/372 (32%, 55 ± 16 years) underwent disopyramide therapy. Twenty-eight (24%) patients responded to therapy, 39 (33%) were incomplete responders, and 51 (43%) did not respond. Responder were mainly patients in functional NYHA class I/II (24/28, 86%), whereas incomplete responders and non-responders were more often in functional NYHA class III/IV (50/54 (93%)). An independent predictor of response to disopyramide treatment was the presence of NYHA I/II at the initiation of therapy (HR 1.5 (95% CI 1.1–4.5), p = 0.03). No major life-threatening arrhythmic events or syncope occurred, despite 19 (16%) patients showing reduced QTc from baseline, 19 (16%) having no difference, while 80 (69%) patients had prolonged QTc interval. Thirty-one (26%) patients experienced side effects, in particular, 29 of the anticholinergic type. **Conclusions:** Disopyramide was underused in oHCM but effective in reducing LVOTO gradients and symptoms in slightly symptomatic patients with less severe disease phenotype with a safe pro-arrhythmic profile.

Keywords: hypertrophic cardiomyopathy; disopyramide; obstructive HCM management

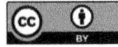

1. Introduction

Hypertrophic cardiomyopathy (HCM) is the most common genetic cardiomyopathy, characterized by heterogeneous phenotype and clinical course [1,2].

Among the earliest functional manifestations of disease are a hyperdynamic ventricular contraction and impaired relaxation. Dynamic left ventricular outflow tract (LVOT) obstruction due to systolic anterior motion (SAM) of the mitral valve and contact with the interventricular septum is a hallmark and one of the determinants of the clinical course in HCM [3]. In recent years, several drugs addressing promising therapeutic targets have been investigated in obstructive HCM, but have failed to demonstrate their efficacy or proved to be poorly tolerated [4]. Therefore, the treatment of symptomatic patients with obstructive

HCM is still mainly based on negative inotropic drugs such as beta-blockers (BB) and/or non-dihydropyridine calcium-channel blockers (CCBs; primarily verapamil) [5]. In patients with resistant symptoms, disopyramide can be employed as a second-line therapy, owing to its strong negative inotropism, increase in systemic resistances, and ability to decrease early LV ejection flow acceleration [5].

Data concerning the safety and efficacy of this disopyramide in obstructive HCM are limited from a few studies [6–9] and still many open questions remain. As an example, patient characteristics associated with treatment response are unclear and incertitude is still present concerning in which disease stage disopyramide would be the most effective [9]. This is of critical relevance since its anti-cholinergic and very rare pro-arrhythmic side effects may limit its use [6,7]. Moreover, the recent development of disease-specific therapies represents not only a major opportunity for HCM patients but also a challenge for the clinician, since the appropriate and timely treatment selection for the correct patient's subgroup is now a priority [10]. Lastly, safety concerns remain, partly due to its anticholinergic effects [8] and its blockage of the rapid delayed rectifier cardiac potassium current (I Kr), with a potential significant QT-prolonging effect [11]. Therefore, we evaluated the real-world use of disopyramide in a large cohort of obstructive HCM, by determining its safety and efficacy in reducing LVOT gradients and symptoms, as to identify possible patient responder sub-groups.

2. Methods

2.1. Study Population

We analyzed the clinical data and management data of 1527 HCM patients consecutively diagnosed at our center from 1980 to 2021. Of these, 372 (25%) had a left ventricular outflow tract obstruction (LVOTO) with active follow-up. Diagnosis was based on two-dimensional echocardiographic evidence of a hypertrophied, non-dilated LV (maximum wall thickness ≥ 15 mm, or the equivalent relative to body surface area in children), in the absence of another cardiac or systemic disease capable of producing the magnitude of hypertrophy evident. The peak LV outflow tract velocity was averaged from 3 to 5 cardiac cycles recorded at a sweep speed of 50 to 100 mm/s. Outflow obstruction was defined using Doppler echocardiography as a systolic anterior motion of the mitral valve and LV outflow tract (subaortic) velocity of >2.7 m/s at rest of >3.5 m/s with provocation, which is respectively comparable to an outflow gradient > 30 mm Hg at rest or >50 mm Hg with provocation. In all cases, particular consideration was given to distinguishing the Doppler signal of LVOTO from that of mitral regurgitation.

2.2. Patient Evaluation and Management

Patients with a diagnosis of HCM presenting with LVOT obstruction were evaluated, according to current ESC Guidelines [5] or up to date best practice, as follows:
1. Patients with a function class NYHA I and symptoms related to LVOT obstruction or NYHA II were treated with non-vasodilating beta-blockers titrated to maximum tolerated dose or, if contraindicated verapamil (starting dose 40 mg three times daily to maximum 480 mg daily);
2. Patients with a function class NYHA I and symptoms related to LVOT obstruction or NYHA II-III, after ineffective 6-month treatment with beta-blockers/verapamil, disopyramide was introduced up to a maximum tolerated dose (usually 400–500 mg/day). Exclusion criteria for disopyramide initiation were glaucoma, men with prostatism, patient with baseline QTc > 550 msec, and those with LVEF < 50%;
3. Patients with an LVOTO gradient ≥ 50 mm Hg, moderate-to-severe symptoms (New York Heart Association (NYHA) functional Class III–IV), and/or recurrent exertional syncope in spite of maximally tolerated negative inotropic therapy were proposed with an invasive management of LVOT gradient.

Disopyramide was initiated at the routine initial dose of 125 mg short-acting disopyramide two times daily. At the day of disopyramide initiation, an electrocardiogram (ECG) and echocardiogram are performed. During each clinical follow-up, patients underwent resting 12-lead ECG, resting echocardiography with provocation, and a questionnaire concerning possible side effects of disopyramide. A 2-, 6-, and 12-month follow-up was scheduled for each patient. From the 6-month visit, according to the clinical response, increasing the disopyramide dose or discontinuation of the drug was considered. Pyridostigmine, which has been demonstrated to attenuate the anticholinergic side effects of disopyramide, was also considered if patients developed such side effects. An intermediate clinical visit was performed at 6 months and the last visit including ECG, and echocardiography was performed at 12 months from therapy initiation. Special care was taken to monitor the side effects of the drug in patients with renal or hepatic impairment attributed to potential effects on drug clearance, in those with atrial fibrillation and atrial flutter because of the potential for disopyramide-induced augmentation of atrioventricular conduction and increased ventricular rate. The decision to initiate disopyramide therapy is taken by the treating physician as is the tailoring of the above-mentioned protocol to the individual patient.

2.3. Twelve-Lead Electrocardiogram Analysis

Each ECG was recorded on the visit day. PR, QRS, and QT intervals were measured manually by a single investigator experienced in ECG interpretation (C.C.). QT intervals were measured using the tangents method using lead II. If measurement in lead II was impossible because of technical limitations, leads V5 or V2 were used in this order. The correction for heart rate was performed using Fridericia's formula. Although Bazett's formula is the most commonly used, it is less accurate in relative tachycardia or bradycardia and therefore less reliable when comparing ECGs with different heart rates. Accordingly, Fridericia's formula is recommended over Bazett's formula for the evaluation of drug-induced QT prolongation (http://www.fda.gov/downloads/drugs/guidancecomplianceregulatoryinformation/guidances/ucm073153.pdf, accessed on 7 March 2023). Patients who were ventricularly paced were excluded from ECG analysis.

2.4. Definition of the Response to Disopyramide

At the 12-month follow-up, patients were categorized based on the clinical and echocardiographic response to negative inotropic agents, specifically:

1. Responders: patients with a functional class NYHA = I and a LVOT gradient < 30 mmHg.
2. Incomplete responders: patients with a functional class NYHA > I and a LVOT gradient < 30 mmHg.
3. Non-responders: symptomatic patients with no change in functional class NYHA and a LVOT gradient > 30 mmHg.

2.5. Statistical Analysis

Continuous variables, reported as means with standard deviations or as medians with interquartile ranges for non-normal distributions, were compared between groups with the Student t tests or non-parametric tests, as appropriate. Categorical variables, reported as counts and percentages, were compared between groups with χ^2 tests or Fisher exact tests when any expected cell count was less than 5.

Cox multivariable regression analysis (variable selection method with backward stepwise elimination) was performed including all candidate variables ($p < 0.10$ at univariate analysis). A 2-sided p-value less than 0.05 was considered statistically significant. All analyses were performed using SPSS Statistics for Macintosh version 25.0 (IBM).

3. Results

3.1. Clinical and Echocardiographic Profile of Patients with Obstructive HCM

Of the 1527 patients diagnosed with HCM in our center from 1981 to 2021, 372 (25%) were diagnosed with obstructive HCM had an active follow-up. Of these, 254 patients (66%)

were in functional class NYHA I/II and 118 (34%) in NYHA class III/IV (Table 1, Figure 1). The mean age at therapy initiation was 43 ± 19 years and 226 (61%) were males. Specifically, among patients in NYHA Class I/II, 185 (75%) were on BB/CCA treatment, 5 (2%) directly underwent septal reduction therapies (SRTs), whereas 64 (26%) were on disopyramide ± BB/CCA treatment (Figure 1). Highly symptomatic patients, in functional class NYHA III/IV, received negative inotropic drugs (25 (19%) on BB/CCA treatment), disopyramide ± BB/CCA (54 (42%)), and direct SRT (49 (14%; Figure 1). Therefore, a total of 118 patients (63 (53%) males, 55 ± 16 years) underwent therapy with disopyramide at the initial 250 mg dose in addition to beta-blocker/calcium channel blocker therapy. One hundred and eleven (94%) patients presented functional limitations (NYHA > I) at the beginning of therapy, and 32 (27%) presented at least an episode of atrial fibrillation. Systolic anterior motion of the mitral valve (SAM) was present in 95 (80%) patients, whereas the mean left atrial diameter was 45 ± 7 mm. A total of 76 (64%) presented a LVOT obstruction > 50 mmHg and mean left ventricular ejection fraction (LV EF) of 66 ± 7 % (Table 1).

Table 1. Baseline characteristics of the cohort at disopyramide therapy initiation.

	Variable	Total Cohort (n = 118)	Responders (n = 28)	Incomplete Responders (n = 39)	Non-Responders (n = 51)
Demographic					
	Age (ys)	55 ± 16	48 ± 9 *	51 ± 11	58 ± 12
	Male sex (n, %)	63 (53%)	16 (57%)	19 (49%)	28 (55%)
Medical History					
	NYHA Class I–II (n, %)	64 (54 %)	24 (86%) *	24 (62%)	16 (31%)
	NYHA Class III (n, %)	53 (46 %)	3 (11%)	15 (38%)	35 (69%) *
	NYHA Class IV (n, %)	1 (1.5%)	1 (3%)	0	0
	Atrial fibrillation (n, %)	32 (27%)	6 (21%)	11 (28%)	15 (29%)
	Syncope (n, %)	27 (0.12 %)	1 (4%) *	12 (31%)	14 (27%)
	PM/ICD (n, %)	11 (9%)	1 (4%) *	3 (8%)	7 (14%)
	NSVT (n, %)	22 (19%)	3 (11%)	6 (15%)	13 (25%)
	Cardiac Arrest (n, %)	1 (0.8%)	0	1 (2.5%)	0
Treatments					
	Beta-blockers (n, %)	99 (84 %)	22 (79%)	35 (90%)	42 (81%)
	Calcium-Antagonist (n, %)	14 (8 %)	2 (8%)	4 (10%)	8 (16%)
	Amiodarone (n, %)	12 (10 %)	1 (4%)	4 (10%)	7 (14%)
Echocardiogram					
	SAM (n, %)	95 (80%)	22 (78%)	33 (85%)	40 (78%)
	Left Atrial diameter (mm)	45 ± 7	42 ± 5 *	44 ± 6	46 ± 7
	LV Maximal Wall Thickness (mm)	22 ± 5	21 ± 4	22 ± 5	22 ± 6
	Resting LVOTO (mmHg)	72 ± 36	69 ± 21	70 ± 18	73 ± 22
	30 mmHg < LVOTO < 50 mmHg (n, %)	42 (36%)	13 (46%)	10 (26%)	19 (37%)
	LVOTO > 50 mmHg (n, %)	76 (64%)	15 (54 %)	29 (74 %) *	32 (63%)
	Maximal LVOTO (mmHg)	88 ± 35	71 ± 12	91 ± 13	85 ± 21
	LV Ejection Fraction (%)	66 ± 7	69 ± 8	66 ± 6	63 ± 8 *

Abbreviations: PM: pacemaker; ICD: implantable cardioverter defibrillator; NSVT: non-sustained ventricular tachycardia; SAM: systolic anterior motion of the mitral valve; LV: left ventricle; LVOTO: left ventricular outflow tract obstruction. * = $p < 0.05$.

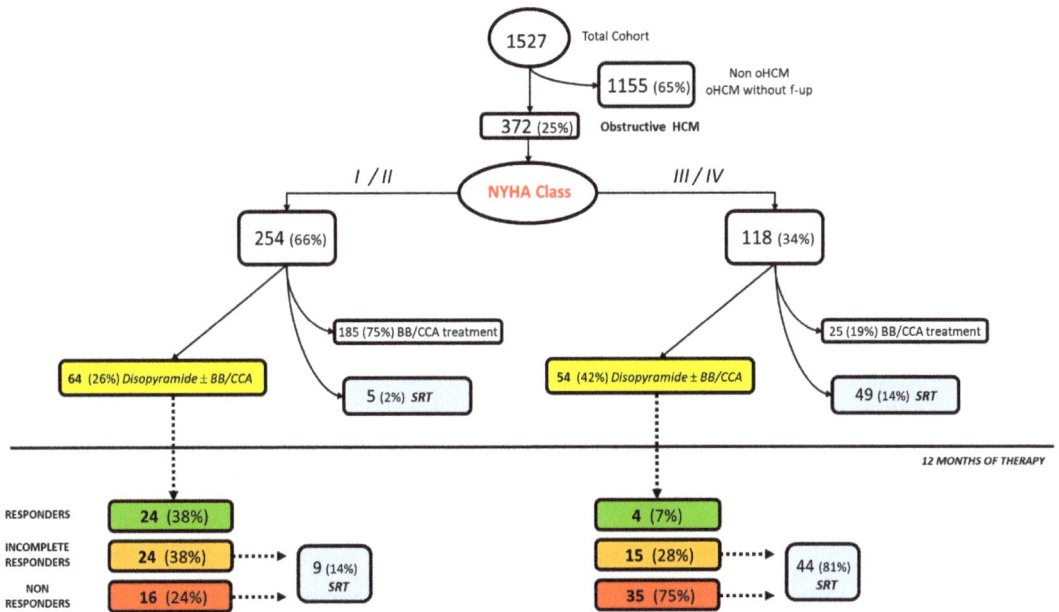

Figure 1. Clinical management of patients with obstructive hypertrophic cardiomyopathy. Abbreviations: oHCM: obstructive hypertrophic cardiomyopathy; f-up: follow-up; BB: beta-blockers; CCA: calcium antagonists; SRT: septal reduction treatments.

Patients who underwent disopyramide therapy presented with, before treatment initiation, a first-degree atrioventricular block (AVB) in 10 (8%) cases, a bundle branch block (BBB) in 14 (11%), a QTc interval > 480 msec in 30 (24%), and a QTc > 500 msec in 14 (11%) (Table 2).

Table 2. Electrocardiographic changes on disopyramide treatment.

Variables	Pre-Treatment	On Treatment	p Values
HR (bpm)	60 ± 8	59 ± 79	0.45
PR (msec)	178 ± 22	183 ± 24	<0.01
AVB I (n)	10 (8%)	22 (17%)	<0.01
QRS (msec)	101 ± 22	109 ± 26	0.10
New Onset Bundle Branch Block (n)	14 (11%)	20 (16%)	0.62
QTc_{max} (msec)	423 ± 29	475 ± 41	0.67
$QTc \geq 480$ msec	30 (24%)	56 (48%)	<0.01
$QTc \geq 500$ msec	14 (11%)	36 (28%)	<0.01

Abbreviations: HR: Heart Rate.

3.2. Efficacy and Criteria of Response to Disopyramide Therapy

After 12 months of therapy, an improvement in the functional class occurred. Five (4%) patients in NYHA II class became asymptomatic; 21 (25%) patients improved their functional class from NYHA III to NYHA II. The symptomatic relief did not differ in patients who took a dose of 250 mg/day vs. higher doses (p = 0.79). The mean LVOTO gradient at rest post-therapy was not abolished but was significantly reduced (72 ± 36 mmHg vs. 49 ± 31 mmHg; $p < 0.001$). Specifically, 28 (24%) were responders to therapy, 39 (33%) were incomplete responders, and 51 (43%) did not respond to therapy. Among the latter, 53 (45%)

underwent subsequent SRT (9/64 (14%) in the NYHA I/II and 44/54 (81%) in the NYHA III/IV group) (Figure 1). Responders were mainly patients in functional NYHA class I/II (24/28, 86%), whereas incomplete responders and non-responders were more often patients in functional NYHA class III/IV (50/54 (93%) (Table 1, Figure 1). Moreover, responders were younger (48 ± 9 mm vs. 51 ± 11 mm and 58 ± 12 mm for incomplete responders and non-responders, p for trend < 0.01), had a smaller left atrium (42 ± 5 mm vs. 44 ± 5 mm and 46 ± 5 mm for incomplete responders and non-responders, p for trend < 0.01), and less severe LVOT gradient (15 (53%) with LVOT > 50 mmHg vs. 29 (74%) and 32 (63%) for incomplete and non-responders, p for trend < 0.01). Non-responders, as compared to the two other groups, had also a lower LV EF (63 ± 8 vs. 66 ± 6 and 69 ± 8 for incomplete responders and responders, p for trend < 0.01) (Table 1).

Factors associated with response to disopyramide therapy were age (per 10 decrease) (HR 1.4 (95% CI 0.5–3.6), p = 0.03), left atrial diameter (per 2 mm decrease) (HR 2.1 (95% CI 0.9–7.8), p < 0.01), LV EF (HR 4.2 (95% CI 1.3–9.9), p < 0.01), and NYHA Class I/II at therapy initiation (HR 5.1 (95% CI 2.3–11.2), p < 0.01). The latter was the only multivariable predictor of response to disopyramide treatment (HR 1.5 (95% CI 1.1–4.5), p = 0.03) (Table 3).

Table 3. Multivariable Predictors of response to disopyramide therapy.

Variable	Univariable Analysis			Multivariable Analysis		
	HR	95% CI	p-Value	HR	95% CI	p-Value
Age (per 10 decrease)	1.4	[0.5–3.6]	0.03			
NYHA Class I-II (n)	5.1	[2.3–11.2]	<0.01	1.5	[1.1–4.5]	0.03
Left atrial diameter (per 2 mm decrease)	2.1	[0.9–7.8]	<0.01			
LV EF (per 5 increase)	4.2	[1.3–9.9]	<0.01	1.9	[0.9–6.4]	0.07

3.3. Safety of Disopyramide Therapy

During the therapy, no major life-threatening arrhythmic events or syncope occurred.

Atrioventricular conduction was prolonged during treatment: the mean PR interval pre-treatment was 178 ± 22 msec in a total of 10 patients (8%) with AVB I vs. 183 ± 24 msec in 22 patients (17%) with AVB I after treatment, p < 0.01. No increase in intraventricular conduction was observed, and the median prolongation of the QTc interval was 21 [2; 32] msec (Table 2).

Specifically, 19 (16%) patients showed reduced QTc from baseline (mean reduction 10 [8; 14] msec), 19 (16%) had no difference, while 80 (68%) patients had a prolonged QTc interval of 27 [19; 37] msec (Figure 2). Patients who presented with a QTc < 480 msec (88/118, 70%) at baseline had a more significant prolongation compared to those with an abnormal baseline QTc (24 [7; 35] vs. 5 [2; 11] msec, p < 0.01). A significantly higher proportion of patients (56, 48%) presented with a QTc > 480 msec after 12 months of treatment (Table 2).

Thirty-one (26%) patients experienced side effects, in particular 29 of the anticholinergic type. Such symptoms led to the reduction of treatment in 5 (4%) patients (Table 4).

At the end of the study period, a total of 67/118 (%) patients suspended the treatment. Specifically, 53 (79%) underwent SRT because of ineffective response, 10 (15%) because of anti-cholinergic collateral effects, and 4 (6%) for QTc prolongation above 550 msec.

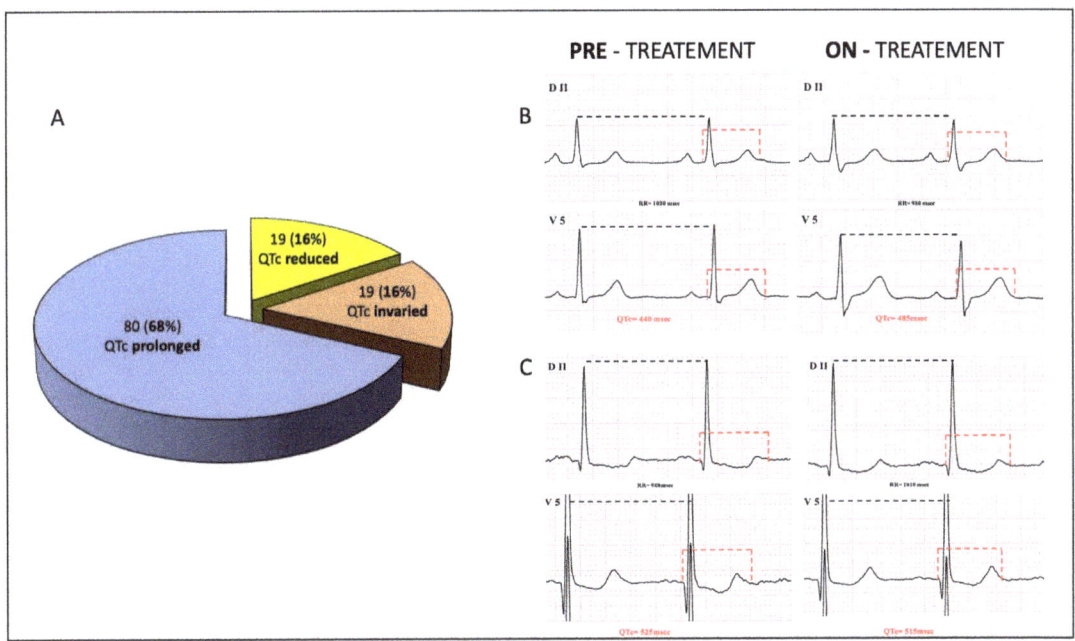

Figure 2. Spectrum of QTc interval changes during disopyramide treatment. In panel (**A**), the spectrum of QT variation following disopyramide therapy is reported. Panel (**B**) shows a case of QT prolongation during treatment, whereas Panel (**C**) represents a patient with QT shortening while on disopyramide.

Table 4. Collateral effects of patients undergoing disopyramide treatment.

	Total Cohort (n = 118)	Treatment Reduction	Treatment Suspension
Anticholinergic collateral effects	29 (24%)	5 (4%)	10 (8%)
Xerostomia/Xerophthalmia	13 (11%)	4 (3%)	8 (7%)
Stypsis	10 (8%)	1 (0.8%)	1 (0.8%)
Blurred vision	2 (2%)	1 (0.8%)	0
Urinary Retention	4 (3%)	0	1
Sustained Ventricular Arrhythmias	0	-	-
Torsade de Pointes	0	-	-

4. Discussion

Despite being largely used since the 1980s for patients with obstructive HCM, the real-world use of disopyramide and the markers of treatment response are still unknown. This is of critical relevance, since the recent development of disease-specific therapies, such as myosin inhibitors, challenges clinicians to find the appropriate sub-group as well as the correct disease stage for each drug [12].

The present study shows that disopyramide was underused since the 1980s in a historical and large cohort of patients with obstructive HCM, being offered to up to one-third of the patients. Such finding reflects several possible limitations related to the use of this treatment. Despite being recommended by scientific societies [5,13], there is a chronic supply shortage of disopyramide in several European countries, being an old medication without important commercial interest. Moreover, a certain lack of confidence by physicians might exist, many of whom are reluctant to use class I anti-arrhythmic agents in structural heart disease and fear possible complications related to disopyramide-induced augmentation of atrioventricular conduction and increased ventricular rate.

In our cohort, the efficacy of disopyramide was present in a quarter of patients, almost exclusively observed in patients who were slightly symptomatic, with a functional class NYHA I or II. Interestingly, responders were younger, had a smaller left atrium, less severe LVOT gradient, and a higher LV EF. These findings are in line with the drug physiopathological effect, mainly driven by its negative inotropic effect, which is the main mechanistic driver of reduction in LVOT gradients; it is less potent in patients who demonstrate less HCM-induced hypercontractility [6,7]. Taken together, these finding suggest that clinicians should not be discouraged from trying disopyramide in patients who are symptomatic and have high LVOT gradients despite administering the maximum doses of other negative inotropic drugs. This may be especially true in those patients with high-normal LVEF and non-enlarged LA, factors that were associated with response to disopyramide therapy in the current study. Moreover, no difference was observed between the maximum drug dose and patients on the minimum effective posology, suggesting that effective reduced dose of the drug might be similarly effective despite limiting adverse effects, which are dose-dependent. Such findings are in accordance with previous smaller reports from Habib et al. [8]. On the contrary, our data highlight that severely symptomatic patients, with a NYHA class III/IV and a remodeled myocardium, would hardly respond to disopyramide. In this subset of patients, direct referral to SRT might probably be the best therapeutic option. At the end of the study period, almost 50% of patients were proposed to be treated with an invasive SRT and almost exclusively in the incomplete and non-responders in the NYHA III/IV group.

Concerning the safety profile, no major sustained arrhythmias occurred during the whole study period. This is in line with current literature that shows freedom from cardiovascular death including sudden cardiovascular death, and with a total mortality similar to the general population [6,7]. QTc prolongation was observed in 68% of patients, and QTc prolongation above 500 msec in up to 28%. This was mainly correlated with an increase in QRS length [14], and only in four cases led to drug discontinuation because of increase in QTc above 550 msec. Interestingly, 32% of patients did not show significant QTc related changes or reduced length of repolarization. This is in line with the in vitro observations from Coppini et al. [11], which showed the multichannel inhibitory effects and the membrane stabilizing actions of disopyramide.

Disopyramide was overall well tolerated, and side effects, mainly anti-cholinergic, led to treatment interruption in 8% of patients. As a limitation and possible bias of the study, investigators did not propose systematic pyridostigmine for patients with severe side effects.

In conclusion, while awaiting approval from the regulatory agencies for disease specific therapies such as myosin inhibitors, HCM experts are evaluating the positioning of each specific therapy in current management algorithms. Despite surgeons' concerns [15], negative inotropic drugs and myosin inhibitors may shape the current practice. Furthermore, as we have recently learned from the case of tafamidis, a progression-slowing drug for transthyretin-related amyloidosis [16], pricing may represent a key issue influencing patients' access to treatment [16], particularly in less-developed economies. Based on the EXPLORER-HCM trial results, symptomatic patients with oHCM not responding fully to (or not tolerating) β-blockers and disopyramide should be considered for mavacamten treatment [17], potentially proposing the drug as a life-long therapy. Therefore, sustainability should be a relevant aspect of all treatments addressing left ventricular obstruction. The present study shows that, in a specific subset of slightly symptomatic patients with oHCM, a relatively inexpensive drug such as disopyramide might still play an important role. This would be a relevant factor for global experts when specific treatment algorithms would be proposed in the Guidelines for patients with symptomatic LVOT. Lastly, further prospective studies would be needed to compare negative inotropic drugs with myosin inhibitors, specifically in the subset of obstructive HCM patients with atrial fibrillation, as mavacamten does not exert any classic antiarrhythmic effect.

5. Limitations

This study was limited by its size and retrospective nature. Accordingly, only the association of the factors studied with response to disopyramide treatment could be investigated. However, the associations demonstrated in this study are in line with our knowledge of disease mechanisms in HCM and the mode of action of disopyramide.

6. Conclusions

Disopyramide was underused in oHCM but effective in reducing symptoms and LVOTO gradients in patients with slightly symptomatic patient with less severe disease phenotype with a safe pro-arrhythmic profile. Further prospective studies would be needed to ascertain the role of negative inotropes in the treatment algorithm of patients with slightly symptomatic obstructive HCM.

Author Contributions: Conceptualization, N.M., C.F., F.C. and I.O.; Methodology, M.T. and R.C.; Validation, N.M.; Formal analysis, S.P.; Investigation, C.C. (Chiara Chiriatti) and A.T.; Writing—original draft, N.M., P.A. and G.B.; Writing—review & editing, I.S., C.C. (Chiara Chiti), S.G. and I.O. All authors have read and agreed to the published version of the manuscript.

Funding: I.O. was supported by the European Union's Horizon 2020 Research and Innovation Programme under Grant Agreement no. 777204: "SILICOFCM-In Silico trials for drug tracing the effects of sarcomeric protein mutations leading to familial cardiomyopathy".

Institutional Review Board Statement: The study was approved by Comitato Etico Area Vasta (SPE 16.211).

Informed Consent Statement: Informed consent was obtained from all subjects involved in the study.

Data Availability Statement: Data would be shared upon reasonable request.

Conflicts of Interest: The authors report no conflicts of interest regarding the topic discussed in the present manuscript.

References

1. Maron, B.J. Clinical course and management of hypertrophic cardiomyopathy. *N. Engl. J. Med.* **2018**, *379*, 655–668. [CrossRef] [PubMed]
2. Maurizi, N.; Olivotto, I.; Maron, M.S.; Bonacchi, G.; Antiochos, P.; Tomberli, B.; Fumagalli, C.; Poggesi, C.; Berteotti, M.; Girolami, F.; et al. Lifetime Clinical Course of Hypertrophic Cardiomyopathy: Outcome of the Historical Florence Cohort over Five Decades. *JACC Adv.* **2023**, in press.
3. Maron, M.S.; Olivotto, I.; Zenovich, A.G.; Link, M.S.; Pandian, N.G.; Kuvin, J.T.; Nistri, S.; Cecchi, F.; Udelson, J.E.; Maron, B.J. Hypertrophic cardiomyopathy is predominantly a disease of left ventricular outflow tract obstruction. *Circulation* **2006**, *114*, 2232–2239. [CrossRef] [PubMed]
4. Maurizi, N.; Ammirati, E.; Coppini, R.; Morrone, A.; Olivotto, I. Clinical and Molecular Aspects of Cardiomyopathies: Emerging Therapies and Clinical Trials. *Heart Fail. Clin.* **2018**, *14*, 161–178. [CrossRef] [PubMed]
5. Elliott, P.M.; Anastasakis, A.; Borger, M.A.; Borggrefe, M.; Cecchi, F.; Charron, P.; Hagege, A.A.; Lafont, A.; Limongelli, G.; Mahrholdt, H. Authors/Task Force members. 2014 ESC Guidelines on diagnosis and management of hypertrophic cardiomyopathy: The Task Force for the Diagnosis and Management of Hypertrophic Cardiomyopathy of the European Society of Cardiology (ESC). *Eur. Heart J.* **2014**, *35*, 2733–2779. [PubMed]
6. Sherrid, M.V.; Barac, I.; McKenna, W.J.; Elliott, P.M.; Dickie, S.; Chojnowska, L.; Casey, S.; Maron, B.J. Multicenter study of the efficacy and safety of disopyramide in obstructive hypertrophic cardiomyopathy. *J. Am. Coll. Cardiol.* **2005**, *45*, 1251–1258. [CrossRef] [PubMed]
7. Sherrid, M.V.; Shetty, A.; Winson, G.; Kim, B.; Musat, D.; Alviar, C.L.; Homel, P.; Balaram, S.K.; Swistel, D.G. Treatment of obstructive hypertrophic cardiomyopathy symptoms and gradient resistant to first-line therapy with beta-blockade or verapamil. *Circ. Heart Fail.* **2013**, *6*, 694–702. [CrossRef] [PubMed]
8. Habib, M.; Hoss, S.; Bruchal-Garbicz, B.; Chan, R.H.; Rakowski, H.; Williams, L.; Adler, A. Markers of responsiveness to disopyramide in patients with hypertrophic cardiomyopathy. *Int. J. Cardiol.* **2019**, *297*, 75–82. [CrossRef] [PubMed]
9. Adler, A.; Fourey, D.; Weissler-Snir, A.; Hindieh, W.; Chan, R.H.; Gollob, M.H.; Rakowski, H. Safety of Outpatient Initiation of Disopyramide for Obstructive Hypertrophic Cardiomyopathy Patients. *J. Am. Heart Assoc.* **2017**, *6*, e005152. [CrossRef] [PubMed]

10. Masri, A.; Olivotto, I. Cardiac Myosin Inhibitors as a Novel Treatment Option for Obstructive Hypertrophic Cardiomyopathy: Addressing the Core of the Matter. *J. Am. Heart Assoc.* **2022**, *11*, e024656. [CrossRef] [PubMed]
11. Coppini, R.; Ferrantini, C.; Pioner, J.M.; Santini, L.; Wang, Z.J.; Palandri, C.; Scardigli, M.; Vitale, G.; Sacconi, L.; Stefàno, P.; et al. Electrophysiological and Contractile Effects of Disopyramide in Patients With Obstructive Hypertrophic Cardiomyopathy: A Translational Study. *JACC Basic Transl. Sci.* **2019**, *4*, 795–813. [CrossRef] [PubMed]
12. Zampieri, M.; Argirò, A.; Marchi, A.; Berteotti, M.; Targetti, M.; Fornaro, A.; Tomberli, A.; Stefàno, P.; Marchionni, N.; Olivotto, I. Mavacamten, a Novel Therapeutic Strategy for Obstructive Hypertrophic Cardiomyopathy. *Curr. Cardiol. Rep.* **2021**, *23*, 79. [CrossRef] [PubMed]
13. Ommen, S.R.; Mital, S.; Burke, M.A.; Day, S.M.; Deswal, A.; Elliott, P.; Evanovich, L.L.; Hung, J.; Joglar, J.A.; Kantor, P.; et al. 2020 AHA/ACC Guideline for the Diagnosis and Treatment of Patients With Hypertrophic Cardiomyopathy: Executive Summary: A Report of the American College of Cardiology/American Heart Association Joint Committee on Clinical Practice Guidelines. *Circulation* **2020**, *142*, e533–e557. [PubMed]
14. Honerjäger, P. The contribution of Na channel block to the negative inotropic effect of antiarrhythmic drugs. *Basic Res. Cardiol.* **1986**, *81* (Suppl. 1), 33–37. [CrossRef] [PubMed]
15. Quintana, E.; Bajona, P.; O Myers, P. Mavacamten for hypertrophic obstructive cardiomyopathy. *Lancet* **2021**, *397*, 369. [CrossRef] [PubMed]
16. Gurwitz, J.H.; Maurer, M.S. Tafamidis—A Pricey Therapy for a Not-So-Rare Condition. *JAMA Cardiol.* **2020**, *5*, 247. [CrossRef] [PubMed]
17. Olivotto, I.; Oreziak, A.; Barriales-Villa, R.; Abraham, T.P.; Masri, A.; Garcia-Pavia, P.; Saberi, S.; Lakdawala, N.K.; Wheeler, M.T.; Owens, A.; et al. Mavacamten for treatment of symptomatic obstructive hypertrophic cardiomyopathy (EXPLORER-HCM): A randomised, double-blind, placebo-controlled, phase 3 trial; EXPLORER-HCM study investigators. *Lancet* **2020**, *396*, 759–769. [CrossRef] [PubMed]

Disclaimer/Publisher's Note: The statements, opinions and data contained in all publications are solely those of the individual author(s) and contributor(s) and not of MDPI and/or the editor(s). MDPI and/or the editor(s) disclaim responsibility for any injury to people or property resulting from any ideas, methods, instructions or products referred to in the content.

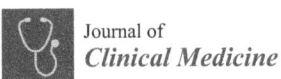

Review

Clinical and Genetic Screening for Hypertrophic Cardiomyopathy in Paediatric Relatives: Changing Paradigms in Clinical Practice

Claire M. Lawley [1,2] and Juan Pablo Kaski [1,3,*]

1. Centre for Inherited Cardiovascular Diseases, Great Ormond Street Hospital, London WC1N 3JH, UK
2. The University of Sydney Children's Hospital Westmead Clinical School, Faculty of Medicine and Health, The University of Sydney, Camperdown, NSW 2006, Australia
3. Centre for Paediatric Inherited and Rare Cardiovascular Disease, University College London Institute of Cardiovascular Science, London WC1E 6DD, UK
* Correspondence: j.kaski@ucl.ac.uk; Tel.: +44-(0)20-7829-8839

Abstract: Hypertrophic cardiomyopathy (HCM) is an important cause of morbidity and mortality in children. While the aetiology is heterogeneous, most cases are caused by variants in the genes encoding components of the cardiac sarcomere, which are inherited as an autosomal dominant trait. In recent years, there has been a paradigm shift in the role of clinical screening and predictive genetic testing in children with a first-degree relative with HCM, with the recognition that phenotypic expression can, and often does, manifest in young children and that familial disease in the paediatric age group may not be benign. The care of the child and family affected by HCM relies on a multidisciplinary team, with a key role for genomics. This review article summarises current evidence in clinical and genetic screening for hypertrophic cardiomyopathy in paediatric relatives and highlights aspects that remain to be resolved.

Keywords: hypertrophic cardiomyopathy; paediatrics; genetics; precision medicine; screening; sudden death

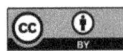

1. Introduction

Hypertrophic cardiomyopathy (HCM) is a clinically and genetically heterogeneous disease characterised by unexplained left ventricular hypertrophy (LVH). While the estimated population prevalence in adults is 1 in 500, it is substantially rarer in the paediatric population, with a reported prevalence of 2.9/100,000 [1] and an estimated annual incidence of 0.3–0.5 per 100.000 [2,3]. A childhood HCM diagnosis may follow a review for cardiac symptoms or the incidental finding of a murmur or an electrocardiogram (ECG) abnormality, or, increasingly, as a result of family screening.

The outcomes of childhood-onset HCM are influenced by aetiology and age at diagnosis. Children diagnosed during infancy or with an inborn error of metabolism (IEM) have a worse prognosis, with a recent study reporting a 5 year survival rate of 80.5% in those diagnosed aged less than one year and 66.4% in those with an IEM at a median of just over 5 years follow-up [4]. In two cohorts with infant diagnoses of HCM, survival beyond the first year was associated with a more favourable natural history [5,6]. In a consortium study including 639 children diagnosed younger than 12 years with non-sarcomeric HCM, almost 10% experienced death or cardiac transplantation, and almost 11% experienced a life-threatening arrhythmic event in a median follow-up of 5.6 years [7]. Importantly, over 50% had a family history of HCM and only 20% were symptomatic, suggesting that adverse outcomes in childhood-onset HCM are not limited to symptomatic probands. Furthermore, children with HCM diagnosed in childhood have been shown to carry a higher risk of life-threatening ventricular arrhythmias and have a greater need for advanced heart failure therapies when compared to those diagnosed in adulthood [8]. Data from the Sarcomeric Human Cardiomyopathy Registry (SHaRe) identified that childhood-onset HCM patients had roughly a 2% per year event rate of serious adverse events, including ventricular arrhythmia, heart failure, and atrial fibrillation, as well as stroke and death, with ventricular arrhythmia being the most common of these adverse events in the first decade following baseline review. From the same registry, work including 4591 individuals with HCM showed that those with pathogenic/likely pathogenic variants in sarcomeric genes had a 2-fold greater risk of adverse outcomes, and those diagnosed before the age of <40 (including 422 paediatric patients) had a higher incidence of the overall composite outcome than those diagnosed at a later age [9].

As in adults, the management of children with HCM and paediatric first-degree relatives of individuals with HCM requires a multidisciplinary team approach. Figure 1 identifies some of the relevant medical teams involved in the care of children and families affected by HCM. Holistic care includes not only symptom management and prevention of disease-related complications (particularly sudden cardiac death) in affected individuals but also well-supported family screening.

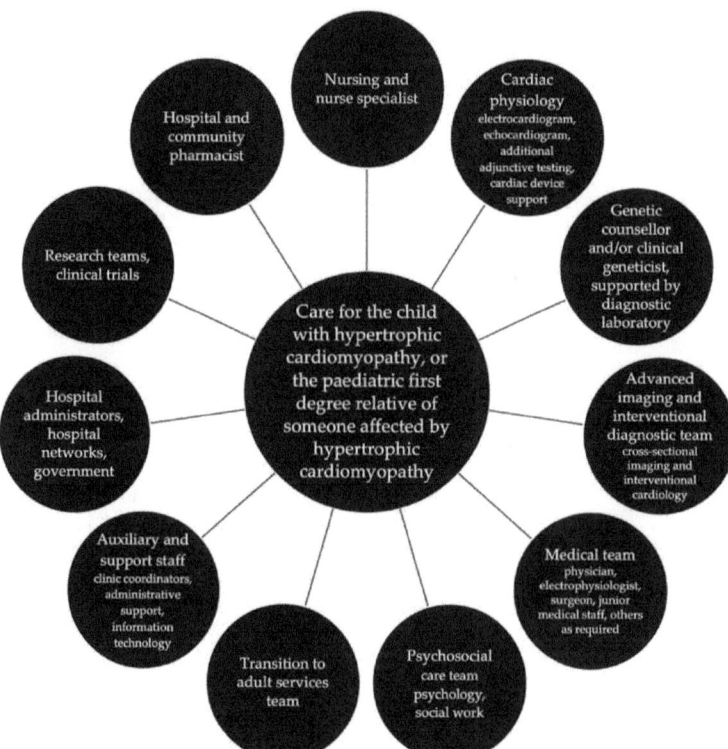

Figure 1. A proposed multidisciplinary approach to caring for the child or adolescent with HCM or a paediatric first-degree relative of someone affected by HCM.

In recent years, there have been important advances in the aetiology-specific management of HCM, particularly in childhood. In infants with HCM in the setting of Pompe disease, a glycogen storage disorder, enzyme replacement therapy has been shown to reduce the degree of LVH and may have a major impact on the natural history of this condition [10]. Similarly, MEK inhibitors are showing some promise in modifying ventricular hypertrophy in infants and children with HCM and a genetic variant in the Ras/MAPK cell signalling pathway (e.g., Noonan syndrome and related disorders) [11,12]. Cardiac myosin inhibitors (mavacamten and the next drug in the class, aficamten) have been shown to improve symptoms and reduce left ventricular outflow tract obstruction in adults with symptomatic obstructive HCM [13–15]. Preclinical studies suggest that their use in mice with sarcomeric gene variants without phenotypic evidence of LVH may prevent the development of the disease [16]. Finally, genetic modification in monogenic HCM is being explored; gene repair in human embryos with a pathogenic *MYBPC3* variant has been shown to be feasible using a variant-specific CRISPR-Cas9 system [17], and 'gene silencing' techniques, initially focusing on *MYH7* variant HCM and using viral vectors, are also being investigated [18,19].

2. Aetiology of Childhood HCM

The aetiology of childhood-onset HCM is heterogeneous and includes cases with genetic variants affecting the Ras/MAPK cell signalling pathway, inborn errors of metabolism (IEM) (including storage disorders), and neuromuscular diseases such as Friedreich's ataxia [6,20]. However, recent data have shown that, in the majority of children with HCM, as in adults, the disease is caused by variants in the sarcomere protein genes, inherited as an autosomal dominant trait [9,21–23]. The list of implicated genetic variants in childhood-onset HCM continues to expand, and there are data to suggest that rates of 'actionable' variants may vary by age of onset of disease and ancestry [21]. Broad categories of paediatric HCM are outlined in Table 1.

Table 1. An approach to classifying paediatric hypertrophic cardiomyopathy.

Category	Example Conditions	Cardiac Features	The Most Common Mode of Inheritance	Example Candidate Genes
"Sarcomeric" HCM [9,22,24,25]	"Thick filament" disease "Thin filament" disease Other	Variable hypertrophy, arrhythmic risk, and patterns of hypertrophy with some genotype-phenotype correlation	Autosomal dominant *	*MYH7, MYBPC3 TNNI3, TNNT2, TPM1, MYL2, MYL3, ACTC1, TNNC1 CSPR3, FLNC ** Additional noncoding variants influencing phenotype*
Non-sarcomeric HCM				
Ras/MAPK disease [26]	Noonan syndrome, Costello syndrome, and cardiofaciocutaneous syndrome	Polyvalvulopathy, biventricular hypertrophy, infancy/early childhood presentation	Autosomal dominant	*RAF1, RIT1, PTPN1, HRAS, MEK1, MEK2*
Inborn errors of metabolism [27,28]	Glycogen storage disorders (Pompe disease, Danon disease, Cori-Forbes disease, and PRKAG2 syndrome) Lysosomal storage disorders (mucopolysaccharidoses)	Disease specific; specific ECG changes (such as short PR, ventricular pre-excitation), variable hypertrophy, polyvavulopathy in some conditions, early childhood onset in some conditions	Autosomal recessive	*GLA LAMP2 PRKAG2*
Neuromuscular disease [12,29]	Mitochondrial disorders (Friedreich's ataxia, Barth syndrome)	Disease specific Friedreich's ataxia—concentric left ventricular hypertrophy, higher rate of atrial arrhythmia, lower risk of sudden death.	Autosomal recessive, X-linked	*FXN TAZ*

HCM: hypertrophic cardiomyopathy; *: compound heterozygosity and homozygosity also identified; ** *FLNC* variants implicated in various cardiomyopathies, including HCM.

3. Screening during Childhood and Adolescence for Those with an Affected First Degree Relative

Traditionally, HCM has been considered a disease of late adolescence and young adulthood. Until very recently, clinical practise guidelines suggested that, in the absence of symptoms, family history of premature death from HCM, competitive athletics, or other clinical suspicion of early LV hypertrophy, children of first-degree relatives with HCM need not be under regular screening until after 10 to 12 years of age [30–32]. Familial HCM was rarely reported in the paediatric literature, with data limited to small series, and there was an assertion that LVH did not develop until adolescence in patients with familial disease [33,34]. It was also felt that diagnosis earlier in childhood would not change outcome [32,35] and that earlier screening would have the potential to increase familial anxiety without any decrease in morbidity or mortality associated with an earlier diagnosis.

More recent data, however, have challenged the paradigm of delayed screening. A large single-centre study of 1198 consecutive children aged 18 years or less with a first-degree relative with HCM referred for clinical screening showed that in almost 10% of families, diagnostic criteria for HCM were met at the first or subsequent evaluation. The majority of these children presented as preadolescents, with a median age at diagnosis of 10 years, including a substantial proportion in infancy [36]. Importantly, the diagnosis of HCM changed the clinical course in nearly one-third of these children, including starting medication for symptoms that previously may have been attributed to non-cardiac disease and proceeding to surgery or an implantable cardiac device. Although patients with a diagnosis made through screening in childhood were more likely to have a family history of childhood disease, this only accounted for half of patients with early-onset disease, and neither the genetic nor the clinical features of those in whom an early diagnosis was made were different from those without childhood-onset disease. These findings were validated in an independent North American cohort, showing that 50% of individuals under the age of 18 diagnosed with HCM during screening were aged less than ten years and that 41% of the major cardiac events occurred in children aged less than ten years. Approximately one-third of the children diagnosed as a result of family screening would not have been screened under the historic guidelines [37]. In addition, patients with disease-causing variants in *MYH7* and *MYBC3* were at the highest risk for developing HCM in childhood and experiencing an adverse event or requiring intervention. Indeed, while previous data had suggested that *MYBPC3* variants in particular were associated with late-onset disease [38], more recent studies have shown that *MYBPC3* variants in heterozygosis can cause severe phenotypic expression of disease in childhood, with a high prevalence of malignant ventricular arrhythmia [39]. Furthermore, there are data to show that, in the context of a multidisciplinary expert setting and with adequate psychological support, clinical screening of paediatric first-degree relatives does not result in psychological harm [40].

The most recent American Heart Association/American College of Cardiology Guidelines for the Diagnosis and Treatment of Patients With Hypertrophic Cardiomyopathy now suggest that clinical screening for HCM should be offered to all first-degree relatives at the time at which the diagnosis is made in the family, regardless of age [41]. In support of this approach, data are also emerging for other cardiomyopathy subtypes, including arrhythmogenic right ventricular cardiomyopathy (ARVC). A recent single-centre cohort study of consecutive ARVC probands and genotype-positive relatives aged ≤18 years found that 40% met diagnostic criteria by age <12 years and that half of the cardiac adverse events occurred in these children [42]. Together, these data herald a need for a screening paradigm shift with the recognition that significant disease exists in pre-adolescents with genetic cardiomyopathies [43].

3.1. The Role of Predictive Genetic Testing in Children in Familial Screening for HCM

In families in which a 'causative' genetic variant (i.e., 'pathogenic' or 'likely pathogenic' variant) has been identified, predictive genetic testing of pre-phenotypic first-degree relatives should be considered, including in children [41]. When considering embarking on genetic testing for HCM in eligible families, pre- and post-test genetic counselling is essential [41]. In the clinically unaffected child, a 'negative' genetic test (whereby the child is found not to carry the familial causative gene variant) offers the opportunity to discharge the child from regular clinical follow-up, placing them at most at the general population risk of developing HCM. A 'positive' genetic test (whereby the child is found to carry the familial causative gene variant) confers a greater lifetime risk of developing HCM. Providing a personal estimate of the lifetime risk of HCM in these individuals remains fraught, but it is estimated that up to 50% of phenotype-negative individuals with disease-causing variants in the sarcomere protein will develop clinical disease within 15 years [44]. Crucially, while some clinical features, such as ECG abnormalities, are predictive of subsequent phenotype development, age at screening is not, and the penetrance of sarcomeric disease is the same regardless of the age at which an individual is assessed.

There are multiple factors that may influence a family's or child's decision to undergo predictive genetic testing. Families may wish to be equipped with the knowledge of who is at a higher risk of HCM or who can be discharged. While not quantified, the family's experience with HCM to date may be a critical factor; severe disease in younger family members may serve as both a reason to test and a psychological deterrent to testing, for example, if there is a preference 'not to know'. Genetic testing may allow for timelier clinical cascade testing, identifying other at-risk individuals who would not previously have been screened. Family preference and societal and cultural norms around consent and parental responsibility may also play a part in determining at what age genetic testing is undertaken. Some families may feel a duty to allow a child to be old enough to 'choose' to have genetic testing, versus the desire or perceived benefit of having a genetic result prior to this age in the best interests of the child [45]. Some health systems only offer pre-implantation genetic diagnosis for HCM to couples where one member has HCM and they do not already have a previously 'unaffected' child [46]. In such instances, while ethically uncertain, this may also serve as a motivator to undertake genetic testing in childhood. Genetic testing in children has been shown, at least in the short term, not to be deleterious to a child's mental health [47–49].

3.2. Challenges and 'the Unknowns' in Familial Screening in Childhood for HCM

While there is now good evidence to support offering clinical and genetic screening to paediatric first-degree relatives of individuals with HCM, uncertainties still remain. Recent data in adult cohorts suggest that in patients with non-genetic HCM, the disease is less likely to be familial [50,51], but whether the same applies in paediatric HCM is unknown. Factors influencing the penetrance of any monogenic variant identified in childhood remain enigmatic. Although there are established monogenic contributions to disease, with mendelian inheritance, penetrance is variable; there are individuals who are identified to carry the familial causative ('pathogenic' or 'likely pathogenic') genetic variant who may never develop a clinical phenotype or only a mild clinical phenotype at a later age [52]. With associated genome-wide studies, the development of polygenic predictors continues to evolve [53]. Increasingly, the role of non-genetic factors as possible contributors to phenotypic expression is being better understood [54]. In adults, well-established risk factors associated with incident HCM include hypertension and obesity. Whether or not these play a role in childhood expression remains to be seen.

Further, in a study by Norrish et al., in those children in whom a childhood diagnosis of HCM was made as a result of family screening, the diagnosis was made during the first clinical visit in 56% of cases, suggesting that ongoing screening, in the context of age-related penetrance, is warranted. The frequency and nature of repeat clinical screenings remain to be determined. It has been shown that penetrance of sarcomeric variants is higher in the presence of an abnormal ECG at the initial screening visit, including in children [44], and more studies are needed to determine if there are additional predictors of subsequent phenotypic expression. Finally, while it is clear that childhood-onset familial HCM exists and that it is not necessarily a benign disease, warranting screening in childhood [36], as in other genetic cardiomyopathies, the survival benefit conferred by an earlier diagnosis needs to be studied systematically [43].

4. Conclusions and Future Directions

In the last decade, data from population-based studies and large international consortia of paediatric HCM have led to an improved understanding of its clinical presentation and natural history. With this has come a recognition that phenotypic expression can, and often does, occur in young children and that early diagnosis is possible with systematic clinical screening strategies. The age-old medical edict of 'first do no harm' must of course underpin the rationale for screening paediatric first-degree relatives of individuals with HCM, with the ultimate aim of identifying children with a potentially life-altering or threatening diagnosis earlier to allow intervention both for the individual and others who would then be identified as at risk through cascade testing. The delicate balance of this goal against the potential harms to individuals, families, and health systems needs to be considered. Current evidence suggests that, in the context of expert multidisciplinary services, clinical and genetic cascade screening should be offered to all children with a first-degree relative with HCM, regardless of their age. Ensuring equitable access to this multidisciplinary care, including genetic and psychological support for children and families affected by HCM, is paramount.

Funding: JPK is funded by a Medical Research Council (MRC) Clinical Academic Research Partnership (CARP) Award.

Conflicts of Interest: The authors declare no conflict of interest.

References

1. Arola, A.; Jokinen, E.; Ruuskanen, O.; Saraste, M.; Pesonen, E.; Kuusela, A.L.; Tikanoja, T.; Paavilainen, T.; Simell, O. Epidemiology of idiopathic cardiomyopathies in children and adolescents: A nationwide study in Finland. *Am. J. Epidemiol.* **1997**, *146*, 385–393. [CrossRef]
2. Lipshultz, S.E.; Sleeper, L.A.; Towbin, J.A.; Lowe, A.M.; Orav, E.J.; Cox, G.F.; Lurie, P.R.; McCoy, K.L.; McDonald, M.A.; Messere, J.E.; et al. The Incidence of Pediatric Cardiomyopathy in Two Regions of the United States. *N. Engl. J. Med.* **2003**, *348*, 1647–1655. [CrossRef] [PubMed]
3. Nugent, A.W.; Daubeney, P.E.; Chondros, P.; Carlin, J.B.; Cheung, M.; Wilkinson, L.C.; Davis, A.M.; Kahler, S.G.; Chow, C.W.; Wilkinson, J.L.; et al. The epidemiology of childhood cardiomyopathy in Australia. *N. Engl. J. Med.* **2003**, *348*, 1639–1646. [CrossRef] [PubMed]
4. Norrish, G.; Field, E.; Mcleod, K.; Ilina, M.; Stuart, G.; Bhole, V.; Uzun, O.; Brown, E.; Daubeney, P.E.F.; Lota, A.; et al. Clinical presentation and survival of childhood hypertrophic cardiomyopathy: A retrospective study in United Kingdom. *Eur. Heart J.* **2018**, *40*, 986–993. [CrossRef]
5. Alexander, P.M.A.; Nugent, A.W.; Daubeney, P.E.F.; Lee, K.J.; Sleeper, L.A.; Schuster, T.; Turner, C.; Davis, A.M.; Semsarian, C.; Colan, S.D.; et al. Long-Term Outcomes of Hypertrophic Cardiomyopathy Diagnosed During Childhood. *Circulation* **2018**, *138*, 29–36. [CrossRef] [PubMed]
6. Norrish, G.; Kolt, G.; Cervi, E.; Field, E.; Dady, K.; Ziółkowska, L.; Olivotto, I.; Favilli, S.; Passantino, S.; Limongelli, G.; et al. Clinical presentation and long-term outcomes of infantile hypertrophic cardiomyopathy: A European multicentre study. *ESC Heart Fail.* **2021**, *8*, 5057–5067. [CrossRef]
7. Norrish, G.; Cleary, A.; Field, E.; Cervi, E.; Boleti, O.; Ziółkowska, L.; Olivotto, I.; Khraiche, D.; Limongelli, G.; Anastasakis, A.; et al. Clinical Features and Natural History of Preadolescent Nonsyndromic Hypertrophic Cardiomyopathy. *J. Am. Coll. Cardiol.* **2022**, *79*, 1986–1997. [CrossRef]
8. Marston, N.A.-O.; Han, L.A.-O.; Olivotto, I.A.-O.; Day, S.A.-O.; Ashley, E.A.-O.; Michels, M.A.-O.; Pereira, A.C.; Ingles, J.A.-O.; Semsarian, C.; Jacoby, D.A.-O.X.; et al. Clinical characteristics and outcomes in childhood-onset hypertrophic cardiomyopathy. *Eur. Heart J.* **2021**, *42*, 1988–1996. [CrossRef]
9. Ho, C.Y.; Day, S.M.; Ashley, E.A.; Michels, M.; Pereira, A.C.; Jacoby, D.; Cirino, A.L.; Fox, J.C.; Lakdawala, N.K.; Ware, J.S.; et al. Genotype and Lifetime Burden of Disease in Hypertrophic Cardiomyopathy. *Circulation* **2018**, *138*, 1387–1398. [CrossRef]
10. van Capelle, C.I.; Poelman, E.; Frohn-Mulder, I.M.; Koopman, L.P.; van den Hout, J.M.P.; Régal, L.; Cools, B.; Helbing, W.A.; van der Ploeg, A.T. Cardiac outcome in classic infantile Pompe disease after 13 years of treatment with recombinant human acid alpha-glucosidase. *Int. J. Cardiol.* **2018**, *269*, 104–110. [CrossRef]
11. Andelfinger, G.; Marquis, C.; Raboisson, M.J.; Théoret, Y.; Waldmüller, S.; Wiegand, G.; Gelb, B.D.; Zenker, M.; Delrue, M.A.; Hofbeck, M. Hypertrophic Cardiomyopathy in Noonan Syndrome Treated by MEK-Inhibition. *J. Am. Coll. Cardiol.* **2019**, *73*, 2237–2239. [CrossRef]

12. Gross, A.M.; Frone, M.; Gripp, K.W.; Gelb, B.D.; Schoyer, L.; Schill, L.; Stronach, B.; Biesecker, L.G.; Esposito, D.; Hernandez, E.R.; et al. Advancing RAS/RASopathy therapies: An NCI-sponsored intramural and extramural collaboration for the study of RASopathies. *Am. J. Med. Genet. Part A* **2020**, *182*, 866–876. [CrossRef] [PubMed]
13. Maron, M.S.; Masri, A.; Choudhury, L.; Olivotto, I.; Saberi, S.; Wang, A.; Garcia-Pavia, P.; Lakdawala, N.K.; Nagueh, S.F.; Rader, F.; et al. Phase 2 Study of Aficamten in Patients With Obstructive Hypertrophic Cardiomyopathy. *J. Am. Coll. Cardiol.* **2023**, *81*, 34–45. [CrossRef]
14. Spertus, J.A.; Fine, J.T.; Elliott, P.; Ho, C.Y.; Olivotto, I.; Saberi, S.; Li, W.; Dolan, C.; Reaney, M.; Sehnert, A.J.; et al. Mavacamten for treatment of symptomatic obstructive hypertrophic cardiomyopathy (EXPLORER-HCM): Health status analysis of a randomised, double-blind, placebo-controlled, phase 3 trial. *Lancet* **2021**, *397*, 2467–2475. [CrossRef] [PubMed]
15. Desai, M.Y.; Owens, A.; Geske, J.B.; Wolski, K.; Naidu, S.S.; Smedira, N.G.; Cremer, P.C.; Schaff, H.; McErlean, E.; Sewell, C.; et al. Myosin Inhibition in Patients With Obstructive Hypertrophic Cardiomyopathy Referred for Septal Reduction Therapy. *J. Am. Coll. Cardiol.* **2022**, *80*, 95–108. [CrossRef] [PubMed]
16. Green, E.M.; Wakimoto, H.; Anderson, R.L.; Evanchik, M.J.; Gorham, J.M.; Harrison, B.C.; Henze, M.; Kawas, R.; Oslob, J.D.; Rodriguez, H.M.; et al. A small-molecule inhibitor of sarcomere contractility suppresses hypertrophic cardiomyopathy in mice. *Science* **2016**, *351*, 617–621. [CrossRef]
17. Ma, H.; Marti-Gutierrez, N.; Park, S.-W.; Wu, J.; Lee, Y.; Suzuki, K.; Koski, A.; Ji, D.; Hayama, T.; Ahmed, R.; et al. Correction of a pathogenic gene mutation in human embryos. *Nature* **2017**, *548*, 413–419. [CrossRef]
18. Dainis, A.; Zaleta-Rivera, K.; Ribeiro, A.; Chang, A.C.H.; Shang, C.; Lan, F.; Burridge, P.W.; Liu, W.R.; Wu, J.C.; Chang, A.C.Y.; et al. Silencing of MYH7 ameliorates disease phenotypes in human iPSC-cardiomyocytes. *Physiol. Genom.* **2020**, *52*, 293–303. [CrossRef]
19. Chai, A.A.-O.; Cui, M.; Chemello, F.A.-O.X.; Li, H.A.-O.; Chen, K.; Tan, W.; Atmanli, A.; McAnally, J.R.; Zhang, Y.A.-O.; Xu, L.A.-O.; et al. Base editing correction of hypertrophic cardiomyopathy in human cardiomyocytes and humanized mice. *Nat. Med.* **2023**, *29*, 401–411. [CrossRef]
20. Monda, E.; Rubino, M.; Lioncino, M.; Di Fraia, F.; Pacileo, R.; Verrillo, F.; Cirillo, A.; Caiazza, M.; Fusco, A.; Esposito, A.; et al. Hypertrophic Cardiomyopathy in Children: Pathophysiology, Diagnosis, and Treatment of Non-sarcomeric Causes. *Front. Pediatr.* **2021**, *9*, 632293. [CrossRef]
21. Ware, S.M.; Bhatnagar, S.; Dexheimer, P.J.; Wilkinson, J.D.; Sridhar, A.; Fan, X.; Shen, Y.; Tariq, M.; Schubert, J.A.; Colan, S.D.; et al. The genetic architecture of pediatric cardiomyopathy. *Am. J. Hum. Genet.* **2022**, *109*, 282–298. [CrossRef] [PubMed]
22. Kaski, J.P.; Syrris, P.; Esteban, M.T.T.; Jenkins, S.; Pantazis, A.; Deanfield, J.E.; McKenna, W.J.; Elliott, P.M. Prevalence of Sarcomere Protein Gene Mutations in Preadolescent Children With Hypertrophic Cardiomyopathy. *Circ. Cardiovasc. Genet.* **2009**, *2*, 436–441. [CrossRef] [PubMed]
23. Erdmann, J.; Moretti, A. *The Genetic Landscape of Cardiomyopathies*; Springer International Publishing AG: Cham, Switzerland, 2019; Volume 7, pp. 45–91.
24. Wilde, A.A.M.; Semsarian, C.; Márquez, M.F.; Sepehri Shamloo, A.; Ackerman, M.J.; Ashley, E.A.; Sternick Eduardo, B.; Barajas-Martinez, H.; Behr, E.R.; Bezzina, C.R.; et al. European Heart Rhythm Association (EHRA)/Heart Rhythm Society (HRS)/Asia Pacific Heart Rhythm Society (APHRS)/Latin American Heart Rhythm Society (LAHRS) Expert Consensus Statement on the state of genetic testing for cardiac diseases. *J. Arrhythmia* **2022**, *38*, 491–553. [CrossRef] [PubMed]
25. Valdés-Mas, R.; Gutiérrez-Fernández, A.; Gómez, J.; Coto, E.; Astudillo, A.; Puente, D.A.; Reguero, J.R.; Álvarez, V.; Morís, C.; León, D.; et al. Mutations in filamin C cause a new form of familial hypertrophic cardiomyopathy. *Nat. Commun.* **2014**, *5*, 5326. [CrossRef] [PubMed]
26. Gelb, B.D.; Roberts, A.E.; Tartaglia, M. Cardiomyopathies in Noonan syndrome and the other RASopathies. *Prog. Pediatr. Cardiol.* **2015**, *39*, 13–19. [CrossRef] [PubMed]
27. Porto, A.G.; Brun, F.; Severini, G.M.; Losurdo, P.; Fabris, E.; Taylor, M.R.G.; Mestroni, L.; Sinagra, G. Clinical Spectrum of PRKAG2 Syndrome. *Circ. Arrhythmia Electrophysiol.* **2016**, *9*, e003121. [CrossRef]
28. Arad, M.; Maron, B.J.; Gorham, J.M.; Johnson, W.H.; Saul, J.P.; Perez-Atayde, A.R.; Spirito, P.; Wright, G.B.; Kanter, R.J.; Seidman, J.G.; et al. Glycogen Storage Diseases Presenting as Hypertrophic Cardiomyopathy. *N. Engl. J. Med.* **2005**, *352*, 362–372. [CrossRef] [PubMed]
29. Finsterer, J. Barth syndrome: Mechanisms and management. *Appl. Clin. Genet.* **2019**, *12*, 95–106. [CrossRef]
30. Elliott, P.M.; Anastasakis, A.; Borger, M.A.; Borggrefe, M.; Cecchi, F.; Charron, P.; Hagege, A.A.; Lafont, A.; Limongelli, G.; Mahrholdt, H.; et al. 2014 ESC Guidelines on diagnosis and management of hypertrophic cardiomyopathy The Task Force for the Diagnosis and Management of Hypertrophic Cardiomyopathy of the European Society of Cardiology (ESC). *Eur. Heart J.* **2014**, *35*, 2733–2779. [CrossRef] [PubMed]
31. Gersh, B.J.; Maron, B.J.; Bonow, R.O.; Dearani, J.A.; Fifer, M.A.; Link, M.S.; Naidu, S.S.; Nishimura, R.A.; Ommen, S.R.; Rakowski, H.; et al. 2011 ACCF/AHA Guideline for the Diagnosis and Treatment of Hypertrophic Cardiomyopathy. *Circulation* **2011**, *124*, e783–e831. [CrossRef]
32. Maron, D.J. Clinical Course and Management of Hypertrophic Cardiomyopathy. *N. Engl. J. Med.* **2018**, *379*, 655–668. [CrossRef]
33. Maron, B.J.; Rowin, E.J.; Casey, S.A.; Maron, M.S. How Hypertrophic Cardiomyopathy Became a Contemporary Treatable Genetic Disease With Low Mortality: Shaped by 50 Years of Clinical Research and Practice. *JAMA Cardiol.* **2016**, *1*, 98–105. [CrossRef]
34. Maron, B.J.; Spirito, P.; Wesley, Y.; Arce, J. Development and Progression of Left Ventricular Hypertrophy in Children with Hypertrophic Cardiomyopathy. *N. Engl. J. Med.* **1986**, *315*, 610–614. [CrossRef]

35. Jensen, M.K.; Havndrup, O.; Christiansen, M.; Andersen, P.S.; Diness, B.; Axelsson, A.; Skovby, F.; KØBer, L.; Bundgaard, H. Penetrance of Hypertrophic Cardiomyopathy in Children and Adolescents: A 12-Year Follow-up Study of Clinical Screening and Predictive Genetic Testing. *Circulation* **2013**, *127*, 48–54. [CrossRef]
36. Norrish, G.; Jager, J.; Field, E.; Quinn, E.; Fell, H.; Lord, E.; Cicerchia, M.N.; Ochoa, J.P.; Cervi, E.; Elliott, P.M.; et al. Yield of Clinical Screening for Hypertrophic Cardiomyopathy in Child First-Degree Relatives. *Circulation* **2019**, *140*, 184–192. [CrossRef]
37. Lafreniere-Roula, M.; Bolkier, Y.; Zahavich, L.; Mathew, J.; George, K.; Wilson, J.; Stephenson, E.A.; Benson, L.N.; Manlhiot, C.; Mital, S. Family screening for hypertrophic cardiomyopathy: Is it time to change practice guidelines? *Eur. Heart J.* **2019**, *40*, 3672–3681. [CrossRef]
38. Page, S.P.; Kounas, S.; Syrris, P.; Christiansen, M.; Frank-Hansen, R.; Andersen, P.S.; Elliott, P.M.; McKenna, W.J. Cardiac myosin binding protein-C mutations in families with hypertrophic cardiomyopathy: Disease expression in relation to age, gender, and long term outcome. *Circ. Cardiovasc. Genet.* **2012**, *1*, 156–166. [CrossRef]
39. Field, E.A.-O.; Norrish, G.; Acquaah, V.; Dady, K.; Cicerchia, M.N.; Ochoa, J.P.; Syrris, P.; McLeod, K.; McGowan, R.; Fell, H.; et al. Cardiac myosin binding protein-C variants in paediatric-onset hypertrophic cardiomyopathy: Natural history and clinical outcomes. *J. Med. Genet.* **2022**, *59*, 768–775. [CrossRef]
40. Spanaki, A.; O'Curry, S.; Winter-Beatty, J.; Mead-Regan, S.; Hawkins, K.; English, J.; Head, C.; Ridout, D.; Tome-Esteban, M.T.; Elliott, P.; et al. Psychosocial adjustment and quality of life in children undergoing screening in a specialist paediatric hypertrophic cardiomyopathy clinic. *Cardiol. Young* **2016**, *26*, 961–967. [CrossRef]
41. Ommen, S.R.; Mital, S.; Burke, M.A.; Day, S.M.; Deswal, A.; Elliott, P.; Evanovich, L.L.; Hung, J.; Joglar, J.A.; Kantor, P.; et al. 2020 AHA/ACC Guideline for the Diagnosis and Treatment of Patients With Hypertrophic Cardiomyopathy. *Circulation* **2020**, *142*, e558–e631. [CrossRef]
42. Smedsrud, M.K.; Chivulescu, M.; Forså, M.I.; Castrini, I.; Aabel, E.W.; Rootwelt-Norberg, C.; Bogsrud, M.P.; Edvardsen, T.; Hasselberg, N.E.; Früh, A.; et al. Highly malignant disease in childhood-onset arrhythmogenic right ventricular cardiomyopathy. *Eur. Heart J.* **2022**, *43*, 4694–4703. [CrossRef]
43. Kaski, J.P. Arrhythmogenic cardiomyopathies in children: Seek and you shall find. *Eur. Heart J.* **2022**, *43*, 4704–4706. [CrossRef]
44. Lorenzini, M.; Norrish, G.; Field, E.; Ochoa, J.P.; Cicerchia, M.; Akhtar, M.M.; Syrris, P.; Lopes, L.R.; Kaski, J.P.; Elliott, P.M. Penetrance of Hypertrophic Cardiomyopathy in Sarcomere Protein Mutation Carriers. *J. Am. Coll. Cardiol.* **2020**, *76*, 550–559. [CrossRef]
45. Arbour, L.; Canadian Paediatric Society; Bioethics Committee. Guidelines for genetic testing of healthy children. *Paediatr. Child Health* **2003**, *8*, 42–45. [CrossRef]
46. NHS Commissioning Board. *Clinical Commissioning Policy: Pre-Implantation Genetic Diagnosis (PGD)*; NHS Commissioning Board: Leeds, UK, 2013.
47. Wakefield, C.E.; Hanlon, L.V.; Tucker, K.M.; Patenaude, A.F.; Signorelli, C.; McLoone, J.K.; Cohn, R.J. The psychological impact of genetic information on children: A systematic review. *Genet. Med.* **2016**, *18*, 755–762. [CrossRef]
48. Ingles, J.; Burns, C.; Barratt, A.; Semsarian, C. Application of Genetic Testing in Hypertrophic Cardiomyopathy for Preclinical Disease Detection. *Circ. Cardiovasc. Genet.* **2015**, *8*, 852–859. [CrossRef]
49. GradDipGenCouns, J.I.; Yeates, L.; O'Brien, L.; McGaughran, J.; Scuffham, P.A.; Atherton, J.; Semsarian, C. Genetic testing for inherited heart diseases: Longitudinal impact on health-related quality of life. *Genet. Med.* **2012**, *14*, 749–752. [CrossRef]
50. de Feria, A.E.; Kott, A.E.; Becker, J.R. Sarcomere mutation negative hypertrophic cardiomyopathy is associated with ageing and obesity. *Open Heart* **2021**, *8*, e001560. [CrossRef]
51. Ko, C.; Arscott, P.; Concannon, M.; Saberi, S.; Day, S.M.; Yashar, B.M.; Helms, A.S. Genetic testing impacts the utility of prospective familial screening in hypertrophic cardiomyopathy through identification of a nonfamilial subgroup. *Genet. Med.* **2018**, *20*, 69–75. [CrossRef]
52. Canepa, M.; Fumagalli, C.; Tini, G.; Vincent-Tompkins, J.; Day, S.M.; Ashley, E.A.; Mazzarotto, F.; Ware, J.S.; Michels, M.; Jacoby, D.; et al. Temporal Trend of Age at Diagnosis in Hypertrophic Cardiomyopathy: An Analysis of the International Sarcomeric Human Cardiomyopathy Registry. *Circ. Heart Fail.* **2020**, *13*, e007230. [CrossRef]
53. Tadros, R.A.-O.; Francis, C.; Xu, X.; Vermeer, A.M.C.; Harper, A.A.-O.; Huurman, R.A.-O.; Kelu Bisabu, K.A.-O.X.; Walsh, R.A.-O.; Hoorntje, E.T.; Te Rijdt, W.P.; et al. Shared genetic pathways contribute to risk of hypertrophic and dilated cardiomyopathies with opposite directions of effect. *Nat. Genet.* **2021**, *53*, 128–134. [CrossRef] [PubMed]
54. Biddinger, K.J.; Jurgens, S.J.; Maamari, D.; Gaziano, L.; Choi, S.H.; Morrill, V.N.; Halford, J.L.; Khera, A.V.; Lubitz, S.A.; Ellinor, P.T.; et al. Rare and Common Genetic Variation Underlying the Risk of Hypertrophic Cardiomyopathy in a National Biobank. *JAMA Cardiol.* **2022**, *7*, 715–722. [CrossRef] [PubMed]

Disclaimer/Publisher's Note: The statements, opinions and data contained in all publications are solely those of the individual author(s) and contributor(s) and not of MDPI and/or the editor(s). MDPI and/or the editor(s) disclaim responsibility for any injury to people or property resulting from any ideas, methods, instructions or products referred to in the content.

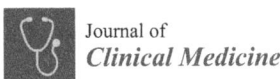

Review

Alcohol Septal Ablation in Patients with Hypertrophic Obstructive Cardiomyopathy: A Contemporary Perspective

Felice Gragnano [1,2,†], Francesco Pelliccia [3,†], Natale Guarnaccia [1,2], Giampaolo Niccoli [4], Salvatore De Rosa [5], Raffaele Piccolo [6], Elisabetta Moscarella [1,2], Enrico Fabris [7], Rocco Antonio Montone [8], Arturo Cesaro [1,2], Italo Porto [9], Ciro Indolfi [5,10], Gianfranco Sinagra [7], Pasquale Perrone Filardi [6], Giuseppe Andò [11] and Paolo Calabrò [1,2,*] on behalf of the Working Group of Interventional Cardiology of the Italian Society of Cardiology

1. Department of Translational Medical Sciences, University of Campania "Luigi Vanvitelli", 83043 Naples, Italy
2. Division of Clinical Cardiology, Azienda Ospedaliera di Rilievo Nazionale "Sant'Anna e San Sebastiano", 81100 Caserta, Italy
3. Department of Cardiovascular Sciences, University Sapienza, 00185 Rome, Italy
4. Department of Medicine and Surgery, University of Parma, 43121 Parma, Italy
5. Division of Cardiology, Department of Medical and Surgical Sciences, Magna Graecia University of Catanzaro, 88100 Catanzaro, Italy
6. Department of Advanced Biomedical Sciences, University of Naples Federico II, 80138 Naples, Italy
7. Cardiothoracovascular Department, Azienda Sanitaria Universitaria Giuliano Isontina (ASUGI), University of Trieste, 34127 Trieste, Italy
8. Department of Cardiovascular Medicine, Fondazione Policlinico Universitario A. Gemelli IRCCS, 00168 Rome, Italy
9. Dipartimento CardioToracoVascolare, Ospedale Policlinico San Martino IRCCS, 16132 Genova, Italy
10. Mediterranea Cardiocentro, 80122 Naples, Italy
11. Department of Clinical and Experimental Medicine, University of Messina, AOU Policlinic "G. Martino", 98122 Messina, Italy

* Correspondence: paolo.calabro@unicampania.it; Tel./Fax: +39-0823-232395
† These authors contributed equally to this work.

Abstract: Alcohol septal ablation is a minimally invasive procedure for the treatment of left ventricular outflow tract (LVOT) obstruction in patients with hypertrophic obstructive cardiomyopathy (HOCM) who remain symptomatic despite optimal medical therapy. The procedure causes a controlled myocardial infarction of the basal portion of the interventricular septum by the injection of absolute alcohol with the aim of reducing LVOT obstruction and improving the patient's hemodynamics and symptoms. Numerous observations have demonstrated the efficacy and safety of the procedure, making it a valid alternative to surgical myectomy. In particular, the success of alcohol septal ablation depends on appropriate patient selection and the experience of the institution where the procedure is performed. In this review, we summarize the current evidence on alcohol septal ablation and highlight the importance of a multidisciplinary approach involving a team of clinical and interventional cardiologists and cardiac surgeons with high expertise in the management of HOCM patients—the Cardiomyopathy Team.

Keywords: alcohol septal ablation; myectomy; hypertrophic cardiomyopathy

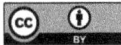

1. Introduction

Alcohol septal ablation is a minimally invasive procedure for treating left ventricular outflow tract obstruction (LVOTO) in patients with hypertrophic obstructive cardiomyopathy (HOCM) who are symptomatic despite optimal medical therapy. The intervention causes a controlled myocardial infarction of the basal portion of the interventricular septum by the injection of absolute alcohol to reduce LVOTO and improve the patient's hemodynamics and symptoms. Numerous studies have demonstrated the efficacy and safety of the procedure, which today represents a valid alternative to surgical myectomy. The success of alcohol septal ablation depends on patient selection and the experience of the operators and institution where it is performed. In this review, we provide an updated overview of available evidence on alcohol septal ablation, focusing on the importance of a multidisciplinary approach involving a team of clinical and interventional cardiologists and cardiac surgeons with high expertise in managing HOCM patients—the Cardiomyopathy Team.

Clinical Characteristics of Hypertrophic Cardiomyopathy

Hypertrophic cardiomyopathy (HCM) is a relatively common genetic cardiomyopathy characterized by increased left ventricular wall thickness that is not solely due to hemodynamic overload [1,2]. More than two decades ago, the CARDIA study estimated the prevalence of the disease in young adults to be around 1:500 [3]. More recently, advances in cardiac imaging and genetic testing have allowed the prevalence of HCM to be redefined to approximately 1:200 in contemporary cohorts [4]. Genetic transmission is mostly autosomal dominant and is caused by mutations in cardiac sarcomeric protein genes, with beta-myosin heavy chain (MYH) and myosin-binding protein C (MYBPC3) involved in 70% of cases. Other less common genes are also involved in the case of metabolic (i.e., Anderson–Fabry disease), mitochondrial, and infiltrative disorders (i.e., hereditary cardiac transthyretin-related amyloidosis) [2,5–7].

In daily practice, HCM is usually suspected when there is a family history of cardiomyopathy or sudden cardiac death (SCD). Commonly reported symptoms include angina, dyspnea, syncope, and palpitations, which may be due to the presence of left ventricular outflow tract obstruction (LVOTO), atrial fibrillation, ventricular arrhythmias, and heart failure [1,2,5,8]. The diagnosis is confirmed by imaging techniques such as echocardiography or cardiac magnetic resonance (CMR) that show left ventricular wall thickness $\geq$ 15 mm (or $\geq$13 in the case of a confirmed gene mutation or affected first-degree relatives) in any myocardial segment. Importantly, these techniques allow the assessment of the left ventricular hypertrophy morphology (i.e., asymmetric, mid-ventricular), LVOTO, concomitant valve disease, and degree of myocardial fibrosis (i.e., CMR with late gadolinium enhancement), which are key features in predicting the risk of SCD [1,9–11]. Noteworthy, although some patients with HCM remain long asymptomatic, a non-negligible proportion of cases may initially manifest with life-threatening arrhythmias and SCD, especially in athletes and the young. Therefore, a systematic assessment of multiple parameters (i.e., using the HCM Risk-SCD score) is crucial to predicting and preventing fatal arrhythmias [9].

2. Diagnostic and Therapeutic Work-Up in Patients with HCM and LVOTO

2.1. Pathophysiology

The presence of LVOTO is a hallmark of HCM manifestation and is a key element in the diagnosis and management of these patients. LVOTO occurs at rest in about 35% of patients with HCM; in approximately 30% of cases, the dynamic obstruction can be provoked during the Valsalva maneuver or exercise [12]. In patients with HOCM, the obstruction is primarily caused by the systolic anterior motion (SAM) of the mitral valve leaflets. This phenomenon is generally attributed to the Venturi effect and the reduction of the mitro-aortic angle and is considered severe when it occupies more than 30% of the systolic phase [1,2,13–15]. Another critical factor in the development of LVOTO is the presence of mitral valve and papillary muscle abnormalities (i.e., mitral leaflets elongation, abnormal chordal attachment, and anterior papillary muscle rotation/displacement) [1,16]. As the LVOTO is often dynamic, it may vary according to loading conditions, left ventricular contractility, and respiratory cycle. Therefore, these aspects should be considered in therapeutic decision-making [13,17,18].

2.2. Diagnosis

The diagnosis of HOCM is usually made by echocardiography and is defined in the presence of a peak LVOT gradient $\geq$ 30 mmHg measured by continuous Doppler (at rest or after the Valsalva maneuver). The LVOT gradient becomes hemodynamically relevant when its peak reaches ≥ 50 mmHg, identifying individuals who are candidates for invasive septal reduction therapies. Notably, when patients with a peak gradient ≤ 50 mmHg at rest present with suggestive symptoms, a physical stress echocardiography is indicated to identify a latent obstruction [1,2]. Pharmacological stress tests with dobutamine or nitrates are usually poorly tolerated and may not reproduce the true mechanism of obstruction; therefore, they are generally discouraged and reserved for selected cases [19,20]. The prognostic value of LVOTO remains controversial, considering that fatal events occur with similar incidence in patients with and without obstruction. Accordingly, whether the presence and the grade of obstruction should only be considered as a clinical/hemodynamic marker or as a prognostic factor remains controversial [21].

2.3. Therapeutic Work-Up

Medical therapy is the first-line treatment for patients with HOCM, with the goal of reducing obstruction and relieving symptoms. Non-vasodilating β-blockers (i.e., propranolol, nadolol, bisoprolol, and metoprolol) are the first choice. In case of intolerance, current guidelines recommend non-dihydropyridine calcium channel blockers (i.e., verapamil and diltiazem). In patients who are intolerant or poor-responders to these drugs, disopyramide should be considered because of its negative inotropic effect. Allosteric myosin inhibitors (i.e., mavacamten and aficamten) have recently been proposed as new therapeutic strategies in HOCM patients to prevent/delay the need for invasive treatment [1,2,22–25]. Specific to mavacamten, the first U.S. Food and Drug Administration (FDA)-approved medication targeting HCM, the EXPLORER-HCM (Clinical Study to Evaluate Mavacamten [MYK-461] in Adults With Symptomatic Obstructive Hypertrophic Cardiomyopathy) trial [26] and the VALOR-HCM (A Study to Evaluate Mavacamten in Adults With Symptomatic Obstructive HCM Who Are Eligible for Septal Reduction Therapy) trial [27] have shown that a significant proportion of HCM patients experience an improvement in clinical endpoints and quality-of-life measures. In a further subgroup of patients, mavacamten significantly reduced the fraction of patients meeting guideline criteria for septal reduction therapy after 16 weeks.

Septal reduction therapy has clearly shown to be effective in reducing LVOTO and should be considered in HOCM patients with LVOT gradient > 50 mmHg, moderate to severe symptoms and/or exertional syncope despite maximally tolerated medical therapy [1]. The septal reduction can be completed by either surgical myomectomy or percutaneous catheter-based intervention. The first percutaneous septal reduction treatment was performed with alcohol septal ablation. Subsequently, nonalcohol agents, including microspheres, have been proposed as an alternative to alcohol. More recently, radiofrequency ablation has been used for non-surgical septal reduction as it is both minimally invasive and independent of coronary anatomy. This novel technique uses echocardiography to guide the transapical placement of an intraseptal radiofrequency electrode that delivers energy to the core of the hypertrophic segment. The authors reported an impressive septal reduction of 11 mm with a resolution of LVOTO and improvements in functional class [28].

3. Alcohol Septal Ablation

3.1. Historical, Clinical, and Procedural Considerations

The concept of alcohol septal ablation in patients with HOCM was first introduced in the 1980s by Gunnar Berghöfer (March 1989, personal communication), based on several studies on the effects of temporary balloon occlusion of coronary arteries on myocardial wall motion and alcohol trans-coronary ablation of ventricular tachycardia [29,30]. In 1995, a German cardiologist, Ulrich Sigwart, first described three cases of HOCM patients who were persistently symptomatic despite optimal medical therapy and were treated with alcohol septal ablation. All patients had a complete resolution of the LVOTO and regression of symptoms from the day after the procedure, showing the potential of this strategy [31].

Current European and American guidelines recommend the use of alcohol septal ablation in patients who remain symptomatic on maximally tolerated medical therapy (i.e., New York

Heart Association [NYHA] class III-IV), with evidence of an LVOT gradient > 50 mmHg and established contraindications to surgery [1,2]. The procedure consists of the injection of a small amount of absolute alcohol into the septal arteries to induce iatrogenic myocardial infarction selectively localized in the basal part of the interventricular septum. Despite the lack of large-scale randomized trials, numerous observational studies in recent decades have provided sufficient evidence to support the use of this strategy as a viable alternative to surgical myectomy, with the advantage of a shorter hospital stay and rapid discharge [1].

The first steps in evaluating symptomatic HOCM patients who are candidates for alcohol septal ablation are careful medical history collection and clinical examination to exclude other conditions that may act as possible confounders (i.e., coronary artery disease, respiratory disease, and anemia). Among demographic factors, age should be considered in the decision-making: although there is no specific age cut-off in current guidelines, alcohol septal ablation is generally not the preferred strategy in children and young adults, given the higher rate of LVOTO recurrence and a lack of long-term data on clinical outcomes [1,32–34]. Other important elements are represented by comorbidities and patient frailty, which may contraindicate surgery in favor of a less invasive approach. The presence of other surgical indications (coronary artery disease and valvular heart disease) also favors surgical myectomy, whereas the history of cardiac surgery favors alcohol septal ablation. The baseline ECG should also be considered as both surgical and non-surgical interventions can be complicated by rhythm disturbances, including complete atrioventricular block. Because the infarct is located near the right bundle branch, the development of a right bundle branch block is common after alcohol septal ablation. Therefore, this procedure is not recommended in the case of pre-existing left bundle branch block (unless a pacemaker has been previously implanted). On the other hand, as surgical myectomy can be associated with the development of a left bundle branch block, alcohol septal ablation is favored in patients with pre-existing right bundle branch block [35–37]. Finally, comprehensive morphological and angiographic assessment by cardiac ultrasound, CMR, CT-angiography, and/or invasive coronary angiography is essential to assess whether the patient can successfully undergo the procedure.

3.2. Pre-Procedural Anatomic Evaluation

Left ventricular and mitral valve anatomy should be carefully assessed before the intervention. Imaging assessment includes LVOT geometry, extent and distribution of myocardial hypertrophy and fibrosis, septal morphology, and mitral valvular and subvalvular anatomy, all crucial in predicting procedural success. In this context, CMR provides high-resolution images and should be used routinely in the pre-procedural anatomic assessment of patients undergoing an invasive treatment for HOCM [38]. Abnormalities of the mitral valve apparatus and papillary muscles can significantly reduce the procedural success of alcohol septal ablation and should be excluded by comprehensive imaging assessment. Conversely, the procedure can be performed in case of posterior mitral regurgitation secondary to systolic anterior motion of the anterior mitral leaflet. The presence of a focal *septal bulge*, a wide angle of the papillary muscles, and chords to the ventricular septum also favor alcohol septal ablation, whereas midventricular hypertrophy leans toward surgical myectomy. A septal thickness of ≥ 17 mm is a widely accepted cut-off to safely perform alcohol septal ablation and minimize the risk of an iatrogenic ventricular septal defect [1,16]. However, the procedure may be suboptimal in the case of severe hypertrophy (>25 mm), possibly because of the need for high-dose alcohol infusion and the subsequent increased risk of complications. Furthermore, high LVOT gradient (>100 mmHg), large left atrial diameter (>40 mm), and low center experience (less than 50 patients) are additional predictors of poor post-procedural outcomes [35,39,40].

The key to successful alcohol septal ablation is suitable coronary anatomy and the correct selection of the septal branches. The diameter of the left anterior descending artery (LAD) has been reported to be an independent predictor of successful ablation, with a smaller vessel being associated with a higher likelihood of success [40]. The first septal branch often perfuses the basal septum (which is commonly involved in LVOTO) and is often the target vessel for ablation. This vessel usually originates from the LAD and runs close to the His bundle and right bundle branch, although, in 15% of cases, it may originate from other arteries such as the diagonal, the ramus intermedius, the left main, or even from the right coronary artery [41–44]. The complex anatomical variability mandates a careful and systematic assessment of the coronary tree for a safe procedure. The most appropriate coronary anatomy consists of a single septal perforator of adequate size supplying the target area. In the case of multiple septal branches supplying the hypertrophic basal septum, all should be ablated during the index or in staged procedures, if necessary. Yet, in 10–15% of patients, a culprit septal branch for ablation cannot be identified, forcing the operator to abandon the procedure [41,45]. Importantly, septal branches may supply other myocardial segments, such as the free walls of the left and right ventricles or papillary muscles. This condition is an absolute contraindication to alcohol injection because of the risk of potentially life-threatening complications such as extensive myocardial infarction. Intracoronary contrast echocardiography performed during the procedure is recommended in all patients undergoing ASA to ensure the size and the localization of iatrogenic myocardial infarct, prevent adverse events, and assess procedural success [36].

3.3. Description of the Procedure

Alcohol septal ablation consists of selective infusion of 95–96% absolute alcohol into the septal perforator branch supplying the left ventricular side of the basal or mid cavitary septum [43,46]. The rationale is to create an alcohol-induced occlusion of the vessel, with a controlled infarct in the basal septum that progressively changes from viable hypertrophic myocardium to a thin akinetic scar, thus reducing LVOTO. Radial and femoral access are both feasible, and the choice mainly depends on operator preference. In fact, the two approaches show similar short- and long-term success rates, although the radial approach has been associated with fewer vascular complications [47]. The main steps of the procedure are shown in Figure 1. After placement of a 6–7 Fr arterial sheath and temporary pacemaker via the femoral or internal jugular vein, analgesics (i.e., morphine) can be administered to control pain caused by alcohol injection and iatrogenic infarction. Coronary angiography is then performed to select the septal branch for ethanol infusion and to assess vessel anatomy, origin, angulation, and size. The course of septal vessels can be appropriately visualized using the right anterior oblique or postero-anterior cranial projections, while the left anterior oblique view allows differentiation of whether the septal branches run along the right or left side of the septum (the selection of left-sided branches reduces the risk of an atrioventricular block) [43,46].

After engaging the left main with a guide catheter providing extra support, a short over-the-wire (OTW) (1.5–2.5 mm in diameter, 6–10 mm long, with a balloon-to-artery ratio of approximately 1.3:1) is passed over a standard 180 cm 0.014″ extra support wire and positioned in the target vessel. OTW balloons are recommended as they allow selective septal branch angiography during balloon inflation (1–2 mL of contrast slowly injected into the proximally occluded vessel) to verify the correct positioning, complete septal occlusion, and absence of contrast reflux into the LAD. During balloon inflation, continuous invasive monitoring may reveal a reduction in LVOT pressure gradient, indicating a good target vessel for ablation [44]. Due to the high degree of collateralization between the left and right coronary arteries, it is imperative to exclude the filling of other coronary arteries by septal collaterals prior to alcohol injection [48]. The target vessel must then be tested using myocardial contrast echocardiography (Figure 2): 1–2 mL of contrast medium should be injected through the OTW balloon to visualize the target area at the basal septum, adjacent to the point of mitral-septal contact, and to rule out contrast enhancement in other regions (i.e., inferior wall, papillary muscles, and right ventricle), which is an absolute contraindication to ethanol infusion and requires interruption of the procedure [49]. In more challenging cases, intracardiac or 3D contrast echocardiography may be helpful for intraprocedural guidance [50]. The operator can then inject ethanol over 1 to 5 min [1]. The amount of alcohol is about 0.7–1 mL per 10 mm of measured septal thickness [51]. During ethanol infusion, the inflated balloon must be firmly placed to completely occlude the vessel and avoid extensive myocardial damage due to reverse flow in the LAD or other coronary vessels [50]. The aggressive injection is discouraged as ethanol may pass through collaterals and cause inferior wall injury. Finally, analgesic infusion (i.e., morphine) is recommended immediately before alcohol infusion to control the pain caused by the alcohol injection and the provoked ischemia. The final coronary angiography should be performed about 20 min after alcohol infusion to exclude possible complications and conclude the procedure.

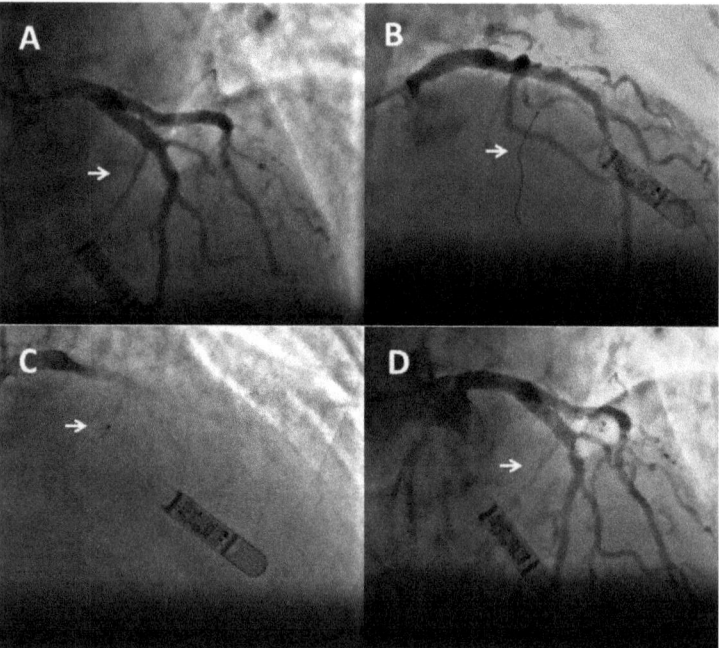

Figure 1. Angiographic sequence of alcohol septal ablation. (**A**) Baseline angiogram of the left coronary artery with estimated target septal branch (arrow). (**B**) Wiring of the target septal branch (arrow). (**C**) Injection of angiographic contrast media through the lumen of the over-the-wire balloon (arrow). (**D**) Occlusion of the distal portion of the septal branch (arrow) after balloon retraction 10 min after the last alcohol injection without damage to the left anterior descending artery.

3.4. How to Assess Procedural Success?

The goal of alcohol septal ablation is to achieve a significant and sustained improvement in symptoms and to reduce LVOT gradient by >50%. Additional beneficial effects include a reduction in mitral regurgitation and left ventricular end-diastolic pressure, which results in a lower incidence of atrial fibrillation and an improvement in pulmonary hypertension [36,52]. Favorable cardiac remodeling is also an important effect of the procedure, particularly in young patients, and may be clinically evident after 12 months [33,53]. Among possible predictors of procedural failure, a total creatine kinase (CK) peak less than 1300 U/L and an immediate residual LVOT gradient greater than 25 mm Hg have been reported in previous studies, although their association with long-term clinical outcomes remains uncertain and requires further investigations [37,54–57]. To date, there is no standardized follow-up pathway after alcohol septal ablation; therefore, the follow-up schedule usually depends on the center's experience. In the case of an uncomplicated post-procedural course, hospital discharge is usually 3–5 days after ablation [58]. After discharge, the patient should preferably be evaluated at one month, three months, and one year to assess changes in LVOT gradient. Notably, while some patients experience "monophasic" success (≥50% gradient reduction at three days and three months), in some cases, "triphasic" success can be observed (<50% gradient reduction at three days but ≥50% gradient reduction at three months or later) [59]. Therefore, serial evaluations should be performed to monitor the short- and long-term evolution of hemodynamic changes after the procedure.

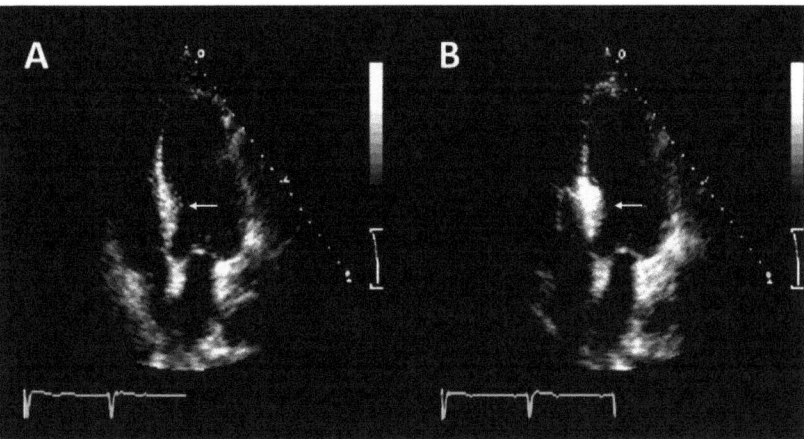

Figure 2. Echocardiographic contrast used for the guidance of alcohol septal. (**A**) Four-chamber echocardiogram shows increased LV wall thickness at basal septum level with no apical aneurysm (arrow). (**B**) Intracoronary echocardiographic contrast injection is localized to the basal septum at the site of greatest hypertrophy (arrow) without extending beyond the point of mitral septal contact, consistent with an appropriate target vessel for alcohol septal ablation.

Numerous studies have shown that approximately 90% of patients undergoing a successful procedure experience an improvement of functional status (i.e., post-procedural NYHA class I-II), and in 80% of cases, there is a significant reduction in LVOTO [53]. CMR can be used during the follow-up to quantify the size and location of the iatrogenic infarct. The use of CMR is also helpful in the case of procedural failure to evaluate the reasons for unsuccess (i.e., the iatrogenic infarct is too small or outside the target area) [60]. In the event of failure, surgical myectomy may be performed as a rescue strategy. Of note, several studies have reported on patients with a previous alcohol septal ablation undergoing surgical myectomy, showing that these patients have a higher risk of complete atrioventricular block and progression to heart failure because of the more extensive conduction system and myocardial injury [60–62].

3.5. Procedural Safety and Possible Complications

A complete atrioventricular block is the most common complication after alcohol septal ablation (transient in about 30% of patients and permanent in about 10%) and is due to the alcoholic injury to the conduction system [36,53]. This adverse event may occur during the procedure or in the first few days after and is more frequent in older patients or those with preexistent conduction disorders [33]. In patients with pre-existing left bundle branch block, a temporary pacemaker could be placed after the procedure, while a permanent pacemaker is indicated if an advanced block persists for more than 24–72 h [43,46]. If a concomitant indication for an implantable cardiac defibrillator exists, device implantation should precede the procedure to simplify the management of post-procedural arrhythmias. Infarction of the left and right ventricle-free walls or papillary muscles is a possible but rare adverse event related to the presence of collateral branches supplying distant myocardial areas and to the reflow of alcohol in the LAD artery. Although there have been concerns in the past about the arrhythmic risk associated with the septal scar, recent studies have demonstrated the long-term safety of the procedure, with a survival rate similar to surgical myectomy [52,63]. The rate of early mortality (up to 30 days) is relatively low and approximates 1.5%. Causes of death include LAD dissection, ventricular fibrillation, cardiac tamponade, cardiogenic shock, and pulmonary embolism. Late mortality is reported in 0.5% of patients and is often due to SCD, heart failure, pulmonary embolism, or other non-cardiac causes [36].

Alternative techniques have been explored to minimize the risks associated with the potential spillover of alcohol outside the target area, including various embolization techniques [64–67]. The most promising is the use of (n-butyl cyanoacrylate), a clear and colorless monomer that polymerizes rapidly on contact with blood [68]. Initial clinical experience with cyanoacrylate for septal ablation in HOCM patients showed an excellent safety profile, paving the way for long-term efficacy studies [69]. In addition, several catheter-based procedures, including the PIMSRA (percutaneous intramyocardial septal radiofrequency ablation) and the SESAME (septal scoring along the midline endocardium), have recently been tested in patients ineligible for surgery and alcohol septal ablation with encouraging results [70,71]. However, these procedures are currently performed in a limited number of centers in the US, Europe and Asia, and further prospective data are needed to safely introduce such novel strategies into practice.

3.6. Comparison between Alcohol Septal Ablation and other Surgical Reduction Therapies

Despite extensive research, the choice of the best option for septal reduction strategy in the individual patient remains challenging and poses numerous clinical dilemmas. To date, there is no current or completed randomized trial comparing surgical myectomy vs. alcohol septal ablation, and all available information is derived from retrospective investigations. Overall, the benefits of alcohol septal ablation are comparable to those seen with surgical myectomy in terms of functional class, exercise capacity, and LVOTO regression. Morbidity and mortality resemble those of surgical intervention. The major complication of alcohol septal ablation compared with surgery is a complete atrioventricular block requiring pacemaker implantation and the need for a re-do procedure. At variance with surgery, there are poor data on the comparison between alcohol septal ablation and other catheter-based interventions or the novel pharmacologic therapy with allosteric myosin inhibitors.

The lack of randomized evidence affects existing recommendations which are primarily based on observational findings and expert consensus. European and American guidelines do not provide class I recommendations for any of the invasive options [1,2] and the choice in the individual patient is largely determined by clinical judgement, local expertise, and patient preference. Specifically, the 2014 European guidelines are not in favor of any procedure but highlight that alcohol septal ablation is controversial in children, adolescents, and young adults for the absence of data on the long-term effects of a myocardial scar in these groups [1]. Conversely, the 2020 American guidelines for the diagnosis and treatment of HOCM state that myectomy should be preferred over alcohol septal ablation [2]. However, they recommend the latter procedure—when feasible and performed in experienced centers—in adult patients with symptomatic HOCM in whom surgery is contraindicated or risk is considered unacceptably high because of serious comorbidities or advanced age.

4. Multidisciplinary Evaluation and Management: The HCM Heart Team

The choice of the optimal septal reduction strategy (i.e., surgical vs. non-surgical) is crucial in the management of HOCM and should be the result of a comprehensive and personalized evaluation, as the success of the intervention depends on the patient's characteristics and center expertise. To date, procedural success and long-term survival are comparable between alcohol septal ablation and surgical myectomy when patients are carefully selected, and the procedures are performed in high-volume centers [72,73]. Importantly, the risks and benefits of both procedures should always be discussed with patients in order to match their expectations and preferences [1].

Given the complexity of clinical and anatomical factors that characterize both surgical and non-surgical strategies, it is crucial that the final decision is made by an experienced team working in centers of excellence for the management of HOCM [14,74]. In analogy with the "Heart Team" approach that is the current standard of care for patients with coronary and valvular heart disease [75–78], the "Cardiomyopathy Team" should represent the standard approach for the management of patients with HOCM. This team should include at least a clinical cardiologist, an interventional cardiologist, and a cardiac surgeon with documented expertise in the treatment of HOCM patients [14,74]. Specifically, the operators should have high experience with a minimum caseload of 10 alcohol septal ablations or surgical myectomies per year, as recommended by current guidelines [1,2]. This concept is supported by the evidence that highly experienced operators/institutions have a lower incidence of complications, a higher success rate, and a lower rate of re-intervention [79]. To date, further studies are needed to define better the role of the Cardiomyopathy Team in clinical practice and inform international guideline recommendations in this regard.

5. Conclusions

Alcohol septal ablation is a minimally invasive procedure for treating patients with HOCM who remain symptomatic despite optimal medical therapy. Available evidence supports the use of this procedure as a valid alternative to surgical myectomy when performed in high-volume centers. The appropriate patient selection remains critical in the decision-making process to maximize procedural success and minimize the risk of complications. Today, a precise and multidisciplinary assessment by the Cardiomyopathy Team appears to be crucial to improving the management and prognosis of patients with HOCM in daily practice.

Funding: This research received no external funding.

Informed Consent Statement: Not applicable.

Data Availability Statement: Not applicable.

Conflicts of Interest: The authors declare no conflict of interest.

References

1. Elliott, P.M.; Anastasakis, A.; Borger, M.A.; Borggrefe, M.; Cecchi, F.; Charron, P.; Hagege, A.A.; Lafont, A.; Limongelli, G.; Mahrholdt, H.; et al. 2014 ESC Guidelines on diagnosis and management of hypertrophic cardiomyopathy: The Task Force for the Diagnosis and Management of Hypertrophic Cardiomyopathy of the European Society of Cardiology (ESC). *Eur. Heart J.* **2014**, *35*, 2733–2779. [PubMed]
2. Ommen, S.R.; Mital, S.; Burke, M.A.; Day, S.M.; Deswal, A.; Elliott, P.; Evanovich, L.L.; Hung, J.; Joglar, J.A.; Kantor, P.; et al. 2020 AHA/ACC Guideline for the Diagnosis and Treatment of Patients with Hypertrophic Cardiomyopathy: Executive Summary: A Report of the American College of Cardiology/American Heart Association Joint Committee on Clinical Practice Guidelines. *Circulation* **2020**, *142*, e533–e557.
3. Maron, B.J.; Gardin, J.M.; Flack, J.M.; Gidding, S.S.; Kurosaki, T.T.; Bild, D.E. Prevalence of hypertrophic cardiomyopathy in a general population of young adults. Echocardiographic analysis of 4111 subjects in the CARDIA Study. Coronary Artery Risk Development in (Young) Adults. *Circulation* **1995**, *92*, 785–789. [CrossRef]
4. Semsarian, C.; Ingles, J.; Maron, M.S.; Maron, B.J. New Perspectives on the Prevalence of Hypertrophic Cardiomyopathy. *J. Am. Coll. Cardiol.* **2015**, *65*, 1249–1254. [CrossRef] [PubMed]
5. Limongelli, G.; Adorisio, R.; Baggio, C.; Bauce, B.; Biagini, E.; Castelletti, S.; Favilli, S.; Imazio, M.; Lioncino, M.; Merlo, M.; et al. Diagnosis and Management of Rare Cardiomyopathies in Adult and Paediatric Patients. A Position Paper of the Italian Society of Cardiology (SIC) and Italian Society of Paediatric Cardiology (SICP). *Int. J. Cardiol.* **2022**, *357*, 55–71. [CrossRef]
6. Monda, E.; Lioncino, M.; Rubino, M.; Passantino, S.; Verrillo, F.; Caiazza, M.; Cirillo, A.; Fusco, A.; Di Fraia, F.; Fimiani, F.; et al. Diagnosis and Management of Cardiovascular Involvement in Friedreich Ataxia. *Heart Fail Clin.* **2022**, *18*, 31–37. [CrossRef] [PubMed]

7. Rubino, M.; Monda, E.; Lioncino, M.; Caiazza, M.; Palmiero, G.; Dongiglio, F.; Fusco, A.; Cirillo, A.; Cesaro, A.; Capodicasa, L.; et al. Diagnosis and Management of Cardiovascular Involvement in Fabry Disease. *Heart Fail Clin.* **2022**, *18*, 39–49. [CrossRef] [PubMed]
8. Monda, E.; Limongelli, G. The hospitalizations in hypertrophic cardiomyopathy: "The dark side of the moon". *Int. J. Cardiol.* **2020**, *318*, 101–102. [CrossRef]
9. O'Mahony, C.; Jichi, F.; Pavlou, M.; Monserrat, L.; Anastasakis, A.; Rapezzi, C.; Biagini, E.; Gimeno, J.R.; Limongelli, G.; McKenna, W.J.; et al. A novel clinical risk prediction model for sudden cardiac death in hypertrophic cardiomyopathy (HCM risk-SCD). *Eur. Heart J.* **2014**, *35*, 2010–2020. [CrossRef]
10. Weng, Z.; Yao, J.; Chan, R.H.; He, J.; Yang, X.; Zhou, Y.; He, Y. Prognostic Value of LGE-CMR in HCM: A Meta-Analysis. *JACC Cardiovasc. Imaging* **2016**, *9*, 1392–1402. [CrossRef]
11. Rowin, E.J.; Maron, M.S. The role of cardiac MRI in the diagnosis and risk stratification of hypertrophic cardiomyopathy. *Arrhythm. Electrophysiol. Rev.* **2016**, *5*, 197–202. [CrossRef] [PubMed]
12. Maron, M.S.; Olivotto, I.; Zenovich, A.G.; Link, M.S.; Pandian, N.G.; Kuvin, J.T.; Nistri, S.; Cecchi, F.; Udelson, J.E.; Maron, B.J. Hypertrophic cardiomyopathy is predominantly a disease of left ventricular outflow tract obstruction. *Circulation* **2006**, *114*, 2232–2239. [CrossRef] [PubMed]
13. Maron, B.J. Clinical Course and Management of Hypertrophic Cardiomyopathy. *N. Engl. J. Med.* **2018**, *379*, 1977. [CrossRef] [PubMed]
14. Pelliccia, F.; Alfieri, O.; Calabrò, P.; Cecchi, F.; Ferrazzi, P.; Gragnano, F.; Kaski, J.P.; Limongelli, G.; Maron, M.; Rapezzi, C.; et al. Multidisciplinary evaluation and management of obstructive hypertrophic cardiomyopathy in 2020: Towards the HCM Heart Team. *Int. J. Cardiol.* **2020**, *304*, 86–92. [CrossRef]
15. Charls, L.M. SAM-systolic anterior motion of the anterior mitral valve leaflet post-surgical mitral valve repair. *Heart Lung* **2003**, *32*, 402–406. [CrossRef]
16. Patel, P.; Dhillon, A.; Popovic, Z.B.; Smedira, N.G.; Rizzo, J.; Thamilarasan, M.; Agler, D.; Lytle, B.W.; Lever, H.M.; Desai, M.Y. Left Ventricular Outflow Tract Obstruction in Hypertrophic Cardiomyopathy Patients without Severe Septal Hypertrophy: Implications of Mitral Valve and Papillary Muscle Abnormalities Assessed Using Cardiac Magnetic Resonance and Echocardiography. *Circ. Cardiovasc. Imaging* **2015**, *8*, e003132. [CrossRef]
17. Geske, J.B.; Sorajja, P.; Ommen, S.R.; Nishimura, R.A. Variability of left ventricular outflow tract gradient during cardiac catheterization in patients with hypertrophic cardiomyopathy. *JACC Cardiovasc. Interv.* **2011**, *4*, 704–709. [CrossRef]
18. Jain, R.; Osranek, M.; Jan, M.F.; Kalvin, L.R.; Olet, S.; Allaqaband, S.Q.; Jahangir, A.; Khandheria, B.K.; Tajik, A.J. Marked respiratory-related fluctuations in left ventricular outflow tract gradients in hypertrophic obstructive cardiomyopathy: An observational study. *Eur. Heart J. Cardiovasc. Imaging* **2018**, *19*, 1126–1133. [CrossRef]
19. Pellikka, P.A.; Oh, J.K.; Bailey, K.R.; Nichols, B.A.; Monahan, K.H.; Tajik, A.J. Dynamic intraventricular obstruction during dobutamine stress echocardiography. A new observation. *Circulation* **1992**, *86*, 1429–1432. [CrossRef]
20. Marwick, T.H.; Nakatani, S.; Haluska, B.; Thomas, J.D.; Lever, H.M. Provocation of latent left ventricular outflow gradients with amyl nitrite and exercise in hypertrophic cardiomyopathy. *Am. J. Cardiol.* **1995**, *75*, 805–809. [CrossRef]
21. Pelliccia, F.; Pasceri, V.; Limongelli, G.; Autore, C.; Basso, C.; Corrado, D.; Imazio, M.; Rapezzi, C.; Sinagra, G.; Mercuro, G.; et al. Long-term outcome of nonobstructive versus obstructive hypertrophic cardiomyopathy: A systematic review and meta-analysis. *Int. J. Cardiol.* **2017**, *243*, 379–384. [CrossRef] [PubMed]
22. Iavarone, M.; Monda, E.; Vritz, O.; Calila Albert, D.; Rubino, M.; Verrillo, F.; Caiazza, M.; Lioncino, M.; Amodio, F.; Guarnaccia, N.; et al. Medical treatment of patients with hypertrophic cardiomyopathy: An overview of current and emerging therapy. *Arch. Cardiovasc. Dis.* **2022**, *115*, 529–537. [CrossRef]
23. Borlaug, B.A.; Omote, K. Beta-Blockers and Exercise Hemodynamics in Hypertrophic Cardiomyopathy. *J. Am. Coll. Cardiol.* **2022**, *79*, 1576–1578. [CrossRef]
24. Ammirati, E.; Contri, R.; Coppini, R.; Cecchi, F.; Frigerio, M.; Olivotto, I. Pharmacological treatment of hypertrophic cardiomyopathy: Current practice and novel perspectives. *Eur. J. Heart Fail.* **2016**, *18*, 1106–1118. [CrossRef] [PubMed]
25. Maron, B.J.; Desai, M.Y.; Nishimura, R.A.; Spirito, P.; Rakowski, H.; Towbin, J.A.; Dearani, J.A.; Rowin, E.J.; Maron, M.S.; Sherrid, M.V. Management of Hypertrophic Cardiomyopathy: JACC State-of-the-Art Review. *J. Am. Coll. Cardiol.* **2022**, *79*, 390–414. [CrossRef]
26. Olivotto, I.; Oreziak, A.; Barriales-Villa, R.; Abraham, T.P.; Masri, A.; Garcia-Pavia, P.; Saberi, S.; Lakdawala, N.K.; Wheeler, M.T.; Owens, A.; et al. Mavacamten for treatment of symptomatic obstructive hypertrophic cardiomyopathy (EXPLORER-HCM): A randomised, double-blind, placebo-controlled, phase 3 trial. *Lancet* **2020**, *396*, 759–769. [CrossRef] [PubMed]
27. Desai, M.Y.; Owens, A.; Geske, J.B.; Wolski, K.; Naidu, S.S.; Smedira, N.G.; Cremer, P.C.; Schaff, H.; McErlean, E.; Sewell, C.; et al. Myosin Inhibition in Patients with Obstructive Hypertrophic Cardiomyopathy Referred for Septal Reduction Therapy. *J. Am. Coll. Cardiol.* **2022**, *80*, 95–108. [CrossRef]
28. Liu, L.; Li, J.; Zuo, L.; Zhang, J.; Zhou, M.; Xu, B.; Hahn, R.T.; Leon, M.B.; Hsi, D.H.; Ge, J.; et al. Percutaneous intramyocardial septal radiofrequency ablation for hypertrophic obstructive cardiomyopathy. *J. Am. Coll. Cardiol.* **2018**, *72*, 1898–1909. [CrossRef]
29. Brugada, P.; de Swart, H.; Smeets, J.L.; Wellens, H.J. Transcoronary chemical ablation of ventricular tachycardia. *Circulation* **1989**, *79*, 475–482. [CrossRef] [PubMed]

30. Sigwart, U.; Grbic, M.; Essinger, A.; Bischof-Delaloye, A.; Sadeghi, H.; Rivier, J.L. Improvement of left ventricular function after percutaneous transluminal coronary angioplasty. *Am. J. Cardiol.* **1982**, *49*, 651–657. [CrossRef]
31. Sigwart, U. Non-surgical myocardial reduction for hypertrophic obstructive cardiomyopathy. *Lancet* **1995**, *346*, 211–214. [CrossRef] [PubMed]
32. Lawin, D.; Lawrenz, T.; Radke, K.; Stellbrink, C. Safety and efficacy of alcohol septal ablation in adolescents and young adults with hypertrophic obstructive cardiomyopathy. *Clin. Res. Cardiol.* **2022**, *111*, 207–217. [CrossRef]
33. Batzner, A.; Aicha, D.; Pfeiffer, B.; Neugebauer, A.; Seggewiss, H. Age-related survival after alcohol septal ablation in hypertrophic obstructive cardiomyopathy. *ESC Heart Fail.* **2022**, *9*, 327–336. [CrossRef] [PubMed]
34. Liebregts, M.; Faber, L.; Jensen, M.K.; Vriesendorp, P.A.; Januska, J.; Krejci, J.; Hansen, P.R.; Seggewiss, H.; Horstkotte, D.; Adlova, R.; et al. Outcomes of Alcohol Septal Ablation in Younger Patients with Obstructive Hypertrophic Cardiomyopathy. *JACC Cardiovasc. Interv.* **2017**, *10*, 1134–1143. [CrossRef] [PubMed]
35. Yuan, J.; Qiao, S.; Zhang, Y.; You, S.; Duan, F.; Hu, F.; Yang, W. Follow-up by cardiac magnetic resonance imaging in patients with hypertrophic cardiomyopathy who underwent percutaneous ventricular septal ablation. *Am. J. Cardiol.* **2010**, *106*, 1487–1491. [CrossRef]
36. Achim, A.; Serban, A.M.; Mot, S.D.C.; Leibundgut, G.; Marc, M.; Sigwart, U. Alcohol septal ablation in hypertrophic cardiomyopathy: For which patients? *ESC Heart Fail.* **2023**. [CrossRef]
37. Veselka, J.; Jensen, M.K.; Liebregts, M.; Januska, J.; Krejci, J.; Bartel, T.; Dabrowski, M.; Hansen, P.R.; Almaas, V.M.; Seggewiss, H.; et al. Long-term clinical outcome after alcohol septal ablation for obstructive hypertrophic cardiomyopathy: Results from the Euro-ASA registry. *Eur. Heart J.* **2016**, *37*, 1517–1523. [CrossRef]
38. Spirito, P.; Binaco, I.; Poggio, D.; Zyrianov, A.; Grillo, M.; Pezzoli, L.; Rossi, J.; Malanin, D.; Vaccari, G.; Dorobantu, L.; et al. Role of Preoperative Cardiovascular Magnetic Resonance in Planning Ventricular Septal Myectomy in Patients with Obstructive Hypertrophic Cardiomyopathy. *Am. J. Cardiol.* **2019**, *123*, 1517–1526. [CrossRef]
39. Cui, H.; Schaff, H.V.; Wang, S.; Lahr, B.D.; Rowin, E.J.; Rastegar, H.; Hu, S.; Eleid, M.F.; Dearani, J.A.; Kimmelstiel, C.; et al. Survival Following Alcohol Septal Ablation or Septal Myectomy for Patients with Obstructive Hypertrophic Cardiomyopathy. *J. Am. Coll. Cardiol.* **2022**, *79*, 1647–1655. [CrossRef]
40. Sorajja, P.; Binder, J.; Nishimura, R.A.; Holmes, D.R., Jr.; Rihal, C.S.; Gersh, B.J.; Bresnahan, J.F.; Ommen, S.R. Predictors of an optimal clinical outcome with alcohol septal ablation for obstructive hypertrophic cardiomyopathy. *Catheter. Cardiovasc. Interv.* **2013**, *81*, E58–E67. [CrossRef]
41. Alkhouli, M.; Sajjad, W.; Lee, J.; Fernandez, G.; Waits, B.; Schwarz, K.Q.; Cove, C.J. Prevalence of Non-Left Anterior Descending Septal Perforator Culprit in Patients with Hypertrophic Cardiomyopathy Undergoing Alcohol Septal Ablation. *Am. J. Cardiol.* **2016**, *117*, 1655–1660. [CrossRef] [PubMed]
42. Singh, M.; Edwards, W.D.; Holmes, D.R., Jr.; Tajil, A.J.; Nishimura, R.A. Anatomy of the first septal perforating artery: A study with implications for ablation therapy for hypertrophic cardiomyopathy. *Mayo Clin. Proc.* **2001**, *76*, 799–802. [CrossRef] [PubMed]
43. Holmes, D.R.; Valeti, U.S.; Nishimura, R.A. Alcohol septal ablation for hypertrophic cardiomyopathy: Indications and technique. *Catheter. Cardiovasc. Interv.* **2005**, *66*, 375–389. [CrossRef]
44. Arévalos, V.; Rodríguez-Arias, J.J.; Brugaletta, S.; Micari, A.; Costa, F.; Freixa, X.; Masotti, M.; Sabaté, M.; Regueiro, A. Alcohol Septal Ablation: An Option on the Rise in Hypertrophic Obstructive Cardiomyopathy. *J. Clin. Med.* **2021**, *10*, 2276. [CrossRef] [PubMed]
45. Angelini, P. The "1st septal unit" in hypertrophic obstructive cardiomyopathy: A newly recognized anatomo-functional entity, identified during recent alcohol septal ablation experience. *Tex. Heart Inst. J.* **2007**, *34*, 336–346. [PubMed]
46. Pelliccia, F.; Niccoli, G.; Gragnano, F.; Limongelli, G.; Moscarella, E.; Andò, G.; Esposito, A.; Stabile, E.; Ussia, G.P.; Tarantini, G.; et al. Alcohol septal ablation for hypertrophic obstructive cardiomyopathy: A contemporary reappraisal. *EuroIntervention* **2019**, *15*, 411–417. [CrossRef]
47. Sawaya, F.J.; Louvard, Y.; Spaziano, M.; Morice, M.C.; Hage, F.; El-Khoury, C.; Roy, A.; Garot, P.; Hovasse, T.; Benamer, H.; et al. Short and long-term outcomes of alcohol septal ablation with the trans-radial versus the trans-femoral approach: A single center-experience. *Int. J. Cardiol.* **2016**, *220*, 7–13. [CrossRef]
48. Koljaja-Batzner, A.; Pfeiffer, B.; Seggewiss, H. Septal Collateralization to Right Coronary Artery in Alcohol Septal Ablation: Solution to a Dangerous Pitfall. *JACC Cardiovasc. Interv.* **2018**, *11*, 2009–2011. [CrossRef]
49. Faber, L.; Seggewiss, H.; Ziemssen, P.; Gleichmann, U. Intraprocedural myocardial contrast echocardiography as a routine procedure in percutaneous transluminal septal myocardial ablation: Detection of threatening myocardial necrosis distant from the septal target area. *Catheter. Cardiovasc. Interv.* **1999**, *47*, 462–466. [CrossRef]
50. Moya Mur, J.L.; Salido Tahoces, L.; Mestre Barceló, J.L.; Rodríguez Muñoz, D.; Hernández, R.; Fernández-Golfín, C.; Zamorano Gómez, J.L. Alcohol septal ablation in hypertrophic cardiomyopathy. 3D contrast echocardiography allows localization and quantification of the extension of intraprocedural vascular recruitment. *Int. J. Cardiol.* **2014**, *174*, 761–762. [CrossRef]
51. Faber, L.; Seggewiss, H.; Welge, D.; Fassbender, D.; Schmidt, H.K.; Gleichmann, U.; Horstkotte, D. Echo-guided percutaneous septal ablation for symptomatic hypertrophic obstructive cardiomyopathy: 7 years of experience. Echo-guided percutaneous septal ablation for symptomatic hypertrophic obstructive cardiomyopathy: 7 years of experience. *Eur. J. Echocardiogr.* **2004**, *5*, 347–355. [CrossRef] [PubMed]

52. Batzner, A.; Pfeiffer, B.; Neugebauer, A.; Aicha, D.; Blank, C.; Seggewiss, H. Survival After Alcohol Septal Ablation in Patients with Hypertrophic Obstructive Cardiomyopathy. *J. Am. Coll. Cardiol.* **2018**, *72*, 3087–3094. [CrossRef]
53. Liebregts, M.; Vriesendorp, P.A.; Mahmoodi, B.K.; Schinkel, A.F.; Michels, M.; ten Berg, J.M. A Systematic Review and Meta-Analysis of Long-Term Outcomes After Septal Reduction Therapy in Patients with Hypertrophic Cardiomyopathy. *JACC Heart Fail.* **2015**, *3*, 896–905. [CrossRef]
54. Veselka, J.; Procházková, S.; Duchonová, R.; Bolomová-Homolová, I.; Páleníčková, J.; Tesar, D.; Cervinka, P.; Honek, T. Alcohol septal ablation for hypertrophic obstructive cardiomyopathy: Lower alcohol dose reduces size of infarction and has comparable hemodynamic and clinical outcome. *Catheter. Cardiovasc. Interv.* **2004**, *63*, 231–235. [CrossRef]
55. Hage, F.G.; Aqel, R.; Aljaroudi, W.; Heo, J.; Pothineni, K.; Hansalia, R.; Lawson, D.; Dubovsky, E.; Iskandrian, A.E. Correlation between serum cardiac markers and myocardial infarct size quantified by myocardial perfusion imaging in patients with hypertrophic cardiomyopathy after alcohol septal ablation. *Am. J. Cardiol.* **2010**, *105*, 261–266. [CrossRef]
56. Aguiar Rosa, S.; Fiarresga, A.; Galrinho, A.; Cacela, D.; Ramos, R.; de Sousa, L.; Gonçalves, A.; Bernardes, L.; Patrício, L.; Branco, L.M.; et al. Short- and long-term outcome after alcohol septal ablation in obstructive hypertrophic cardiomyopathy: Experience of a reference center. *Rev. Port. Cardiol.* **2019**, *38*, 473–480. (In English, Portuguese) [CrossRef] [PubMed]
57. Nguyen, A.; Schaff, H.V.; Hang, D.; Nishimura, R.A.; Geske, J.B.; Dearani, J.A.; Lahr, B.D.; Ommen, S.R. Surgical myectomy versus alcohol septal ablation for obstructive hypertrophic cardiomyopathy: A propensity score-matched cohort. *J. Thorac. Cardiovasc. Surg.* **2019**, *157*, 306–315.e3. [CrossRef]
58. Veselka, J. Ten Tips and Tricks for Performing Alcohol Septal Ablation in Patients with Hypertrophic Obstructive Cardiomyopathy. *Int. J. Angiol.* **2020**, *29*, 180–182. [CrossRef]
59. Yoerger, D.M.; Picard, M.H.; Palacios, I.F.; Vlahakes, G.J.; Lowry, P.A.; Fifer, M.A. Time course of pressure gradient response after first alcohol septal ablation for obstructive hypertrophic cardiomyopathy. *Am. J. Cardiol.* **2006**, *97*, 1511–1514. [CrossRef] [PubMed]
60. Yang, Q.; Zhu, C.; Cui, H.; Tang, B.; Wang, S.; Yu, Q.; Zhao, S.; Song, Y.; Wang, S. Surgical septal myectomy outcome for obstructive hypertrophic cardiomyopathy after alcohol septal ablation. *J. Thorac. Dis.* **2021**, *13*, 1055–1065. [CrossRef]
61. Quintana, E.; Sabate-Rotes, A.; Maleszewski, J.J.; Ommen, S.R.; Nishimura, R.A.; Dearani, J.A.; Schaff, H.V. Septal myectomy after failed alcohol ablation: Does previous percutaneous intervention compromise outcomes of myectomy? *J. Thorac. Cardiovasc. Surg.* **2015**, *150*, 159–167.e1. [CrossRef] [PubMed]
62. Rudenko, K.V.; Lazoryshynets, V.V.; Nevmerzhytska, L.O.; Tregubova, M.O.; Danchenko, P.A. Septal myectomy with mitral valve surgery in patients after alcohol septal ablation. *Interact. Cardiovasc. Thorac. Surg.* **2022**, *34*, 723–730. [CrossRef]
63. Rigopoulos, A.G.; Daci, S.; Pfeiffer, B.; Papadopoulou, K.; Neugebauer, A.; Seggewiss, H. Low occurrence of ventricular arrhythmias after alcohol septal ablation in high-risk patients with hypertrophic obstructive cardiomyopathy. *Clin. Res. Cardiol.* **2016**, *105*, 953–961. [CrossRef] [PubMed]
64. Lafont, A.; Durand, E.; Brasselet, C.; Mousseaux, E.; Hagege, A.; Desnos, M. Percutaneous transluminal septal coil embolisation as an alternative to alcohol septal ablation for hypertrophic obstructive cardiomyopathy. *Heart* **2005**, *91*, 92. [CrossRef]
65. Gross, C.M.; Schulz-Menger, J.; Krämer, J.; Siegel, I.; Pilz, B.; Waigand, J.; Friedrich, M.G.; Uhlich, F.; Dietz, R. Percutaneous transluminal septal artery ablation using polyvinyl alcohol foam particles for septal hypertrophy in patients with hypertrophic obstructive cardiomyopathy: Acute and 3-year outcomes. *J. Endovasc. Ther.* **2004**, *11*, 705–711. [CrossRef]
66. Lawrenz, T.; Kuhn, H.; Endocardial Radiofrequency Ablation of Septal Hypertrophy. A new catheter-based modality of gradient reduction in hypertrophic obstructive cardiomyopathy. *Z. Kardiol.* **2004**, *93*, 493–499.
67. Llamas-Esperón, G.A.; Sandoval-Navarrete, S. Percutaneous septal ablation with absorbable gelatin sponge in hypertrophic obstructive cardiomyopathy. *Catheter. Cardiovasc. Interv.* **2007**, *69*, 231–235. [CrossRef] [PubMed]
68. Okutucu, S.; Aytemir, K.; Oto, A. Glue septal ablation: A promising alternative to alcohol septal ablation. *JRSM Cardiovasc. Dis.* **2016**, *5*, 1–8. [CrossRef]
69. Oto, A.; Aytemir, K.; Okutucu, S.; Kaya, E.B.; Deniz, A.; Cil, B.; Peynircioglu, B.; Kabakci, G. Cyanoacrylate for septal ablation in hypertrophic cardiomyopathy. *J. Interv. Cardiol.* **2011**, *24*, 77–84. [CrossRef]
70. Zhou, M.; Ta, S.; Hahn, R.T.; Hsi, D.H.; Leon, M.B.; Hu, R.; Zhang, J.; Zuo, L.; Li, J.; Wang, J.; et al. Percutaneous Intramyocardial Septal Radiofrequency Ablation in Patients with Drug-Refractory Hypertrophic Obstructive Cardiomyopathy. *JAMA Cardiol.* **2022**, *7*, 529–538. [CrossRef]
71. Greenbaum, A.B.; Khan, J.M.; Bruce, C.G.; Hanzel, G.S.; Gleason, P.T.; Kohli, K.; Inci, E.K.; Guyton, R.A.; Paone, G.; Rogers, T.; et al. Transcatheter Myotomy to Treat Hypertrophic Cardiomyopathy and Enable Transcatheter Mitral Valve Replacement: First-in-Human Report of Septal Scoring Along the Midline Endocardium. *Circ. Cardiovasc. Interv.* **2022**, *15*, e012106. [CrossRef]
72. Singh, K.; Qutub, M.; Carson, K.; Hibbert, B.; Glover, C. A meta analysis of current status of alcohol septal ablation and surgical myectomy for obstructive hypertrophic cardiomyopathy. *Catheter. Cardiovasc. Interv.* **2016**, *88*, 107–115. [CrossRef] [PubMed]
73. Kim, L.K.; Swaminathan, R.V.; Looser, P.; Minutello, R.M.; Wong, S.C.; Bergman, G.; Naidu, S.S.; Gade, C.L.; Charitakis, K.; Singh, H.S.; et al. Hospital Volume Outcomes After Septal Myectomy and Alcohol Septal Ablation for Treatment of Obstructive Hypertrophic Cardiomyopathy: US Nationwide Inpatient Database, 2003–2011. *JAMA Cardiol.* **2016**, *1*, 324–332. [CrossRef] [PubMed]

74. Gragnano, F.; Pasceri, V.; Limongelli, G.; Tanzilli, G.; Calabrò, P.; Pelliccia, F. L'alcolizzazione del setto interventricolare nella cardiomiopatia ipertrofica ostruttiva: Il ruolo emergente del Cardiomyopathy Team [Alcohol septal ablation for hypertrophic obstructive cardiomyopathy: The emerging role of the Cardiomyopathy Team]. *G. Ital. Cardiol.* **2021**, *22*, 25S–31S.
75. Lawton, J.S.; Tamis-Holland, J.E.; Bangalore, S.; Bates, E.R.; Beckie, T.M.; Bischoff, J.M.; Bittl, J.A.; Cohen, M.G.; DiMaio, J.M.; Don, C.W.; et al. 2021 ACC/AHA/SCAI Guideline for Coronary Artery Revascularization: Executive Summary: A Report of the American College of Cardiology/American Heart Association Joint Committee on Clinical Practice Guidelines. *J. Am. Coll. Cardiol.* **2022**, *79*, 197–215. [CrossRef]
76. Lee, G.; Chikwe, J.; Milojevic, M.; Wijeysundera, H.C.; Biondi-Zoccai, G.; Flather, M.; Gaudino, M.F.L.; Fremes, S.E.; Tam, D.Y. ESC/EACTS vs. ACC/AHA guidelines for the management of severe aortic stenosis. *Eur. Heart J.* **2023**, *44*, 796–812. [CrossRef] [PubMed]
77. Gragnano, F.; Mehran, R.; Branca, M.; Franzone, A.; Baber, U.; Jang, Y.; Kimura, T.; Hahn, J.Y.; Zhao, Q.; Windecker, S.; et al. P2Y12 Inhibitor Monotherapy or Dual Antiplatelet Therapy After Complex Percutaneous Coronary Interventions. *J. Am. Coll. Cardiol.* **2023**, *81*, 537–552. [CrossRef]
78. Calabrò, P.; Gragnano, F.; Niccoli, G.; Marcucci, R.; Zimarino, M.; Spaccarotella, C.; Renda, G.; Patti, G.; Andò, G.; Moscarella, E.; et al. Antithrombotic Therapy in Patients Undergoing Transcatheter Interventions for Structural Heart Disease. *Circulation* **2021**, *144*, 1323–1343. [CrossRef]
79. Veselka, J.; Faber, L.; Jensen, M.K.; Cooper, R.; Januska, J.; Krejci, J.; Bartel, T.; Dabrowski, M.; Hansen, P.R.; Almaas, V.M.; et al. Effect of Institutional Experience on Outcomes of Alcohol Septal Ablation for Hypertrophic Obstructive Cardiomyopathy. *Can. J. Cardiol.* **2018**, *34*, 16–22. [CrossRef]

Disclaimer/Publisher's Note: The statements, opinions and data contained in all publications are solely those of the individual author(s) and contributor(s) and not of MDPI and/or the editor(s). MDPI and/or the editor(s) disclaim responsibility for any injury to people or property resulting from any ideas, methods, instructions or products referred to in the content.

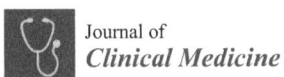

Article

Sex-Related Differences among Adults with Hypertrophic Obstructive Cardiomyopathy Undergoing Transcoronary Ablation of Septal Hypertrophy

Emyal Alyaydin *, Julia Kirsten Vogel, Peter Luedike, Tienush Rassaf, Rolf Alexander Jánosi and Maria Papathanasiou

Department of Cardiology and Vascular Medicine, West German Heart and Vascular Center, University Hospital Essen, Hufelandstrasse 55, 45147 Essen, Germany
* Correspondence: emyal.alyaydin@uk-essen.de; Tel.: +49-201-723-82072

Abstract: (1) Background: The transcoronary ablation of septal hypertrophy (TASH) is an established therapy for hypertrophic obstructive cardiomyopathy (HOCM). Previous studies on this topic are characterised by a consistent male predominance and show a worse prognosis in females. (2) Methods: This study is a retrospective analysis of all TASH procedures conducted between 2006 and 2021 at a tertiary academic centre. A solution of 75 µm microspheres (Embozene®, Boston Scientific, Marlborough, MA, USA) was used as an embolising agent. The outcomes of interest were left ventricular outflow tract (LVOT) gradient reduction and symptom improvement among males vs. that among females. Secondarily, we analysed the sex-related differences in procedural safety outcomes and mortality. (3) Results: The study population consisted of 76 patients, with a median age of 61 years. Females comprised 57% of the cohort. We observed no sex-related differences in the baseline LVOT gradients at rest or under provocation ($p = 0.560$ and $p = 0.208$, respectively). Females were significantly older at the time of the procedure ($p < 0.001$), had lower tricuspid annular systolic excursion (TAPSE) ($p = 0.009$), presented a worse clinical status according to the NYHA functional classification (for NYHA ≥ 3, $p < 0.001$), and were more often on diuretics ($p < 0.001$). We did not observe sex-related differences in absolute gradient reduction at rest ($p = 0.147$) and under provocation ($p = 0.709$). There was a reduction in the NYHA class by a median value of 1 ($p = 0.636$) at follow-up for both sexes. Postprocedural access site complications were documented in four cases (two of which concerned females), and complete atrioventricular block was noted in five patients (three of which concerned females). The 10-year survival rates were comparable between the sexes (85% in females and 88% in males). The female sex was not associated with enhanced mortality according to multivariate analysis after adjusting for the confounding variables (HR 0.94; 95% CI 0.376–2.350; $p = 0.895$), but we observed age-related differences in long-term mortality (HR 1.035; 95% CI 1.007–1.063; $p = 0.015$). (4) Conclusions: TASH is safe and effective in both sexes, irrespective of their clinical differences. Women present at an advanced age and with more severe symptoms. An advanced age at the time of the intervention is an independent predictor of mortality.

Keywords: hypertrophic cardiomyopathy; transcoronary ablation of septal hypertrophy; sex-related differences; outcome; prognosis

Citation: Alyaydin, E.; Vogel, J.K.; Luedike, P.; Rassaf, T.; Jánosi, R.A.; Papathanasiou, M. Sex-Related Differences among Adults with Hypertrophic Obstructive Cardiomyopathy Undergoing Transcoronary Ablation of Septal Hypertrophy. *J. Clin. Med.* **2023**, *12*, 3024. https://doi.org/10.3390/jcm12083024

Academic Editors: Emanuele Monda and Francesco Pelliccia

Received: 31 March 2023
Revised: 15 April 2023
Accepted: 19 April 2023
Published: 21 April 2023

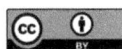

Copyright: © 2023 by the authors. Licensee MDPI, Basel, Switzerland. This article is an open access article distributed under the terms and conditions of the Creative Commons Attribution (CC BY) license (https://creativecommons.org/licenses/by/4.0/).

1. Introduction

The current level of awareness of cardiomyopathies in women is insufficient, leading to under-recognition, delayed identification, and treatment disparities compared to their male counterparts [1]. Studies reporting sex-related differences in the outcomes of hypertrophic obstructive cardiomyopathy (HOCM) are characterised by male predominance, and the results regarding disease manifestation and outcomes remain contradictory [2–6]. While some results indicate more pronounced obstruction, higher prevalence of heart failure, and worse cardiopulmonary exercise tolerance, which is associated with inferior survival in women [2–4], in other cases, the sex-related differences in the disease phenotype are considered to have no impact on mortality [6]. Irrespective of the patient's sex, the transcoronary ablation of septal hypertrophy (TASH) and surgical septal myectomy (SSM) are the therapies of choice for patients resistant to pharmacological treatment [7–10].

This study aimed to investigate the effect of sex-related differences in clinical phenotypes on procedural outcomes in patients undergoing TASH using microspheres.

2. Materials and Methods

2.1. Study Population and Design

This is a retrospective analysis of sex differences in the clinical characteristics and outcomes of adult patients who have undergone TASH at the West German Heart and Vascular Centre. Data were retrieved from the patients' electronic health records. We included all subjects who had undergone TASH over the last 15 years (April 2006 to July 2021). Figure 1 depicts the derivation of the study cohort. Incomplete follow-up, age < 18 years, and prior interventional or surgical therapy for septal reduction were the study's exclusion criteria. The study population comprised 87 patients. Nine patients were excluded because they underwent prior TASH or SSM before referral to our centre. Additionally, two patients were excluded due to unfavourable anatomy of the septal perforators, rendering the intervention unsuccessful. The remaining 76 patients were stratified into two groups according to their sex (males: $n = 33$, 43%; females: $n = 43$, 57%). Indications for TASH were LVOT gradient at rest ≥ 30 mmHg and/or with Valsalva manoeuvre ≥ 50 mmHg in combination with clinical symptoms (dyspnoea, syncope, cardiac arrest, and arrhythmia). The predefined inclusion criteria were age ≥ 18 years at the time of intervention and complete assessment, including initial investigations, periprocedural data, and follow-up results encompassing clinical, echocardiographic, and laboratory data.

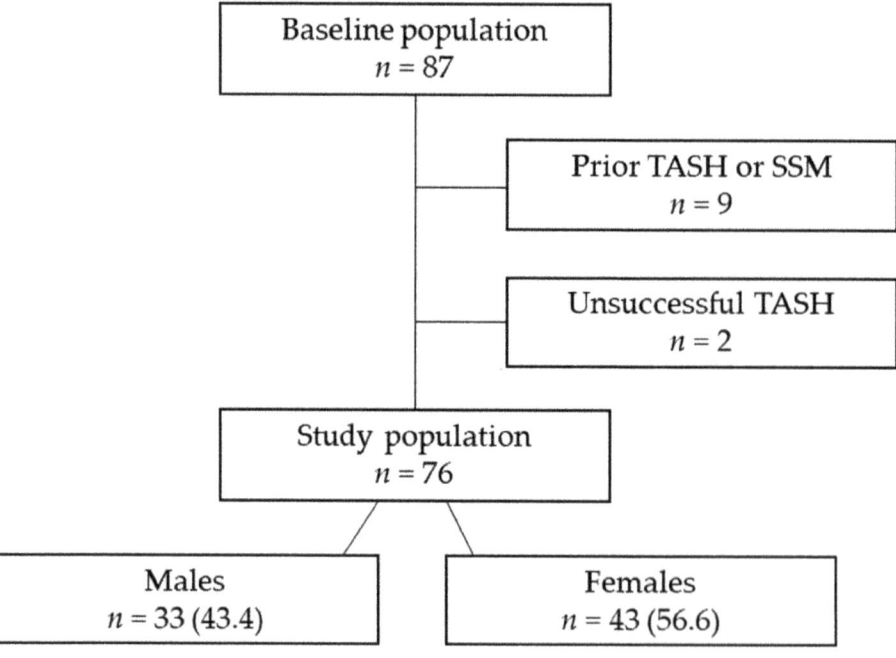

Figure 1. Derivation of the analytic cohort. TASH—transcoronary ablation of septal hypertrophy using alcohol; SSM—surgical septal myectomy. Data are presented as n (%).

The primary endpoint was the difference in peak left ventricular outflow tract gradients (Δ left ventricular outflow tract (LVOT)) among men and women, considering the echocardiographically derived peak gradients before the intervention and at the first scheduled follow-up. Secondary endpoints were major adverse cardiovascular events, including stroke and cardiovascular death, and high-degree atrioventricular (AV) block, access site complications, arrhythmias, the need for redo-procedures, and long-term mortality with regard to patient sex.

2.2. TASH Protocol and Non-Invasive Investigations

LVOT gradients were estimated using transthoracic echocardiography at rest and under Valsalva provocation before and after the intervention. The interventricular septal diameter (IVSd), systolic anterior motion (SAM) of the mitral valve, and the left atrial (LA) diameter were evaluated in M-mode. The biplane Simpson's method was used to estimate left ventricular ejection fraction. Daily echocardiographic monitoring was performed after a successful procedure. According to a predefined institutional protocol, patients were scheduled for a follow-up assessment three to six months after the TASH procedure. Additionally, blood tests were performed concerning coagulation, complete blood count, liver and renal function, and N-terminal prohormone of B-type natriuretic peptide (NT-proBNP). The cardiac enzymes were measured at six-hour intervals after TASH to determine the peak value and further assessed until reaching 50% of the peak values.

All septal reduction procedures were conducted by embolization of the septal perforator of interest using a solution of 75 μm microspheres (Embozene®, Boston Scientific) [11]. This medium is implemented for the treatment of hyper-vascular tumours. The higher viscosity and non-resorbable nature of the microspheres offer potential advantages over alcohol. Since 2005, microspheres have been the medium of choice for TASH procedures at our centre [12]. All procedures were performed by experienced professionals. Over the fifteen years encompassed by our study, four interventional cardiologists mastered the TASH technique, and the procedures were conducted in the presence of at least two of them. All interventions were performed via the femoral approach. A temporary pacemaker lead was advanced using a venous sheath. Simultaneous LVOT gradient assessment was conducted by inserting two pigtail catheters into the left ventricle (LV) and the ascending aorta. After wiring the target septal branch, an over-the-wire balloon was used to occlude the vessel. Subsequently, the application of microspheres was performed under fluoroscopic guidance until angiographic evidence of vessel occlusion was obtained. After the procedure, patients were admitted to the intermediate care unit for at least 24 h.

2.3. Statistical Analysis

All statistical analyses were performed using IBM SPSS Statistics software (version 29). The Shapiro–Wilk test was used to determine the normality of the data distribution. Continuous variables are given as mean ± standard deviation (mean ± SD) if normally distributed and median and interquartile range (IQR) if skewed. Normally distributed data were further assessed using Student's t-test. Otherwise, the non-parametric Mann–Whitney U test was used. Categorical variables are presented as numbers (percentages) and were analysed using the chi-square test. Assessment of factors associated with long-term mortality in patients undergoing TASH was performed using Cox regression analysis with stepwise backward selection. Variables for which $p < 0.10$ were included in the final model. Statistical significance was set at $p < 0.05$.

3. Results

3.1. Baseline Characteristics

The study cohort comprised 76 patients. Females constituted more than half of the population ($n = 43$, 57%) and were older at admission for TASH compared to their male counterparts (median age 68 years in females vs. 54 years in males; $p < 0.001$) (Table 1). Severe dyspnoea was the leading symptom upon initial presentation (NYHA ≥ 3 in 86%

of the patients), for which there were significant differences between both sexes (93% in females and 76% in males; $p = 0.049$). A fifth of the patients had syncope, for which there no sex-related differences (24% in males and 14% in females; $p = 0.371$). Previous cardiac arrest or sustained ventricular tachycardia with hemodynamic instability were reported in 4% of the population (6% in males and 2% in females; $p = 0.576$). One fifth of the study population had undergone previous device implantation, for which there was a non-significant predominance of implantable cardiac defibrillators (ICDs) in males ($n = 5$, 12% in females vs. $n = 8$, 24% in males; $p = 0.219$). Hypertension was the most common comorbidity irrespective of patient sex ($n = 37$, 86% in females vs. $n = 28$, 85% in males; $p = 1.000$). Diabetes and atrial fibrillation had an overall prevalence of 17%, for which there were no sex-related differences ($p = 0.766$ and $p = 1.000$, respectively). We observed a non-significant difference in the rate of coronary artery disease, with 35% of females affected compared to 21% of males ($p = 0.214$). Inter- or intraventricular conduction disturbances not requiring pacemaker implantation were observed in less than 10% of the overall cohort, for which there were no sex-related differences (Table 1).

Table 1. Baseline characteristics of the patient population.

Patient Characteristics	Overall Population $n = 76$	Male $n = 33$ (43.4)	Female $n = 43$ (56.6)	p Value
1. Demographics				
Age, years	60.5 [26.0]	54.0 [22.0]	68.0 [21.0]	<0.001
BMI, kg/m^2	28.2 ± 4.8	28.6 ± 4.8	27.9 ± 4.9	0.509
BSA, m^2	1.9 ± 0.3	2.0 ± 0.3	1.8 ± 0.2	<0.001
NYHA $\geq$ 3, n (%)	65 (85.5)	25 (75.8)	40 (93.0)	0.049
Previous syncope, n (%)	14 (18.4)	8 (24.2)	6 (14.0)	0.371
Family history of SCD, n (%)	11 (14.5)	6 (18.2)	5 (11.6)	0.517
Previous cardiac arrest or sustained VT, n (%)	3 (3.9)	2 (6.1)	1 (2.3)	0.576
ICD, n (%)	13 (17.1)	8 (24.2)	5 (11.6)	0.219
Pacemaker, n (%)	2 (2.6)	1 (3.0)	1 (2.3)	1.000
CRT, n (%)	1 (1.3)	0 (0.0)	1 (2.3)	1.000
2. Comorbidities				
HTN, n (%)	65 (85.5)	28 (84.8)	37 (86.0)	1.000
Diabetes mellitus, n (%)	13 (17.1)	5 (15.2)	8 (18.6)	0.766
Atrial fibrillation, n (%)	13 (17.1)	6 (18.2)	7 (16.3)	1.000
CAD, n (%)	22 (28.9)	7 (21.2)	15 (34.9)	0.214
COPD, n (%)	6 (7.9)	3 (9.1)	3 (7.0)	1.000
AV block, n (%)	5 (6.7)	1 (3.0)	4 (9.3)	0.381
LAFB, n (%)	5 (6.6)	3 (9.1)	2 (4.7)	0.647
LBBB, n (%)	6 (7.9)	2 (6.1)	4 (9.3)	0.692
RBBB, n (%)	6 (7.9)	5 (15.2)	1 (2.3)	0.080
nsVT, n (%)	8 (10.5)	3 (9.1)	5 (11.6)	1.000
3. Echocardiography				
LVEF, %	61 [11.0]	63 [14.0]	60 [8.0]	0.113
LVOT gradient at rest, mmHg	41.0 [27.0]	40.0 [28.0]	42.0 [32.0]	0.560
LVOT gradient (Valsalva), mmHg	95.0 [71.0]	95.0 [75.0]	85.0 [60.0]	0.208
SAM, n (%)	62 (81.6)	29 (87.9)	33 (76.7)	0.248
MR $\geq$ 2 grade, n (%)	35 (46.1)	16 (48.5)	19 (44.2)	0.817
LA diameter/m^2, mm	22.0 [4.6]	21.5 [4.7]	23.7 [5.3]	0.040
LAVI/m^2, mL	38.9 [20.0]	34.8 [4.7]	40.1 [20.5]	0.283
TAPSE, mm	19 [4.0]	21 [5.0]	19 [3.0]	0.009
sPAP > 35 mmHg, n (%)	22 (28.9)	9 (27.3)	13 (30.2)	0.805
4. Laboratory results				
NTproBNP, pg/mL	388.0 [737.0]	318.0 [562.0]	430.7 [1142.0]	0.099
Creatinine, mg/dL	1.1 [0.2]	1.1 [0.3]	1.1 [0.2]	0.146
CK, U/L	75.0 [53.5]	77.0 [33.0]	69.0 [67.0]	0.052
TroponinI, ng/L	20.0 [30.0]	20.0 [48.5]	20.0 [30.0]	0.577

Table 1. Cont.

Patient Characteristics	Overall Population n = 76	Male n = 33 (43.4)	Female n = 43 (56.6)	p Value
Medical treatment				
Betablockers, n (%)	62 (81.6)	29 (87.9)	33 (76.7)	0.248
Verapamil, n (%)	16 (21.1)	6 (18.2)	10 (23.3)	0.778
Diltiazem, n (%)	1 (1.3)	1 (3.1)	0 (0.0)	0.427
Diuretics, n (%)	45 (59.2)	12 (36.4)	33 (76.7)	<0.001
NOACs, n (%)	4 (5.3)	2 (6.1)	2 (4.7)	1.000
Vitamin K antagonists, n (%)	8 (10.5)	4 (12.1)	4 (9.3)	0.721
Antiplatelet agents, n (%)	42 (55.3)	17 (51.5)	25 (58.1)	0.644

Data are presented as mean ± (SD), median (IQR), or n (%). BMI—Body Mass Index, BSA—body surface area (Du Bois Method), NYHA—New York Heart Association (NYHA) Classification, SCD—sudden cardiac death, VT—ventricular tachycardia, ICD—implantable cardioverter defibrillator, CRT—cardiac resynchronization therapy, HTN—hypertension, CAD—coronary artery disease, COPD—chronic obstructive pulmonary disease, AV block—atrioventricular block, LAFB—left anterior fascicular block, LBBB—left bundle branch block, RBBB—right bundle branch block, nsVT—non-sustained ventricular tachycardia, LVEF—left ventricular ejection fraction, LVOT—left ventricular outflow tract, SAM—systolic anterior motion of the mitral valve, MR—mitral regurgitation, LA—left atrium, LAVI—left atrial volume index, TAPSE—tricuspid annular plane systolic excursion, sPAP—systolic pulmonary artery pressure, NT-proBNP—N-terminal prohormone of brain natriuretic peptide, CK—creatine kinase, and NOACs—novel oral anticoagulants.

The median left ventricular ejection fraction (LVEF) was 61.0 [11.0]%. The median LVOT gradients at rest (42 [32.0] mmHg in females vs. 40 [28.0] mmHg in males; $p = 0.560$) and during Valsalva provocation (85 [60.0] mmHg in females vs. 95 [75.0] mmHg in males; $p = 0.208$) were comparable in both sexes. There was no sex-related difference in the rate of systolic anterior motion (SAM) of the mitral valve ($n = 33$, 77%, in females vs. $n = 29$, 88%, in males; $p = 0.248$). Females presented with lower tricuspid annular systolic excursion (TAPSE) (19 mm in females vs. 21 mm in males; $p = 0.009$). As depicted in Table 1, beta-blockers were the most utilised agent in the overall population irrespective of sex ($n = 62$, 82%), whereas verapamil was the drug of second choice ($n = 16$, 21%). Significantly more females were on diuretics ($n = 33$, 77%, for females vs. $n = 12$, 36%, for males; $p < 0.001$). NT-proBNP levels were non-significantly elevated in females compared to their male counterparts (431 [1142.0] pg/mL in females vs. 318 [562.0] pg/mL in males; $p = 0.099$). Additionally, more than half of the patients were taking antiplatelet agents ($n = 42$, 55%), whereas oral anticoagulation was implemented in 16% of the population (Table 1).

3.2. Periprocedural Outcomes

As shown in Table 2, there were no significant differences in the volume of microspheres used to occlude the septal perforator of interest (2 [2.0] mL in females vs. 3 [3.0] mL in males; $p = 0.306$).

We observed no differences in the maximal postprocedural levels of Troponin I levels between the study groups (2659 [2889.0] ng/L in females vs. 2311 [2908.0] ng/L in males; $p = 0.506$). There were no significant differences in the incidence of postprocedural complete atrioventricular (AV) block, left bundle branch block (LBBB), or right bundle branch block (RBBB) (Table 2). When considering AV and interventricular conduction disturbances as a composite entity, the overall incidence of conduction disturbances was 14% in females and 9% in males ($p = 0.518$). We did not observe an impact of age on the incidence of complete AV block after TASH in our cohort of patients (OR 1.02; 95% CI 0.957–1.084; $p = 0.564$). Access site complications were observed in four patients ($n = 2$ in females; $p = 0.786$). Intraprocedural death occurred in one case of urgent TASH, which was performed as a rescue procedure following haemodynamic instability immediately after the deployment of an aortic valve prosthesis during transcatheter aortic valve replacement (TAVR) with a multifactorial aetiology. This is a rare indication, as previously mentioned in the medical literature [13,14]. We did not observe any periprocedural stroke events or arrhythmias.

Table 2. Procedural characteristics and complications.

Peri- and Postprocedural Outcomes	Overall Population n = 76	Male n = 33	Female n = 43	p Value
Volume of microspheres, mL	2.0 [2.0]	3.0 [3.0]	2.0 [2.0]	0.306
ICU stay, days	1.0 [0.0]	1.0 [0.0]	1.0 [1.0]	0.133
Hospitalisation, days	12.5 [10.0]	12.0 [8.0]	13.0 [11.0]	0.449
CK max, U/L	926.0 [949.0]	1018.0 [1537.0]	897 [947.0]	0.234
Troponin I, ng/L	2485.0 [2874.0]	2311.0 [2908.0]	2659.0 [2889.0]	0.506
Complications				
AV block, n (%)	5 (6.6)	2 (6.1)	3 (7.0)	1.000
New LBBB, n (<%)	1 (1.3)	0 (0.0)	1 (2.3)	1.000
New RBBB, n (%)	3 (3.9)	1 (3.0)	2 (4.7)	1.000
Access site complications, n (%)	4 (5.3)	2 (6.1)	2 (4.7)	1.000
Postprocedural death, n (%)	1 (1.3)	1 (3.0)	0 (0.0)	0.434

ICU—intensive care unit, CK—creatine kinase, AV block—atrioventricular block, LBBB—left bundle branch block, and RBBB—right bundle branch block. Data are presented as n (%) or median (IQR).

As depicted in Table 3, the routine follow-up assessment of the patients after a median period of 4 [8.0] months revealed a significant reduction in LVOT gradients at rest and after Valsalva provocation ($p < 0.001$ for both sexes), without differences between the study groups (females vs. males; $p = 0.147$ at rest and $p = 0.709$ under provocation). LVOT gradient < 30 mmHg at rest was achieved in 88% of the patients, without differences between the sexes ($p = 0.948$). Provoked gradient < 50 mmHg was reported in 70% of males and 79% of females ($p = 0.353$). Furthermore, we observed a significant reduction in the prevalence of severe dyspnoea according to the New York Heart Association (NYHA) functional classification (NYHA ≥ 3: 76% at baseline assessment to 3% following TASH in males, $p < 0.001$, and 93% to 5% in females, $p < 0.001$) irrespective of patients' sex ($p = 0.636$). There was a significant reduction in NT-proBNP levels at follow-up in females (431 pg/mL to 281 pg/mL; $p = 0.009$) compared with males (318 pg/mL to 189 pg/mL; $p = 0.073$) (Table 3).

Table 3. Short-term outcomes after TASH (initial assessment and first clinical follow-up at 4 [8.0] months).

Characteristics	Males (n = 33)			Females (n = 43)			Males vs. Females
	Pre-TASH	Post-TASH	p Value	Pre-TASH	Post-TASH	p Value	p Value for Δ
LVOT gradient at rest, mmHg	40 [22.0]	16.0 [14.0]	<0.001	42.0 [32.0]	15.0 [17.0]	<0.001	0.147
Provoked LVOT gradient, mmHg	95.0 [75.0]	25.0 [41.0]	<0.001	85.0 [60.0]	24.0 [42.0]	<0.001	0.709
NT-proBNP, pg/mL	318.0 [562.0]	189.0 [367.0]	0.073	430.7 [1142.0]	281.0 [408.0]	0.009	0.338
NYHA ≥ 3, n (%)	25 (75.8)	1 (3.0)	<0.001	40 (93.0)	2 (4.7)	<0.001	0.636
IVSd > 20 mm, n (%)	16 (48.5)	4 (12.1)	<0.001	21 (48.8)	3 (7.0)	<0.001	0.583

LVOT—left ventricular outflow tract, NYHA—Ney York Heart Association functional classification, IVSd—Interventricular septum thickness in diastole, and TASH—transcoronary ablation of septal hypertrophy. Data are presented as median (IQR) and n (%).

3.3. Long-Term Follow-up

The 10-year survival rates were comparable in both sexes (85% in females and 88% in males). The female sex was not associated with enhanced mortality according to multivariate analysis after adjustment for the confounding variables (TAPSE, use of diuretics, left atrial diameter, age at TASH, and NYHA class) (HR 0.94; 95% CI 0.38–2.35; $p = 0.895$), but there were age-related differences in mortality (HR 1.035; 95% CI 1.007–1.063; $p = 0.015$) (Table 4).

Table 4. Multivariate Cox regression analysis.

Characteristics	HR	95% CI	p Value
Age at TASH, years	1.035	1.007–1.063	0.015
NYHA ≥ 3	1.256	0.359–4.395	0.722
Female sex	0.940	0.376–2.350	0.895
TAPSE, mm	1.921	0.802–1.057	0.240
Diuretics	1.703	0.707–4.101	0.235
LA diameter, mm	1.007	0.974–1.040	0.697

TASH—transcoronary ablation of septal hypertrophy, NYHA—New York Heart Association, TAPSE—Tricuspid annular systolic excursion, and LA dimeter—left atrial diameter in parasternal long-axis view.

We did not observe a significant impact of the estimated gradient measures, family history of SCD, a previous pacemaker or ICD implantation, LVEF, IVSd ≥ 20 mm, or sex-related differences on the primary outcome measures. The male sex was associated with a non-significantly elevated rate of redo procedures at follow-up (25% in males vs. 13.6% in females; p = 0.445).

4. Discussion

In contrast to previous studies, our cohort is characterised by female predominance [9–11]. As we report on the results of a tertiary referral centre with well-established experience in treating patients with cardiomyopathies, the study cohort may have included some high-risk individuals. For a disease considered equally prevalent among males and females, the female predominance of patients referred for TASH may be due to the more pronounced disease manifestations in women, resistance to conservative treatment, more obstructive physiology, or even lack of disease awareness among females [2–4]. A potential indicator in favour of the latter is that females were significantly older at admission for TASH, with a median age difference of 14 years. A recent analysis of registry data reported a similar age distribution [5]. The significantly higher rate of severe dyspnoea in females is an alarming sign of a potential failure to recognise the isolated disease symptoms and comorbidities, contributing to the more advanced impairment of their physical capacity. The higher rate of diuretic treatment also suggests an advanced disease stage with signs of congestion. This is in accordance with previous studies reporting a higher risk of developing severe heart failure in females with HOCM [2,15]. The more pronounced disease manifestation in females may also be due to the higher burden of sarcomere variants [15].

We did not observe any differences in the prevalence of a positive family history of sudden cardiac death or previous syncope. There was a non-significant male predominance in the cardiac defibrillator implantation rate. Previous studies have reported a higher risk of exercise-induced non-sustained and sustained ventricular tachycardias in males with HCM compared to females [16]. Additionally, females with HOCM are known to have a lower left ventricular mass, fewer fibrotic changes, and a lower rate of electrocardiographic abnormalities [17,18]. Due to the retrospective nature of this analysis, we do not have sufficient data regarding disease history or exercise-related electrocardiographic abnormalities.

The median LVEF was within the normal range in our patient population, and we observed no significant differences in the LVOT gradients at rest or under Valsalva provocation. The larger diameter of the left atrium in females may indicate more pronounced diastolic dysfunction and elevated filling pressure due to disease progression [19]. Combined with the finding of a lower TAPSE, this may be a warning sign of worsening heart failure. Recent studies based on a magnetic-resonance-guided assessment of the biventricular function in HOCM found that right ventricular function declines prior to that of the LV as assessed by LVEF during the course of disease [20]. Our observations are consistent with those of previous studies reporting that heart failure is the most common feature leading to the diagnosis of HCM in females. In contrast, in males, diagnosis often follows a routine medical assessment with the identification of an abnormal electrocardiogram or heart murmur [6]. There are still relevant sex disparities in terms of the percentage of subjects undergoing routine health risk assessments, with males more often being the focus of preventive care [21].

Despite sex-related differences in the baseline characteristics, the TASH procedure was associated with a significant reduction in LVOT gradients at rest and under provocation, without differences between the study groups. Relief from LVOT obstruction led to a significant symptomatic improvement irrespective of sex. Additionally, there was a significant reduction in NT-proBNP in females, which was potentially due to advanced disease and more pronounced congestion. Advanced age has been previously reported to be associated with a higher rate of conduction disturbance following TASH using alcohol [22]. We did not observe correlation between age and AV block. This may be attributed to the advantages of microspheres over alcohol for septal reduction. On the one hand, the higher viscosity of microspheres may reduce the risk of accidental off-target coronary embolization. Their inability to be resorbed reduces the risk of cardiotoxicity compared with alcohol [23]. The rate of complete AV block in our population was lower than the incidence reported for TASH with alcohol [24]. The volume of microspheres was non-significantly higher in males. The amount of injected medium was much lower than that in TASH using alcohol, where an association between alcohol volume and postprocedural conduction disturbances has been reported [25]. We observed no differences in the rate of access site complications between the sexes, and the overall incidence was lower than that previously reported for TASH using the femoral approach [26].

Regarding long-term prognosis, the 10-year survival rates were comparable between the sexes. The female sex was not associated with enhanced mortality in the multivariate analysis after adjusting for the confounding variables, and age was the only independent predictor of mortality. This is in line with the results reported to date, indicating a higher mortality risk at advanced age, which is potentially related to disease progression and higher comorbidity burden of the patients [25].

It remains unknown whether there are any sex-related differences in the rates of recurrent LVOT obstruction after TASH using microspheres, an outcome that is not specifically addressed in the current analysis. There were no differences in the rates of redo procedures in our patient population. However, in the era of disease-modifying therapies using myosin inhibitors, it is of profound interest to identify whether sex could be a confounder of outcomes beyond LVOT gradient reduction [27,28]. The female sex is associated with a higher rate of sarcomere mutations [15,21]; potential sex-related differences in the long-term effectiveness of myosin inhibitors remain yet to be investigated.

Our study has inherent limitations associated with its retrospective design. We reported on all-cause mortality, but we did not have data regarding the specific cause of death of all patients. Long-term outcomes of gradient reduction and symptom severity after TASH were not consistently available. The microsphere solution for septal embolization is not directly comparable to alcohol, and its utility is limited because of its higher cost. Compared to radiofrequency ablation, TASH using microspheres is associated with a comparable reduction in LVOT gradients at rest and under provocation [29]. The complete AV block and periprocedural complication rates are higher in radiofrequency ablation, and there are no data regarding the rate of recurrent obstruction. Due to the limited experience and small sample size of studies concerning radiofrequency ablation, this result should be interpreted with caution. Nevertheless, it remains a medium with potential advantages in terms of complication rates.

5. Conclusions

Women with HOCM present at a more advanced age, with more severe symptoms and a poor clinical status. TASH using microspheres is safe and effective in both sexes irrespective of their clinical differences. Age was an independent predictor of long-term mortality after TASH regardless of sex.

Author Contributions: Conceptualization, E.A. and M.P.; methodology, E.A.; software, E.A.; validation, P.L., M.P., R.A.J. and T.R.; formal analysis, E.A.; investigation, E.A. and M.P.; resources, E.A. and M.P.; data curation, E.A. and J.K.V.; writing—original draft preparation, E.A.; writing—review and editing, J.K.V., P.L., R.A.J., M.P. and T.R.; visualization, E.A.; supervision, M.P.; project administration, E.A. and M.P.; funding acquisition, M.P. and T.R. All authors have read and agreed to the published version of the manuscript.

Funding: This work was supported by the University Medicine Essen Clinician Scientist Academy (UMEA) and the German Research Foundation (DFG, Deutsche Forschungsgemeinschaft) [Research grant FU356/12-1 to M.P.].

Institutional Review Board Statement: The study was conducted in accordance with the Declaration of Helsinki and approved by the Institutional Review Board of the University of Duisburg-Essen (No: 22-10972-BO, 22 November 2022).

Informed Consent Statement: Patient consent was waived due to the retrospective design of the study.

Data Availability Statement: The data presented in this study are available on reasonable request from the corresponding author. The data are not publicly available due to data confidentiality regulation.

Conflicts of Interest: The authors declare no conflict of interest related to this manuscript.

References

1. Pelliccia, F.; Limongelli, G.; Autore, C.; Gimeno-Blanes, J.R.; Basso, C.; Elliott, P. Sex-related differences in cardiomyopathies. *Int. J. Cardiol.* **2019**, *286*, 239–243. [CrossRef]
2. Geske, J.B.; Ong, K.C.; Siontis, K.C.; Hebl, V.B.; Ackerman, M.J.; Hodge, D.O.; Miller, V.M.; Nishimura, R.A.; Oh, J.K.; Schaff, H.V.; et al. Women with hypertrophic cardiomyopathy have worse survival. *Eur. Heart J.* **2017**, *38*, 3434–3440. [CrossRef] [PubMed]
3. Kim, M.; Kim, B.; Choi, Y.J.; Lee, H.J.; Lee, H.; Park, J.B.; Lee, S.P.; Han, K.D.; Kim, Y.J.; Kim, H.K. Sex differences in the prognosis of patients with hypertrophic cardiomyopathy. *Sci. Rep.* **2021**, *11*, 4854. [CrossRef]
4. Kubo, T.; Kitaoka, H.; Okawa, M.; Hirota, T.; Hayato, K.; Yamasaki, N.; Matsumura, Y.; Yabe, T.; Doi, Y.L. Gender-specific differences in the clinical features of hypertrophic cardiomyopathy in a community-based Japanese population: Results from Kochi RYOMA study. *J. Cardiol.* **2010**, *56*, 314–319. [CrossRef]
5. Preveden, A.; Golubovic, M.; Bjelobrk, M.; Miljkovic, T.; Ilic, A.; Stojsic, S.; Gajic, D.; Glavaski, M.; Maier, L.S.; Okwose, N.; et al. Gender Related Differences in the Clinical Presentation of Hypertrophic Cardiomyopathy-An Analysis from the SILICOFCM Database. *Medicina* **2022**, *58*, 314. [CrossRef] [PubMed]
6. Rowin, E.J.; Maron, M.S.; Wells, S.; Patel, P.P.; Koethe, B.C.; Maron, B.J. Impact of Sex on Clinical Course and Survival in the Contemporary Treatment Era for Hypertrophic Cardiomyopathy. *J. Am. Heart Assoc.* **2019**, *8*, e012041. [CrossRef]
7. Ommen, S.R.; Mital, S.; Burke, M.A.; Day, S.M.; Deswal, A.; Elliott, P.; Evanovich, L.L.; Hung, J.; Joglar, J.A.; Kantor, P.; et al. 2020 AHA/ACC Guideline for the Diagnosis and Treatment of Patients With Hypertrophic Cardiomyopathy: Executive Summary: A Report of the American College of Cardiology/American Heart Association Joint Committee on Clinical Practice Guidelines. *Circulation* **2020**, *142*, e533–e557.
8. Elliott, P.M.; Anastasakis, A.; Borger, M.A.; Borggrefe, M.; Cecchi, F.; Charron, P.; Hagege, A.A.; Lafont, A.; Limongelli, G.; Mahrholdt, H.; et al. 2014 ESC Guidelines on diagnosis and management of hypertrophic cardiomyopathy: The Task Force for the Diagnosis and Management of Hypertrophic Cardiomyopathy of the European Society of Cardiology (ESC). *Eur. Heart J.* **2014**, *35*, 2733–2779.
9. Spirito, P.; Rossi, J.; Maron, B.J. Alcohol septal ablation: In which patients and why? *Ann. Cardiothorac. Surg.* **2017**, *6*, 369–375. [CrossRef] [PubMed]
10. Affronti, A.; Pruna-Guillen, R.; Sandoval, E.; Pereda, D.; Alcocer, J.; Castellà, M.; Quintana, E. Surgery for Hypertrophic Obstructive Cardiomyopathy. Comprehensive LVOT Management beyond Septal Myectomy. *J. Clin. Med.* **2021**, *10*, 4397. [CrossRef]
11. Embozene™ Color-Advanced Microspheres. Available online: https://www.bostonscientific.com/content/dam/Manuals/bz/current-rev-pt/50913186-01A_Embozene_eDFU_bz_s.pdf (accessed on 20 February 2023).
12. Dickmann, B.; Baars, T.; Heusch, G.; Erbel, R. Transcoronary septal ablation in hypertrophic obstructive cardiomyopathy by embolizing microspheres. *Eur. Heart J.* **2013**, *34*, 2489. [CrossRef]
13. Bandyopadhyay, D.; Chakraborty, S.; Amgai, B.; Kapadia, S.R.; Braunwald, E.; Naidu, S.S.; Kalra, A. Association of Hypertrophic Obstructive Cardiomyopathy With Outcomes Following Transcatheter Aortic Valve Replacement. *JAMA Netw. Open* **2020**, *3*, e1921669. [CrossRef]
14. Desai, M.Y.; Alashi, A.; Popovic, Z.B.; Wierup, P.; Griffin, B.P.; Thamilarasan, M.; Johnston, D.; Svensson, L.G.; Lever, H.M.; Smedira, N.G. Outcomes in Patients With Obstructive Hypertrophic Cardiomyopathy and Concomitant Aortic Stenosis Undergoing Surgical Myectomy and Aortic Valve Replacement. *J. Am. Heart Assoc.* **2021**, *10*, e018435. [CrossRef] [PubMed]

15. Lakdawala, N.K.; Olivotto, I.; Day, S.M.; Han, L.; Ashley, E.A.; Michels, M.; Ingles, J.; Semsarian, C.; Jacoby, D.; Jefferies, J.L.; et al. Associations Between Female Sex, Sarcomere Variants, and Clinical Outcomes in Hypertrophic Cardiomyopathy. *Circ. Genom. Precis. Med.* **2021**, *14*, e003062. [CrossRef]
16. Gimeno, J.R.; Tomé-Esteban, M.; Lofiego, C.; Hurtado, J.; Pantazis, A.; Mist, B.; Lambiase, P.; McKenna, W.J.; Elliott, P.M. Exercise-induced ventricular arrhythmias and risk of sudden cardiac death in patients with hypertrophic cardiomyopathy. *Eur. Heart J.* **2009**, *30*, 2599–2605. [CrossRef] [PubMed]
17. McLeod, C.J.; Ackerman, M.J.; Nishimura, R.A.; Tajik, A.J.; Gersh, B.J.; Ommen, S.R. Outcome of patients with hypertrophic cardiomyopathy and a normal electrocardiogram. *J. Am. Coll. Cardiol.* **2009**, *54*, 229–233. [CrossRef]
18. Varnava, A.M.; Elliott, P.M.; Sharma, S.; McKenna, W.J.; Davies, M.J. Hypertrophic cardiomyopathy: The interrelation of disarray, fibrosis, and small vessel disease. *Heart* **2000**, *84*, 476–482. [CrossRef]
19. Yang, H.; Woo, A.; Monakier, D.; Jamorski, M.; Fedwick, K.; Wigle, E.D.; Rakowski, H. Enlarged left atrial volume in hypertrophic cardiomyopathy: A marker for disease severity. *J. Am. Soc. Echocardiogr.* **2005**, *18*, 1074–1082. [CrossRef] [PubMed]
20. Mahmod, M.; Raman, B.; Chan, K.; Sivalokanathan, S.; Smillie, R.W.; Samat, A.H.A.; Ariga, R.; Dass, S.; Ormondroyd, E.; Watkins, H.; et al. Right ventricular function declines prior to left ventricular ejection fraction in hypertrophic cardiomyopathy. *J. Cardiovasc. Magn. Reson.* **2022**, *24*, 36. [CrossRef] [PubMed]
21. Butters, A.; Lakdawala, N.K.; Ingles, J. Sex Differences in Hypertrophic Cardiomyopathy: Interaction With Genetics and Environment. *Curr. Heart Fail. Rep.* **2021**, *18*, 264–273. [CrossRef] [PubMed]
22. Lawrenz, T.; Lieder, F.; Bartelsmeier, M.; Leuner, C.; Borchert, B.; Meyer zu Vilsendorf, D.; Strunk-Mueller, C.; Reinhardt, J.; Feuchtl, A.; Stellbrink, C.; et al. Predictors of complete heart block after transcoronary ablation of septal hypertrophy: Results of a prospective electrophysiological investigation in 172 patients with hypertrophic obstructive cardiomyopathy. *J. Am. Coll. Cardiol.* **2007**, *49*, 2356–2363. [CrossRef]
23. Vriesendorp, P.A.; Van Mieghem, N.M.; Vletter, W.B.; Ten Cate, F.J.; de Jong, P.L.; Schinkel, A.F.; Michels, M. Microsphere embolisation as an alternative for alcohol in percutaneous transluminal septal myocardial ablation. *Neth. Heart J.* **2013**, *21*, 245–248. [CrossRef] [PubMed]
24. Nguyen, A.; Schaff, H.V.; Hang, D.; Nishimura, R.A.; Geske, J.B.; Dearani, J.A.; Lahr, B.D.; Ommen, S.R. Surgical myectomy versus alcohol septal ablation for obstructive hypertrophic cardiomyopathy: A propensity score-matched cohort. *J. Thorac. Cardiovasc. Surg.* **2019**, *157*, 306–315.e3. [CrossRef] [PubMed]
25. Nguyen, A.; Schaff, H.V.; Hang, D.; Nishimura, R.A.; Geske, J.B.; Dearani, J.A.; Lahr, B.D.; Ommen, S.R. Long-term clinical outcome after alcohol septal ablation for obstructive hypertrophic cardiomyopathy: Results from the Euro-ASA registry. *Eur. Heart J.* **2016**, *37*, 1517–1523.
26. Sawaya, F.J.; Louvard, Y.; Spaziano, M.; Morice, M.C.; Hage, F.; El-Khoury, C.; Roy, A.; Garot, P.; Hovasse, T.; Benamer, H. Short and long-term outcomes of alcohol septal ablation with the trans-radial versus the trans-femoral approach: A single center-experience. *Int. J. Cardiol.* **2016**, *220*, 7–13. [CrossRef]
27. Saberi, S.; Cardim, N.; Yamani, M.; Schulz-Menger, J.; Li, W.; Florea, V.; Sehnert, A.J.; Kwong, R.Y.; Jerosch-Herold, M.; Masri, A. Mavacamten Favorably Impacts Cardiac Structure in Obstructive Hypertrophic Cardiomyopathy: EXPLORER-HCM Cardiac Magnetic Resonance Substudy Analysis. *Circulation* **2021**, *143*, 606–608. [CrossRef]
28. Marian, A.J.; Braunwald, E. Hypertrophic cardiomyopathy: Genetics, pathogenesis, clinical manifestations, diagnosis, and therapy. *Circ. Res.* **2017**, *121*, 749–770. [CrossRef] [PubMed]
29. Yang, H.; Yang, Y.; Xue, Y.; Luo, S. Efficacy and safety of radiofrequency ablation for hypertrophic obstructive cardiomyopathy: A systematic review and meta-analysis. *Clin. Cardiol.* **2020**, *43*, 450–458. [CrossRef] [PubMed]

Disclaimer/Publisher's Note: The statements, opinions and data contained in all publications are solely those of the individual author(s) and contributor(s) and not of MDPI and/or the editor(s). MDPI and/or the editor(s) disclaim responsibility for any injury to people or property resulting from any ideas, methods, instructions or products referred to in the content.

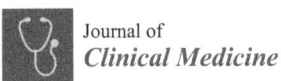

Review

Arrhythmic Risk Stratification among Patients with Hypertrophic Cardiomyopathy

Francesco Santoro [1,*], Federica Mango [1], Adriana Mallardi [1], Damiano D'Alessandro [1], Grazia Casavecchia [1], Matteo Gravina [2] Michele Correale [1] and Natale Daniele Brunetti [1]

[1] Cardiology Unit, Department of Medical and Surgical Sciences, University of Foggia, 71122 Foggia, Italy
[2] Radiology Unit, University Polyclinic Hospital of Foggia, 71100 Foggia, Italy
* Correspondence: dr.francesco.santoro.it@gmail.com; Tel.: +39-3802695183

Abstract: Hypertrophic cardiomyopathy (HCM) is a cardiac muscle disorder characterized by generally asymmetric abnormal hypertrophy of the left ventricle without abnormal loading conditions (such as hypertension or valvular heart disease) accounting for the left ventricular wall thickness or mass. The incidence of sudden cardiac death (SCD) in HCM patients is about 1% yearly in adults, but it is far higher in adolescence. HCM is the most frequent cause of death in athletes in the Unites States of America. HCM is an autosomal-dominant genetic cardiomyopathy, and mutations in the genes encoding sarcomeric proteins are identified in 30–60% of cases. The presence of this genetic mutation carries more than 2-fold increased risk for all outcomes, including ventricular arrhythmias. Genetic and myocardial substrate, including fibrosis and intraventricular dispersion of conduction, ventricular hypertrophy and microvascular ischemia, increased myofilament calcium sensitivity and abnormal calcium handling, all play a role as arrhythmogenic determinants. Cardiac imaging studies provide important information for risk stratification. Transthoracic echocardiography can be helpful to evaluate left ventricular (LV) wall thickness, LV outflow-tract gradient and left atrial size. Additionally, cardiac magnetic resonance can evaluate the prevalence of late gadolinium enhancement, which when higher than 15% of LV mass is a prognostic maker of SCD. Age, family history of SCD, syncope and non-sustained ventricular tachycardia at Holter ECG have also been validated as independent prognostic markers of SCD. Arrhythmic risk stratification in HCM requires careful evaluation of several clinical aspects. Symptoms combined with electrocardiogram, cardiac imaging tools and genetic counselling are the modern cornerstone for proper risk stratification.

Keywords: arrhythmias; genetic testing; hypertrophic cardiomyopathy; HCM; risk score; sudden cardiac death

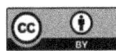

1. Introduction

Hypertrophic cardiomyopathy (HCM) is a cardiac muscle disorder characterized by generally asymmetric abnormal hypertrophy of the left ventricle without abnormal loading conditions (such as hypertension or valvular heart disease) accounting for the left ventricular wall thickness or mass [1,2]. In most of the cases, mutations in the genes encoding sarcomeric proteins are an autosomal dominant trait, responsible for the observed abnormality [1,2]. It is a quite common disease with an estimated prevalence of 1:500 in the general population, whereas in children the prevalence is much lower [3–5].

Sudden cardiac death (SCD), mainly caused by potentially fatal and unpredictable malignant ventricular arrhythmias (VAs) is the most adverse complication of HCM [6,7], with an annual incidence of SCD of approximately 1% in adult HCM patients and far higher in subgroups, such as pediatric HCM patients [8]. It may occur as the initial disease presentation, frequently in asymptomatic or mildly symptomatic young people and even athletes [9].

Several mechanisms predispose HCM patients to re-entrant VA. Genetic and myocardial substrate, including fibrosis and intraventricular dispersion of conduction, disruption of intercalated discs and myofibrillar disarray, ventricular hypertrophy and microvascular ischemia, increased myofilament calcium sensitivity and abnormal calcium handling all play a role as arrhythmogenic determinants [10–12]. Precipitating factors include intense physical exertion and participation in competitive sport or intrinsic features of the disease, such as left ventricular outflow obstruction, which can trigger life-threatening ventricular tachyarrhythmias [7].

Pharmacologic therapy has not proved to be effective alone in providing protection from SCD if compared to implantable cardioverter defibrillators (ICDs). If ICD implantation in secondary prevention is a well-established practice, the real challenge stands in identifying a special subset of HCM patients who are at high risk of SCD prior to a first event and would benefit from an ICD [13]. Therefore, systematic arrhythmic risk stratification at initial evaluation and then periodically is strongly recommended by current clinical guidelines [14]. The aim of this review is to highlight and discuss the most important factors associated with SCD in HCM to guide more comprehensive and exhaustive arrhythmic risk stratification.

2. Demographic and Clinical Characteristics

SCD can occur independently both in male and female HCM patients. However, the role of gender is still a matter of debate. While male patients more frequently show fibrosis on histological examination and consequently usually suffer more often from VA, no study has succeeded in proving a significant association between sex and SCD [2]. Age is a crucial point in SCD related to HCM. Given the potential lifetime risk of SCD in HCM patients, the incidence of SCD is far higher in adolescence and early adulthood, especially in those under the age of 35, with HCM being the most frequent cause of death in athletes in the US [15]. It is generally infrequent in patients older than 60 years as proved by Spirito et al., who demonstrated a significant reduction in SCD risk with increasing age [16].

Family history of SCD (FHSCD) is one of the major factors associated with arrhythmic risk in HCM patients. Personal anamnesis positive for FHSCD events, especially if multiple or occurring at a younger age, carries an increased risk of SCD among individuals of approximately 20% if compared to family without an obvious family history [17]. Nonetheless, definitions of FHSCD may vary considerably—with FHSCD generally considered when one or more first-degree relatives under 40 or 50 years of age dies incidentally within 1 h (witnessed) or 24 h (asymptomatic observation) after the symptom appears—thus influencing the effective individual's risk [18]. However, the average hazard ratio of FHSCD (irrespective of definition) was 1.27 (95% confidence interval (CI) 1.16–1.38) in a systematic review [19]. Different mechanisms responsible for FHSCD have been pointed out, although it is often a dilemma to identify the exact cause of death in the relatives. Considering the genetic nature of the disease, with affected relatives sharing the same genetic defect and with specific mutations associated with a worse prognosis, the extent of the environmental exposure cannot be adequately measured, all translating into a significant variability as to the genotype-phenotype correlation [20,21].

Syncope is defined as a temporary loss of consciousness secondary to transient global cerebral hypoperfusion. Spirito et al. defined unexplained syncope as syncope "of unknown origin, when it occurred in circumstances not clearly consistent with a neurally mediated event, i.e., without apparent explanation at rest or during ordinary daily activities, or during an intense effort" [16]. Multiple studies have shown that there is a significant association between unexplained syncope and SCD. In addition, since there are several causes of syncope in HCM including arrhythmias (sustained ventricular arrhythmias, supraventricular tachycardias, atrial fibrillation, brady-arrhythmias), exercise-related left ventricular outflow-tract obstruction (LVOTO), mitral regurgitation, ischemia and microvascular angina, although even neurally mediated syncope (vasovagal and situational) and orthostatic hypotension are possible, it is very important to deeply analyze the clinical context in which the syncope takes place [22,23]. Given such a high possibility of causes, clues from the patient and the witnesses may help. Additional attention should also be paid to exertional or recurrent syncope if it occurs in the young and in the recent past (<6 months) [24].

There is no particular association between NYHA functional class and the risk of SCD, with SCD being reported in all NYHA classes [25]. However, several factors are involved in functional limitations in HCM including the degree of diastolic dysfunction, LVOTO, cardiac ischemia and microvascular angina and atrial arrhythmias, especially atrial fibrillation (Table 1) [26].

Table 1. Demographic and clinical characteristics associated with the risk of sudden cardiac death. Legend: CMR = cardiac magnetic resonance, FHSCD = family history of sudden cardiac death, LVOTO = left ventricular outflow-tract obstruction, NHYA = New York Heart Association, VA = ventricular arrhythmias.

Sex	no significant association	🟡 male patients show more fibrosis on CMR and experience VA more often
Age	strong association	🟠 especially in adolescence and early adulthood
FHSCD	strong association	🟠 particularly if multiple or occurring at younger ages
Unexplained syncope	strong association	🟠 additional attention required if exertional or recurrent
NYHA class	no particular association	🟡 consider functional limitations, including degree of diastolic dysfunction, LVOTO, microvascular angina and atrial fibrillation

3. Non-Invasive Markers (ECG, Systolic Blood Pressure (SBP) Response to Exercise, Cardiopulmonary Exercise Test)

3.1. Electrocardiogram and Holter ECG

The twelve-lead electrocardiogram (ECG) has been used to evaluate electrophysiological abnormalities in HCM, and some of the ECG parameters including microvolt T-wave alternans, T-peak/T-end interval, fragmented QRS complexes and QT duration were found to be well correlated with myocardial fibrosis and arrhythmic events [27,28]. Given its fast and easy-to-perform evaluation, surface ECG analysis should always be included in each patient evaluation.

The microvolt T-wave alternans (MTWA) consists of microscopic alternans measured in microvolts on every heartbeat and is evidenced in the amplitude or the morphology of the T-wave. The alternation of T-waves in patients with HCM may possibly be explained as a result of inhomogeneous action, potential propagation and heterogeneous repolarization due to abnormal cell-to-cell conduction [29]. Özyılmaz S et al. tried to assess the relationship between the presence of MTWA and the predicted 5-year risk of SCD among patients with hypertrophic cardiomyopathy (HCM). Authors found that patients with MTWA on a Holter ECG had higher risk of ventricular arrhythmias [30].

Akboğa et al. [31] tried to evaluate the electrocardiographic T-wave peak to end interval (Tp–e) and Tp–e/QT corrected (QTc) ratio among patients with HCM. The patients were divided into two groups: those with VA (n = 26) and those without VA (n = 40). Tp–e interval was significantly longer and Tp–e/QTc ratio were significantly higher in HCM patients with VA.

The fragmented QRS (fQRS) complex reflects intraventricular conduction delay and may then be a superficial marker for myocardial fibrosis. Myocardial fibrosis in HCM patients usually has a patchy distribution, and it may not always be detected by pathological Q-waves on a 12-lead ECG. Konno T. et al. demonstrated that fQRS may have a substantially higher sensitivity and diagnostic accuracy if compared to pathological QRS in detecting myocardial fibrosis in HCM patients [32]. Considering its strong association with myocardial fibrosis, according to Ki-Woon Kang et al., fQRS may be a good candidate marker for prediction of VA in HCM patients [33].

Non-sustained ventricular tachycardia (NSVT), defined as three or more consecutive ventricular beats with a frequency of at least 120 beats per minute (bpm) lasting for less than 30 s, and not causing hemodynamic instability, is a very common finding in HCM patients and is often documented in Holter monitoring [34].

NSVT is more frequent with increasing hypertrophy, which may automatically reflect an increased grade of fibrosis and myofibrillar disarray, which themselves are useful predictors of the intrinsic arrhythmic risk of the disease [35,36].

Maron et al. [37] and McKenna et al. [38] showed that in HCM patients NSVT is more common in SCD patients. However, several studies examined the relationship between NSVT and SCD in HCM patients with a prevalence of NSVT ranging between 17% and 32% due to a non-uniform NSVT definition [39,40]. Even though a high incidence rate of NSVT (approximately 20–30%) in HCM patients over the age of 40 is reported, the risk of SCD linked to NSVT seems to be lower in older patients. According to Monserrat et al., a 4-fold increase in the risk of SCD was observed in patients aged ≤30 years with NSVT, (univariable HR, 4.35; 95% CI, 1.54–12.28; $p = 0.006$), but no effects were observed in older patients (univariable HR, 2.16; 95% CI, 0.82–5.69; $p = 0.1$), with frequency, duration and rate of NSVT not having predictive value [41].

3.2. Systolic Blood Pressure (SBP) Response to Exercise

An abnormal blood pressure response to exercise testing, defined as either a drop of at least 20 mmHg during effort or a failure to increase from rest to peak exercise by at least 20 mmHg, is a quite common finding in HCM patients, occurring in more than one out of three HCM patients [42].

Several mechanisms have been studied and are believed to be responsible for this phenomenon, including a hemodynamic hypothesis with an inappropriate drop in systemic vascular resistance, despite an appropriate increase in cardiac output, and/or LVOTO [43,44]. Although the prognostic role of systemic blood pressure response to exercise is still debated [45], it has been introduced as an additional risk factor from the European society of Cardiology (ESC) SCD 2022 guidelines and should be evaluated among patients with an intermediate SCD risk.

3.3. Cardiopulmonary Exercise Test

Cardiopulmonary exercise testing (CPET) data have been shown to improve the risk stratification of patients with heart failure. In the context of hypertrophic cardiomyopathy, a reduced oxygen consumption peak, an increased ventilation/carbon dioxide production slope and chronotropic incompetence correlate with a worse prognosis [46].

Two research groups of Magri et al. [47] and Masri et al. [48] showed that a reduced VO2 peak (i.e., <50%) and high VE/VCO2 slope are associated with overall mortality and SCD in HCM. Recently, the 2020 Guidelines on sports cardiology from ESC included in the indications for the execution of CPET the evaluation of exercise-induced symptoms or arrhythmias and the assessment of systolic blood pressure changes during exercise [49] (Table 2).

Table 2. Non-invasive test and prognostic role in patients with hypertrophic cardiomyopathy.

Type of Test	Evaluation	Prognostic Role
Holter ECG	Non-sustained ventricular tachycardia	🔴 Can stratify arrhythmic risk
Exercise Testing	Systolic blood pressure during exercise test	🟡 Prognostic role is still debated
Cardiopulmonary Exercise Test	Vo2 peak$Ve/Vco2	🔴 Reduced Vo2 peak (<50%); High Ve/Vco2 slope is associated with overall mortality

4. Role of Genetics

HCM is an autosomal-dominant genetic cardiomyopathy, and mutations in the genes encoding sarcomeric proteins are identified in 30–60% of index cases. Eight sarcomeric gene mutations are the most common described in literature for HCM: *MYBPC3*, *MYH7b*, *MYL2*, *MYL3*, *TNNT2*, *TNNI3*, *TPM1* and *ACTC1* (Table 3) [14]. The rate of major adverse cardiovascular events (MACEs) and premature death is significantly higher in patients carrying mutations in the genes encoding sarcomeric proteins than in negative ones [50]. Several analyses have shown that the presence of a mutation in the gene encoding sarcomeric proteins carries a more than 2-fold increased risk for all outcomes, including ventricular arrhythmias, which are more frequent in this group of patients [51]. Mutation of the MYH7 gene is associated with a more aggressive phenotype, characterized by younger onset age, higher degree of left ventricular hypertrophy and higher risk of SCD, resulting in a poor prognosis [52]. This group of patients also suffers from a higher incidence of atrial fibrillation (AF), which is associated with other risk factors such as left atrium (LA) enlargement, left ventricle (LV) wall thickness and LV outflow-tract obstruction. Compared with MYH7 gene mutation, patients with MYBPC3 mutation usually develop the disease at a later age and have a favorable progression of the disease although they are associated with a non-negligible risk of SCD compared to the healthy population. Because of the high risk, intense exercise should be routinely discouraged, especially in patients with the MYH7 gene mutation. Mutations in the TNNT2 gene may manifest with mild LV wall thickening but have more severe myocyte disarray, younger patients and a high incidence of SCD [53]. Given the clinical profile, patients carrying mutations in the genes encoding sarcomeric proteins should benefit from more intensive clinical surveillance. The ESC 2022 guidelines recommend genetic counselling and testing in all HCM patients (Class I, Level B), emphasizing the value of the genotype in guiding clinical management and determining prognosis [14]. They also represent an additional risk factor for HCM patients at intermediate SCD risk [14].

Table 3. Sarcomeric gene mutation described in hypertrophic cardiomyopathy.

Gene	Population Frequency	Protein
		Thick Myofilament Protein
MYBPC3	25%	Myosin binding protein-
MYH7B	20%	Myosin heavy chain
MYL2	<1%	Regulatory myosin light chain
MYL3	<1%	Essential myosin light chain

Table 3. Cont.

Gene	Population Frequency	Protein
		Thin Myofilament protein:
TNNT2	1.3%	Cardiac troponin T
TNNI3	1.3%	Cardiac troponin I
TPM1	>5%	Tropomyosin
ACTC1	<1%	Cardiac α-actin

5. Cardiac Imaging (Echocardiogram and Cardiac Magnetic Resonance)

Cardiac imaging plays a crucial role in management of HCM patients. The gold standard for diagnosis of HCM, assessment of treatment efficacy and prognosis is transthoracic echocardiography supported by cardiac magnetic resonance (CMR) imaging, which plays a central role in the diagnostic process. In 2014, the ESC validated an SCD risk prediction model that provides a 5-year SCD risk score for HCM patients. Echocardiography provides three of the seven parameters required in the 5-year SCD risk stratification score (LV wall thickness, LA size, LVOT gradient) [54]. LV hypertrophy is associated with increasing prevalence of NSVT and exercise-induced VAs. Several studies showed a significant correlation between severe hypertrophy of LV and SCD. Severe left ventricular hypertrophy (LVH) may contribute to SCD due to its effects on myocardial architecture, intramural small vessel disease and mass-to-coronary flow mismatch. A cut-off of maximum wall thickness $\geq$30 mm was used to indicate severe hypertrophy and was seen to be independently associated with SCD [2]. The LV wall thickness must be measured accurately at end-diastole, and elements attached to but not incorporated in the septum, such as papillary muscles, false tendons and right ventricular (RV) trabeculation, should be excluded because wall thickness could be overestimated. Left atrial diameter, quantified with echocardiography in the parasternal long axis, has been associated with SCD in HCM. AF and left atrial size may reflect the risk of SCD, as they may both relate to atrial remodeling secondary to increasing ventricular fibrosis, which makes the myocardium more susceptible to arrhythmias [7]. Diastolic dysfunction is common in HCM and results in elevated filling pressures and left atrial dilatation, so it is also a predictor of arrhythmic events. Patients with a restrictive diastolic filling pattern have adverse outcomes and should be observed closely. LVOTO is caused by systolic anterior movement of the mitral valve into the outflow tract, which creates a physical barrier impeding the flow of blood from the ventricle to the aorta during systole. Significant dynamic obstruction is defined as the presence of an instantaneous peak basal gradient $\geq$30 mmHg or after provocative maneuvers (Valsalva, standing and exercise) $\geq$50 mmHg [55]. Several studies reported a significant association between SCD and LVOTO. LVOTO can cause SCD either through a severe reduction in cardiac output or by myocardial ischemia due to the increase in left ventricular filling pressure, thus creating a substrate for ventricular arrhythmias. Although not included in the ESC risk calculator, additional factors, including LV systolic dysfunction, apical aneurysm, extensive LGE on CMR and presence of sarcomeric mutations, should be considered as possible modifiers of SCD risk [14]. Approximately 2–5% of patients with HCM, typically those with mid-ventricular hypertrophy, develop a left ventricular apical aneurysm associated with regional scarring. A higher incidence of clinical events during follow-up have been reported in this subgroup, including SCD and ventricular arrhythmia [6]. CMR allows accurate measurement of LV wall thickness, LV mass and LV ejection fraction and is the gold standard method for tissue characterization and volumetric evaluation of cardiac chambers. The extent of myocardial scarring on CMR has been shown to predict HCM-related adverse events. Myocardial fibrosis plays a central role in the genesis of arrhythmias through mechanisms of dispersion of electrical activity and formation of re-entry circuits that are responsible for the genesis of ventricular arrhythmias; this, as assessed by CMR, is independently associated with the occurrence of NSVT [56]. LGE is present in 65% of

HCM patients, typically in a patchy mid-wall pattern in areas of hypertrophy and at the anterior and posterior RV insertion points (Figures 1 and 2). A multicenter study found a linear correlation between the risk of SCD and amount of LGE. Extensive LGE on CMR defined as ≥15% of LV mass has been suggested as good predictor of SCD and appropriate ICD therapies in adults [57].

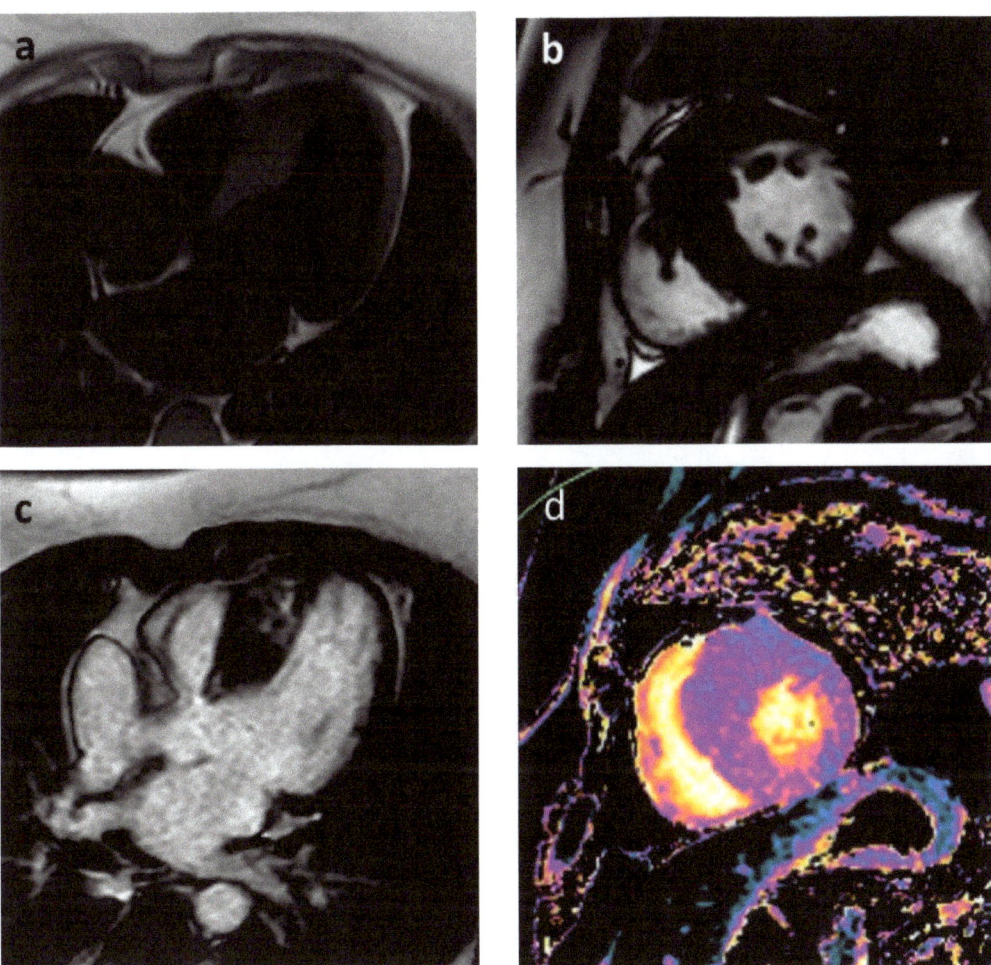

Figure 1. Asymmetric hypertrophic cardiomyopathy; thickening of the interventricular septum which can be evaluated with the T1-TSE four-chamber sequences (**a**); no evident edema in the short axis T2-STIR sequence (**b**); irregular deposits of mesocardial paramagnetic contrast medium in PSIR-TFE sequences in four chambers for the study of "late gadolinium enhancement" (**c**); T1 mapping analysis showing a diffuse increase in signal of the various segments of the walls of the left ventricle as from minimal diffuse interstitial fibrotic deposits (**d**).

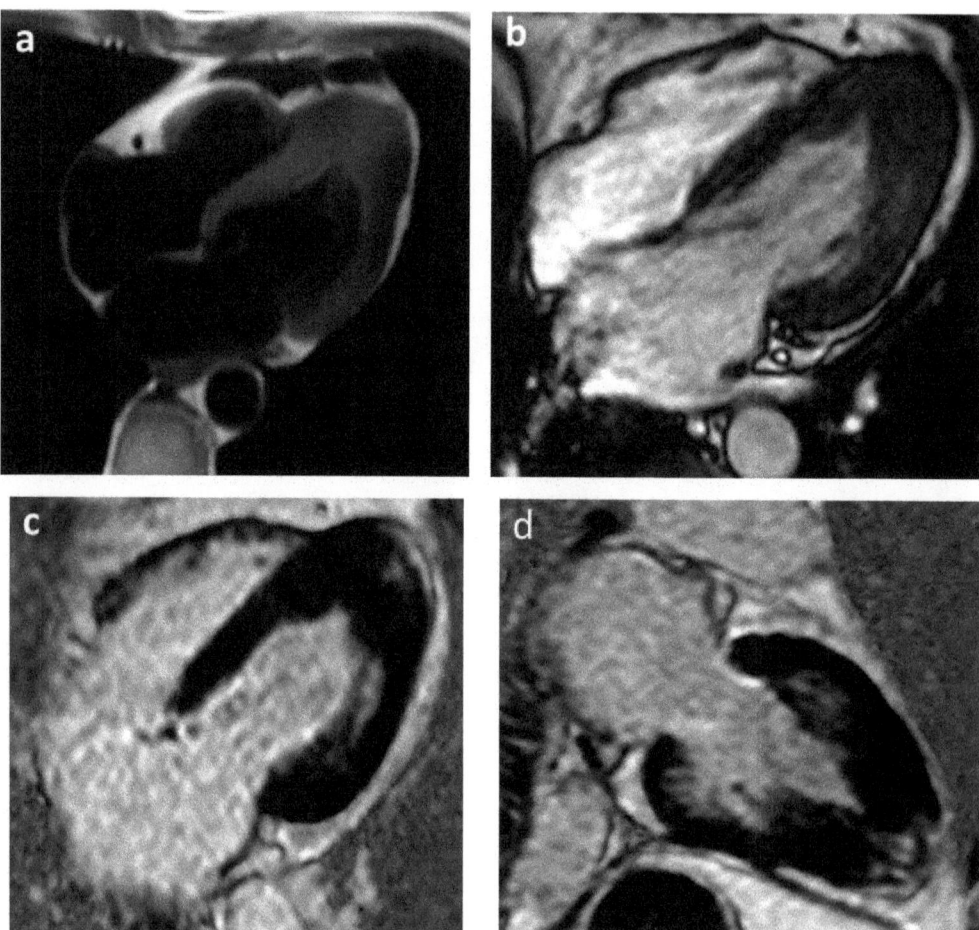

Figure 2. Apical hypertrophic cardiomyopathy with concentric thickening of the left ventricular wall at four-chamber T1-TSE sequences (**a**); absence of edema at four-chamber view T2-STIR sequence (**b**); slight increase in meso-subendocardial signal evident in PSIR-TFE sequences in four and two chambers for the study of "late gadolinium enhancement" (**c**,**d**) compatible with minimal fibrotic deposits.

6. Programmed Electrical Stimulation for Risk Stratification

The role of programmed electrical stimulation (PES) to stratify arrhythmic risk in HCM patients is still controversial. Moreover, most of the studies on the topic date back to the 1980s and are difficult to apply nowadays as most of the studied patients undergoing PES would now be considered high risk by current guidelines and thus already eligible for ICD implantation [58].

The largest study, performed in the late 1980s, proved that induction of ventricular arrhythmias with aggressive PES resulted in a 5-year survival decrease [59]. Aggressive stimulation protocol was able to induce polymorphic ventricular tachycardia (VT) in 76% of inducible patients, with polymorphic VT being the most commonly induced arrhythmia. Geibel et al. studied the effect of PES in HCM patients with or without documented VA through a standardized stimulation protocol [60]. In HCM patients, a stimulation protocol with up to two extra stimuli was sufficient to identify patients with documented sustained monomorphic VT, although there may be some problems with specificity. The sample was very small, which prevented further conclusions from being drawn.

On the other hand, more recently, according to Gatzoulis et al., inducibility at PES predicts SCD or appropriate device therapy in HCM and non-inducibility is associated with prolonged event-free survival [61].

At the moment, no explicit consensus on when to perform PES in HCM patients for arrhythmic risk stratification has been approved, and PES is not considered for arrhythmic risk stratification in current guidelines due to its invasiveness and also due to the fact that VAs induced by PES are still considered non-specific [14].

7. Clinical Score

Despite the fact that SCD in HCM patients is a rare event, it still remains the most adverse and fearsome complication, especially considering that it often occurs in asymptomatic patients and without premonitory symptoms. As a result, identifying a special subset of HCM patients at increased risk for SCD in primary prevention is to be considered a great clinical challenge, and several studies over decades have tried to recognize major clinical risk markers to stratify HCM patients at high risk for SCD who would benefit from an implantable cardioverter defibrillator (ICD) [62]. In addition, both the risk stratification strategy and the spread of ICDs into clinical practice have contributed to cutting disease-related mortality rates. Therefore, the need for arrhythmic risk stratification became a prevalent issue and led the scientific community to develop clinical risk scores. Over the past 20 years, two major risk stratification systems have been incorporated in the clinical practice according to the American College of Cardiology/American Heart Association (ACC/AHA) [63] and the ESC [54] (Table 4).

Table 4. Clinical score proposed by European society of cardiology (HCM RISK-SCD) and American heart association (AHA-HCM-SCD) for sudden cardiac death risk stratification. Legend: CMR = cardiac magnetic resonance, LV = left ventricle, LA = left atrium, LVOT = left ventricular outflow tract, NSVT = non-sustained ventricular tachycardia, LGE = late gadolinium enhancement, SCD = sudden cardiac death.

Clinical Score for SCD in HCM	HCM RISK-SCD (2014)	AHA-HCM-SCD (2020)
Age	✓	✓
Family History Of SCD	✓	✓
Syncope	✓	✓
LV Apical Aneurysm		✓
LV Systolic Dysfunction		✓
Maximal LV Wall Thickness	✓	✓
LA Size	✓	✓
LVOT Gradient	✓	✓
NSVT at Holter ECG	✓	✓
LGE at CMR		✓

ACC/AHA guidelines focus on a comprehensive analysis of non-invasive risk markers to identify patients most likely to benefit from an ICD in primary prevention, which is recommended to be performed at initial evaluation and every 1 to 2 years thereafter [63].

The American guidelines identify major risk factors for SCD: sudden death judged definitively or likely attributable to HCM in ≥ 1 first-degree or close relatives who are ≤ 50 years of age; massive LVH ≥ 30 mm in any LV segment; ≥ 1 recent episodes of syncope suspected by clinical history to be arrhythmic (i.e., unlikely to be of neurocardiogenic (vasovagal) etiology or related to LVOTO); LV apical aneurysm, independent of size; LV systolic dysfunction (EF <50%). According to these guidelines, if any of these major risk factors is present, ICD implantation is reasonable (class 2a indication).

If the decision to proceed to ICD implantation is still uncertain or the HCM patient does not seem to have increased risk of SCD after assessment of the previous risk factors, ICD may be considered in patients with extensive LGE determined by contrast-enhanced CMR imaging or NSVT present on ambulatory monitoring (class 2b indication in HCM patients aged $\geq$ 16 years; class 2a indication in HCM patients aged <16 years).

Moreover, additional parameters, including left atrial diameter and maximal LVOT gradient, may be considered to calculate an estimated 5-year SCD risk through a predictive risk score calculator available online (https://professional.heart.org/en/guidelines-and-statements/hcm-risk-calculator accessed on 15 February 2023) to assist shared decision-making between the physician and the patient for HCM patients $\geq$16 years old.

ESC guidelines [54] propose a more quantitative approach to SCD prediction through a score that predicts the 5-year risk for SCD. Seven factors have been included: age, LV wall thickness, LA size, LVOT gradient, NSVT, unexplained syncope and family history of SCD. Using a multivariable regression model, an online calculator has been created, and HCM patients are therefore stratified into a low (<4%), intermediate (with a risk of 4 to less than 6%) and high ($\geq$6%) 5-year risk of SCD.

According to ESC Guidelines, in patients with a low 5-year risk of SCD, an ICD is generally not indicated, whereas in patients with a high 5-year risk, an ICD should be considered. In patients at intermediate risk, an ICD may be considered, taking into account the risks and benefits of ICD implantation as well as the patient preferences in a view of a more individualized approach.

The ESC risk score was later validated with variable results by several research groups [64,65].

Neither the AHA-HCM-SCD calculator nor the ESC-HCM Risk-SCD score have been validated in the following cohorts of patients and therefore should not be used in pediatric patients (<16 years), elite/competitive athletes, HCM associated with metabolic diseases (e.g., Anderson–Fabry disease) and syndromes (e.g., Noonan syndrome).

Regarding risk stratification for SCD in pediatric patients, important news came from the ESC guidelines of 2022 [14]. These guidelines introduce The HCM Risk-Kids score [66] that has been developed and externally validated [67] for children with HCM (1–16 years of age). It includes unexplained syncope, maximal LV wall thickness, large left atrial diameter, low LVOT gradient and NSVT (https://hcmriskkids.org accessed on 15 February 2023). In contrast to adults' risk score, the age and family history of SCD did not improve its performance.

The American guidelines, however, do not yet accept a pediatric risk score. For the AHA/ACC 2020 guidelines on HCM, the decisions of ICD placement in pediatric patients must be based on individual judgment for each patient, taking into account all age-appropriate risk markers.

8. Future Perspectives

The increasing knowledge in several fields will provide additional insight for better risk stratification. Indeed, several novel approaches for left ventricular outflow tract may reduce arrhythmic risk. Apart from interventional therapy with surgery or radiofrequency [68], novel pharmacological treatment with selective and reversible inhibitors of the cardiac myosin ATPase have been demonstrated to provide improvement in exercise capacity, NYHA functional class and reduction in LVOT gradient [69]. Moreover, apart from cardiac magnetic resonance quantification of LV scars, novel software that evaluate scar features including border zone and conducting channels mass can better predict ICD intervention and therefore could be included in arrhythmic risk stratification [70]. All these data will be combined through artificial intelligence that could stratify different risk phenotypes [71].

9. Conclusions

Arrhythmic risk stratification in HCM requires careful evaluation of several clinical aspects. Symptoms combined with electrocardiogram, cardiac imaging tools and genetic counselling are the modern cornerstone for proper risk stratification.

Author Contributions: Conceptualization, F.S. and N.D.B.; methodology, F.S.; software, F.S.; validation, M.C.; formal analysis, F.S.; investigation, F.M., A.M. and D.D.; resources, N.D.B.; data curation, F.S.; writing—original draft preparation, F.M., D.D. and A.M.; writing—review and editing, F.S.; visualization, G.C. and M.G.; supervision, G.C. and M.G.; project administration, N.D.B.; funding acquisition, N.D.B. All authors have read and agreed to the published version of the manuscript.

Funding: This research received no external funding.

Institutional Review Board Statement: Not applicable.

Informed Consent Statement: Not applicable.

Data Availability Statement: Not applicable.

Conflicts of Interest: The authors declare no conflict of interest.

Abbreviations

AF = atrial fibrillation; ACC/AHA = American College of Cardiology/American Heart Association; CMR = cardiac magnetic resonance; CPET = cardiopulmonary exercise testing; ESC = European Society of Cardiology; FHSCD = family history of SCD; fQRS = fragmented QRS; ECG = electrocardiogram; HCM = hypertrophic cardiomyopathy; ICD = implantable cardioverter defibrillator; LA = left atrium, LGE = late gadolinium enhancement; LV = left ventricle; LVH = left ventricular hypertrophy; LVOTO = left ventricular outflow-tract obstruction; MACE = major adverse cardiovascular events; MTWA= microvolt T-wave alternans; PES = programmed electrical stimulation; NSVT = non-sustained ventricular tachycardia; NYHA = New York Heart Association; SCD = sudden cardiac death; Tp–e = T-wave peak to end interval; VA = ventricular arrhythmia; VT = ventricular tachycardia

References

1. Elliott, P.; Andersson, B.; Arbustini, E.; Bilinska, Z.; Cecchi, F.; Charron, P.; Dubourg, O.; Kuhl, U.; Maisch, B.; McKenna, W.J.; et al. Classification of the cardiomyopathies: A position statement from the european society of cardiology working group on myocardial and pericardial diseases. *Eur. Heart J.* **2008**, *29*, 270–276. [CrossRef] [PubMed]
2. O'Mahony, C.; Elliott, P.; McKenna, W. Sudden Cardiac Death in Hypertrophic Cardiomyopathy. *Circ. Arrhythm. Electrophysiol.* **2013**, *6*, 443–451. [CrossRef] [PubMed]
3. Fananapazir, L.; Epstein, N.D. Prevalence of Hypertrophic Cardiomyopathy and Limitations of Screening Methods. *Circulation* **1995**, *92*, 700–704. [CrossRef] [PubMed]
4. Zou, Y.; Song, L.; Wang, Z.; Ma, A.; Liu, T.; Gu, H.; Lu, S.; Wu, P.; Zhang, Y.; Shen, L.; et al. Prevalence of idiopathic hypertrophic cardiomyopathy in China: A population-based echocardiographic analysis of 8080 adults. *Am. J. Med.* **2004**, *116*, 14–18. [CrossRef] [PubMed]
5. Semsarian, C.; Ingles, J.; Maron, M.S.; Maron, B.J. New Perspectives on the Prevalence of Hypertrophic Cardiomyopathy. *J. Am. Coll. Cardiol.* **2015**, *65*, 1249–1254. [CrossRef] [PubMed]
6. Yinga, H.; Su, W.W.; Xiaoping, L. Risk factors of sudden cardiac death in hypertrophic cardiomyopathy. *Curr. Opin. Cardiol.* **2022**, *37*, 15–21.
7. Jordà, P.; García-Álvarez, A. Hypertrophic cardiomyopathy: Sudden cardiac death risk stratification in adults. *Glob. Cardiol. Sci. Pract.* **2018**, *2018*, 25. [CrossRef]
8. Elliott, P.M.; Poloniecki, J.; Dickie, S.; Sharma, S.; Monserrat, L.; Varnava, A.; Mahon, N.G.; McKenna, W.J. Sudden death in hypertrophic cardiomyopathy: Identification of high risk patients. *J. Am. Coll. Cardiol.* **2000**, *36*, 2212–2218. [CrossRef]
9. Maron, B.J.; Doerer, J.J.; Haas, T.S.; Tierney, D.M.; Mueller, F.O. Sudden deaths in young competitive athletes: Analysis of 1866 deaths in the United States, 1980–2006. *Circulation* **2009**, *199*, 1085–1092. [CrossRef]
10. Baudenbacher, F.; Schober, T.; Pinto, J.R.; Sidorov, V.Y.; Hilliard, F.; Solaro, R.J.; Potter, J.D.; Knollmann, B.C. Myofilament Ca^{2+} sensitization causes susceptibility to cardiac arrhythmia in mice. *J. Clin. Investig.* **2008**, *118*, 3893–3903. [CrossRef]
11. Sepp, R.; Severs, N.J.; Gourdie, R.G. Altered patterns of cardiac intercellular junction distribution in hypertrophic cardiomyopathy. *Heart* **1996**, *76*, 412–417. [CrossRef] [PubMed]

12. Bahrudin, U.; Morikawa, K.; Takeuchi, A.; Kurata, Y.; Miake, J.; Mizuta, E.; Adachi, K.; Higaki, K.; Yamamoto, Y.; Shirayoshi, Y.; et al. Impairment of ubiquitin-proteasome system by E334K cMyBPC modifies channel proteins, leading to electrophysiological dysfunction. *J. Mol. Biol.* **2011**, *413*, 857–878. [CrossRef] [PubMed]
13. Maron, B.J.; Haas, T.S.; Shannon, K.M.; Almquist, A.K.; Hodges, J.S. Long-term survival after cardiac arrest in hypertrophic cardiomyopathy. *Heart Rhythm* **2009**, *6*, 993–997. [CrossRef] [PubMed]
14. Zeppenfeld, K.; Tfelt-Hansen, J.; de Riva, M.; Winkel, B.G.; Behr, E.R.; Blom, N.A.; Charron, P.; Corrado, D.; Dagres, N.; de Chillou, C.; et al. 2022 ESC Guidelines for the management of patients with ventricular arrhythmias and the prevention of sudden cardiac death. *Eur. Heart J.* **2022**, *43*, 3997–4126. [CrossRef]
15. Gersh, B.J.; Maron, B.J.; Bonow, R.O.; Dearani, J.A.; Fifer, M.A.; Link, M.S.; Naidu, S.S.; Nishimura, R.A.; Ommen, S.R.; Rakowski, H.; et al. 2011 ACCF/AHA guideline for the diagnosis and treatment of hypertrophic cardiomyopathy: Executive summary: A report of the American College of Cardiology Foundation/American Heart Association Task Force on Practice Guidelines. *Circulation* **2011**, *124*, 2761–2796. [CrossRef]
16. Spirito, P.; Autore, C.; Rapezzi, C.; Bernabò, P.; Badagliacca, R.; Maron, M.S.; Bongioanni, S.; Coccolo, F.; Estes, N.M.; Barillà, C.S.; et al. Syncope and Risk of Sudden Death in Hypertrophic Cardiomyopathy. *Circulation* **2009**, *119*, 1703–1710. [CrossRef]
17. McKenna, W.; Deanfield, J.; Faruqui, A.; England, D.; Oakley, C.; Goodwin, J. Prognosis in hypertrophic cardiomyopathy: Role of age and clinical, electrocardiographic and hemodynamic features. *Am. J. Cardiol.* **1981**, *47*, 532–538. [CrossRef]
18. Geske, J.B.; Ommen, S.R.; Gersh, B.J. Hypertrophic cardiomyopathy: Clinical update. *JACC Heart Fail.* **2018**, *6*, 364–375. [CrossRef]
19. Christiaans, I.; Van Engelen, K.; Van Langen, I.M.; Birnie, E.; Bonsel, G.J.; Elliott, P.; Wilde, A.A. Risk stratification for sudden cardiac death in hypertrophic cardiomyopathy: Systematic review of clinical risk markers. *Europace* **2010**, *12*, 313–321. [CrossRef]
20. Charron, P.; Dubourg, O.; Desnos, M.; Bennaceur, M.; Carrier, L.; Camproux, A.-C.; Isnard, R.; Hagege, A.; Langlard, J.M.; Bonne, G.; et al. Clinical Features and Prognostic Implications of Familial Hypertrophic Cardiomyopathy Related to the Cardiac Myosin-Binding Protein C Gene. *Circulation* **1998**, *97*, 2230–2236. [CrossRef]
21. Niimura, H.; Bachinski, L.L.; Sangwatanaroj, S.; Watkins, H.; Chudley, A.E.; McKenna, W.; Kristinsson, A.; Roberts, R.; Sole, M.; Maron, B.J.; et al. Mutations in the Gene for Cardiac Myosin-Binding Protein C and Late-Onset Familial Hypertrophic Cardiomyopathy. *N. Engl. J. Med.* **1998**, *338*, 1248–1257. [CrossRef] [PubMed]
22. Schiavone, W.A.; Maloney, J.D.; Lever, H.M.; Castle, L.W.; Sterba, R.; Morant, V. Electrophysiologic Studies of Patients with Hypertrophic Cardiomyopathy Presenting with Syncope of Undetermined Etiology. *Pacing Clin. Electrophysiol.* **1986**, *9*, 476–481. [CrossRef] [PubMed]
23. Barriales-Villa, R.; Centurión-Inda, R.; Fernández-Fernández, X.; Ortiz, M.F.; Pérez-Alvarez, L.; Rodríguez García, I.; Hermida-Prieto, M.; Monserrat, L. Severe cardiac conduction disturbances and pacemaker implantation in patients with hypertrophic cardiomyopathy. *Rev. Esp. Cardiol.* **2010**, *63*, 985–988. [CrossRef] [PubMed]
24. Maron, B.J.; Shen, W.-K.; Link, M.S.; Epstein, A.E.; Almquist, A.K.; Daubert, J.P.; Bardy, G.H.; Favale, S.; Rea, R.F.; Boriani, G.; et al. Efficacy of Implantable Cardioverter–Defibrillators for the Prevention of Sudden Death in Patients with Hypertrophic Cardiomyopathy. *N. Engl. J. Med.* **2000**, *342*, 365–373. [CrossRef] [PubMed]
25. Monserrat, L.; Elliott, P.M.; Gimeno, J.R.; Sharma, S.; Penas-Lado, M.; McKenna, W.J. Non-sustained ventricular tachycardia in hypertrophic cardiomyopathy: An independent marker of sudden death risk in young patients. *J. Am. Coll. Cardiol.* **2003**, *42*, 873–879. [CrossRef]
26. Maron, B.J.; McKenna, W.J.; Danielson, G.K.; Kappenberger, L.J.; Kuhn, H.J.; Seidman, C.E.; Shah, P.M.; Spencer, W.H.; Spirito, P.; Cate, F.J.T.; et al. American College of Cardiology/European Society of Cardiology Clinical Expert Consensus Document on Hypertrophic Cardiomyopathy A report of the American College of Cardiology Foundation Task Force on Clinical Expert Consensus Documents and the European Society of Cardiology Committee for Practice Guidelines. *Eur. Heart J.* **2003**, *24*, 1965–1991. [CrossRef]
27. Konno, T.; Hayashi, K.; Fujino, N.; Oka, R.; Nomura, A.; Nagata, Y.; Hodatsu, A.; Sakata, K.; Furusho, H.; Takamura, M.; et al. Electrocardiographic QRS Fragmentation as a Marker for Myocardial Fibrosis in Hypertrophic Cardiomyopathy. *J. Cardiovasc. Electrophysiol.* **2015**, *26*, 1081–1087. [CrossRef]
28. Femenía, F.; on behalf of Fragmented QRS in Hypertrophic Obstructive Cardiomyopathy (FHOCM) Study Investigators; Arce, M.; Van Grieken, J.; Trucco, E.; Mont, L.; Abello, M.; Merino, J.L.; Rivero-Ayerza, M.; Gorenek, B.; et al. Fragmented QRS as a predictor of arrhythmic events in patients with hypertrophic obstructive cardiomyopathy. *J. Interv. Card. Electrophysiol.* **2013**, *38*, 159–165. [CrossRef]
29. Nienaber, C.A.; Gambhir, S.S.; Mody, F.V.; Ratib, O.; Huang, S.C.; Phelps, M.E.; Schelbert, H.R. Regional myocardial blood flow and glucose utilization in symptomatic patients with hypertrophic cardiomyopathy. *Circulation* **1993**, *87*, 1580–1590. [CrossRef]
30. Zyılmaz, S.; Püşüroğlu, H. Assessment of the relationship between the ambulatory electrocardiography-based micro T-wave alternans and the predicted risk score of sudden cardiac death at 5 years in patients with hypertrophic cardiomyopathy. *Anatol. J. Cardiol.* **2018**, *20*, 165–173. [CrossRef]
31. Akboğa, M.K.; Gülcihan Balcı, K.; Yılmaz, S.; Aydın, S.; Yayla, Ç.; Ertem, A.G.; Ünal, S.; Balcı, M.M.; Balbay, Y.; Aras, D.; et al. Tp-e interval and Tp-e/QTc ratio as novel surrogate markers for prediction of ventricular arrhythmic events in hypertrophic cardiomyopathy. *Anatol. J. Cardiol.* **2017**, *18*, 48–53. [CrossRef] [PubMed]

32. Bi, X.; Yang, C.; Song, Y.; Yuan, J.; Cui, J.; Hu, F.; Qiao, S. Quantitative fragmented QRS has a good diagnostic value on myocardial fibrosis in hypertrophic obstructive cardiomyopathy based on clinical-pathological study. *BMC Cardiovasc. Disord.* **2020**, *20*, 298. [CrossRef] [PubMed]
33. Kang, K.-W.; Janardhan, A.H.; Jung, K.T.; Lee, H.S.; Lee, M.-H.; Hwang, H.J. Fragmented QRS as a candidate marker for high-risk assessment in hypertrophic cardiomyopathy. *Heart Rhythm* **2014**, *11*, 1433–1440. [CrossRef]
34. Savage, D.D.; Seides, S.F.; Maron, B.J.; Myers, D.J.; Epstein, S.E. Prevalence of arrhythmias during 24-hour electrocardiographic monitoring and exercise testing in patients with obstructive and nonobstructive hypertrophic cardiomyopathy. *Circulation* **1979**, *59*, 866–875. [CrossRef] [PubMed]
35. Elliott, P.M.; Gimeno Blanes, J.R.; Mahon, N.G.; Poloniecki, J.D.; McKenna, W.J. Relation between severity of left-ventricular hypertrophy and prognosis in patients with hypertrophic cardiomyopathy. *Lancet* **2001**, *357*, 420–424. [CrossRef]
36. Spirito, P.; Rapezzi, C.; Autore, C.; Bruzzi, P.; Bellone, P.; Ortolani, P.; Fragola, P.V.; Chiarella, F.; Zoni-Berisso, M.; Branzi, A. Prognosis of asymptomatic patients with hypertrophic cardiomyopathy and nonsustained ventricular tachycardia. *Circulation* **1994**, *90*, 2743–2747. [CrossRef]
37. Maron, B.J.; Savage, D.D.; Wolfson, J.K.; Epstein, S.E. Prognostic significance of 24 hour ambulatory electrocardiographic monitoring in patients with hypertrophic cardiomyopathy: A prospective study. *Am. J. Cardiol.* **1981**, *48*, 252–257. [CrossRef]
38. McKenna, W.J.; England, D.; Doi, Y.L.; Deanfield, J.E.; Oakley, C.; Goodwin, J.F. Arrhythmia in hypertrophic cardiomyopathy. I: Influence on prognosis. *Br. Heart J.* **1981**, *46*, 168–172. [CrossRef]
39. Greulich, S.; Seitz, A.; Herter, D.; Günther, F.; Probst, S.; Bekeredjian, R.; Gawaz, M.; Sechtem, U.; Mahrholdt, H. Long-term risk of sudden cardiac death in hypertrophic cardiomyopathy: A cardiac magnetic resonance outcome study. *Eur. Heart J. Cardiovasc. Imaging* **2021**, *22*, 732–741. [CrossRef]
40. Efthimiadis, G.K.; Parcharidou, D.G.; Giannakoulas, G.; Pagourelias, E.D.; Charalampidis, P.; Savvopoulos, G.; Ziakas, A.; Karvounis, H.; Styliadis, I.H.; Parcharidis, G.E. Left Ventricular Outflow Tract Obstruction as a Risk Factor for Sudden Cardiac Death in Hypertrophic Cardiomyopathy. *Am. J. Cardiol.* **2009**, *104*, 695–699. [CrossRef]
41. Wang, W.; Lian, Z.; Rowin, E.J.; Maron, B.J.; Maron, M.S.; Link, M.S. Prognostic Implications of Nonsustained Ventricular Tachycardia in High-Risk Patients with Hypertrophic Cardiomyopathy. *Circ. Arrhythm. Electrophysiol.* **2017**, *10*, e004604. [CrossRef] [PubMed]
42. Sadoul, N.; Prasad, K.; Elliott, P.M.; Bannerjee, S.; Frenneaux, M.P.; McKenna, W.J. Prospective prognostic assessment of blood pressure response during exercise in patients with hypertrophic cardiomyopathy. *Circulation* **1997**, *96*, 2987–2991. [CrossRef] [PubMed]
43. Counihan, P.J.; Frenneaux, M.P.; Webb, D.J.; McKenna, W.J. Abnormal vascular responses to supine exercise in hypertrophic cardiomyopathy. *Circulation* **1991**, *84*, 686–696. [CrossRef] [PubMed]
44. Elliott, P.M.; Gimeno, J.R.; Tomé, M.T.; Shah, J.; Ward, D.; Thaman, R.; Mogensen, J.; McKenna, W.J. Left ventricular outflow tract obstruction and sudden death risk in patients with hypertrophic cardiomyopathy. *Eur. Heart J.* **2006**, *27*, 1933–1941. [CrossRef]
45. Wang, R.S.; Rowin, E.J.; Maron, B.J.; Maron, M.S.; Maron, B.A. A novel patient-patient network medicine approach to refine hypertrophic cardiomyopathy subgrouping: Implications for risk stratification. *Cardiovasc. Res.* **2023**, *119*, e125–e127. [CrossRef]
46. Sinagra, G.; Carriere, C.; Clemenza, F.; Minà, C.; Bandera, F.; Zaffalon, D.; Gugliandolo, P.; Merlo, M.; Guazzi, M.; Agostoni, P. Risk stratification in cardiomyopathy. *Eur. J. Prev. Cardiol.* **2020**, *27* (Suppl. S2), 52–58. [CrossRef]
47. Magrì, D.; Limongelli, G.; Re, F.; Agostoni, P.; Zachara, E.; Correale, M.; Mastromarino, V.; Santolamazza, C.; Casenghi, M.; Pacileo, G.; et al. Cardiopulmonary exercise test and sudden cardiac death risk in hypertrophic cardiomyopathy. *Heart* **2016**, *102*, 602–609. [CrossRef]
48. Masri, A.; Pierson, L.M.; Smedira, N.G.; Agarwal, S.; Lytle, B.W.; Naji, P.; Thamilarasan, M.; Lever, H.M.; Cho, L.S.; Desai, M.Y. Predictors of long-term outcomes in patients with hypertrophic cardiomyopathy undergoing cardiopulmonary stress testing and echocardiography. *Am. Heart J.* **2015**, *169*, 684–692.e1. [CrossRef]
49. Pelliccia, A.; Sharma, S.; Gati, S.; Bäck, M.; Börjesson, M.; Caselli, S.; Collet, J.-P.; Corrado, D.; Drezner, J.A.; Halle, M.; et al. 2020 ESC Guidelines on sports cardiology and exercise in patients with cardiovascular disease. *Eur. Heart J.* **2021**, *42*, 17–96. [CrossRef]
50. Ho, C.Y.; Day, S.M.; Ashley, E.A.; Michels, M.; Pereira, A.C.; Jacoby, D.; Cirino, A.L.; Fox, J.C.; Lakdawala, N.K.; Ware, J.S.; et al. Genotype and Lifetime Burden of Disease in Hypertrophic Cardiomyopathy: Insights from the Sarcomeric Human Cardiomyopathy Registry (SHaRe). *Circulation* **2018**, *138*, 1387–1398. [CrossRef]
51. Kim, H.Y.; Park, J.E.; Lee, S.-C.; Jeon, E.-S.; On, Y.K.; Kim, S.M.; Choe, Y.H.; Ki, C.-S.; Kim, J.-W.; Kim, K.H. Genotype-Related Clinical Characteristics and Myocardial Fibrosis and Their Association with Prognosis in Hypertrophic Cardiomyopathy. *J. Clin. Med.* **2020**, *9*, 1671. [CrossRef] [PubMed]
52. Dimitrow, P.P.; Chojnowska, L.; Rudzinski, T.; Piotrowski, W.; Ziółkowska, L.; Wojtarowicz, A.; Wycisk, A.; Dabrowska-Kugacka, A.; Nowalany-Kozielska, E.; Sobkowicz, B.; et al. Sudden death in hypertrophic cardiomyopathy: Old risk factors re-assessed in a new model of maximalized follow-up. *Eur. Heart J.* **2010**, *31*, 3084–3093. [CrossRef] [PubMed]
53. Velicki, L.; Jakovljevic, D.G.; Preveden, A.; Golubovic, M.; Bjelobrk, M.; Ilic, A.; Stojsic, S.; Barlocco, F.; Tafelmeier, M.; Okwose, N.; et al. Genetic determinants of clinical phenotype in hypertrophic cardiomyopathy. *BMC Cardiovasc. Disord.* **2020**, *20*, 516. [CrossRef] [PubMed]

54. Elliott, P.M.; Anastasakis, A.; Borger, M.A.; Borggrefe, M.; Cecchi, F.; Charron, P.; Hagege, A.A.; Lafont, A.; Limongelli, G.; Mahrholdt, H.; et al. 2014 ESC Guidelines on diagnosis and management of hypertrophic cardiomyopathy: The Task Force for the Diagnosis and Management of Hypertrophic Cardiomyopathy of the European Society of Cardiology (ESC). *Eur. Heart J.* **2014**, *35*, 2733–2779.
55. Turvey, L.; Augustine, D.X.; Robinson, S.; Oxborough, D.; Stout, M.; Smith, N.; Harkness, A.; Williams, L.; Steeds, R.P.; Bradlow, W. Transthoracic echocardiography of hypertrophic cardiomyopathy in adults: A practical guideline from the British Society of Echocardiography. *Echo Res. Pract.* **2021**, *8*, G61–G86. [CrossRef]
56. Habib, M.; Hoss, S.; Rakowski, H. Evaluation of Hypertrophic Cardiomyopathy: Newer Echo and MRI Approaches. *Curr. Cardiol. Rep.* **2019**, *21*, 75. [CrossRef]
57. Weissler-Snir, A.; Dorian, P.; Rakowski, H.; Care, M.; Spears, D. Primary prevention implantable cardioverter-defibrillators in hypertrophic cardiomyopathy-Are there predictors of appropriate therapy? *Heart Rhythm* **2021**, *18*, 63–70. [CrossRef]
58. Watson, R.M.; Schwartz, J.L.; Maron, B.J.; Tucker, E.; Rosing, D.R.; Josephson, M.E. Inducible polymorphic ventricular tachycardia and ventricular fibrillation in a subgroup of patients with hypertrophic cardiomyopathy at high risk for sudden death. *J. Am. Coll. Cardiol.* **1987**, *10*, 761–774. [CrossRef]
59. Kuck, K.-H.; Kunze, K.-P.; Schluter, M.; Nienaber, C.A.; Costard, A. Programmed electrical stimulation in hypertrophic cardiomyopathy. Results in patients with and without cardiac arrest or syncope. *Eur. Heart J.* **1988**, *9*, 177–185. [CrossRef]
60. Geibel, A.; Brugada, P.; Zehender, M.; Stevenson, W.; Waldecker, B.; Wellens, H.J. Value of programmed electrical stimulation using a standardized ventricular stimulation protocol in hypertrophic cardiomyopathy. *Am. J. Cardiol.* **1987**, *60*, 738–739. [CrossRef]
61. Gatzoulis, K.A.; Georgopoulos, S.; Antoniou, C.-K.; Anastasakis, A.; Dilaveris, P.; Arsenos, P.; Sideris, S.; Tsiachris, D.; Archontakis, S.; Sotiropoulos, E.; et al. Programmed ventricular stimulation predicts arrhythmic events and survival in hypertrophic cardiomyopathy. *Int. J. Cardiol.* **2018**, *254*, 175–181. [CrossRef] [PubMed]
62. Efthimiadis, G.K.; Pliakos, C.; Pagourelias, E.D.; Parcharidou, D.G.; Giannakoulas, G.; Kamperidis, V.; Hadjimiltiades, S.; Karvounis, C.; Gavrielidis, S.; Styliadis, I.H.; et al. Identification of high risk patients with hypertrophic cardiomyopathy in a northern Greek population. *Cardiovasc. Ultrasound* **2009**, *7*, 37. [CrossRef] [PubMed]
63. Ommen, S.R.; Mital, S.; Burke, M.A.; Day, S.M.; Deswal, A.; Elliott, P.; Evanovich, L.L.; Hung, J.; Joglar, J.A.; Kantor, P.; et al. 2020 AHA/ACC Guideline for the Diagnosis and Treatment of Patients with Hypertrophic Cardiomyopathy: A Report of the American College of Cardiology/American Heart Association Joint Committee on Clinical Practice Guidelines. *Circulation* **2020**, *142*, e558–e631.
64. Maron, B.J.; Casey, S.A.; Chan, R.H.; Garberich, R.F.; Rowin, E.J.; Maron, M.S. Independent Assessment of the European Society of Cardiology Sudden Death Risk Model for Hypertrophic Cardiomyopathy. *Am. J. Cardiol.* **2015**, *116*, 757–764. [CrossRef]
65. Vriesendorp, P.A.; Schinkel, A.F.; Liebregts, M.; Theuns, D.A.; van Cleemput, J.; Ten Cate, F.J.; Willems, R.; Michels, M. Validation of the 2014 European Society of Cardiology guidelines risk prediction model for the primary prevention of sudden cardiac death in hypertrophic cardiomyopathy. *Circ. Arrhythm. Electrophysiol.* **2015**, *8*, 829–835. [CrossRef] [PubMed]
66. Norrish, G.; Ding, T.; Field, E.; Ziółkowska, L.; Olivotto, I.; Limongelli, G.; Anastasakis, A.; Weintraub, R.; Biagini, E.; Ragni, L.; et al. Development of a novel risk prediction model for sudden cardiac death in childhood hypertrophic cardiomyopathy (HCM risk-kids). *JAMA Cardiol.* **2019**, *4*, 918–927. [CrossRef] [PubMed]
67. Norrish, G.; Qu, C.; Field, E.; Cervi, E.; Khraiche, D.; Klaassen, S.; Ojala, T.H.; Sinagra, G.; Yamazawa, H.; Marrone, C.; et al. External validation of the HCM Risk-Kids model for predicting sudden cardiac death in childhood hypertrophic cardiomyopathy. *Eur. J. Prev. Cardiol.* **2022**, *29*, 678–686. [CrossRef] [PubMed]
68. Sorajja, P. Alcohol Septal Ablation for Obstructive Hypertrophic Cardiomyopathy: Alcohol Septal Ablation for Obstructive Hypertrophic Cardiomyopath. *J. Am. Coll. Cardiol.* **2017**, *70*, 489–494. [CrossRef] [PubMed]
69. Olivotto, I.; Oreziak, A.; Barriales-Villa, R.; Abraham, T.P.; Masri, A.; Garcia-Pavia, P.; Saberi, S.; Lakdawala, N.K.; Wheeler, M.T.; Owens, A.; et al. Mavacamten for treatment of symptomatic obstructive hypertrophic cardiomyopathy (EXPLORER-HCM): A randomised, double-blind, placebo-controlled, phase 3 trial. *Lancet* **2020**, *396*, 759–769. [CrossRef]
70. Sánchez-Somonte, P.; Quinto, L.; Garre, P.; Zaraket, F.; Alarcón, F.; Borràs, R.; Caixal, G.; Vázquez, S.; Prat, S.; Ortiz-Perez, J.T.; et al. Scar channels in cardiac magnetic resonance to predict appropriate therapies in primary prevention. *Heart Rhythm* **2021**, *18*, 1336–1343. [CrossRef]
71. Mancio, J.; Pashakhanloo, F.; El-Rewaidy, H.; Jang, J.; Joshi, G.; Csecs, I.; Ngo, L.; Rowin, E.; Manning, W.; Maron, M.; et al. Machine learning phenotyping of scarred myocardium from cine in hypertrophic cardiomyopathy. *Eur. Heart J. Cardiovasc. Imaging* **2022**, *23*, 532–542. [CrossRef] [PubMed]

Disclaimer/Publisher's Note: The statements, opinions and data contained in all publications are solely those of the individual author(s) and contributor(s) and not of MDPI and/or the editor(s). MDPI and/or the editor(s) disclaim responsibility for any injury to people or property resulting from any ideas, methods, instructions or products referred to in the content.

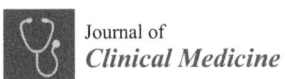

Review

Revisiting Diagnosis and Treatment of Hypertrophic Cardiomyopathy: Current Practice and Novel Perspectives

Andrea Ottaviani [1,†], Davide Mansour [1,†], Lorenzo V. Molinari [1,†], Kristian Galanti [1], Cesare Mantini [1], Mohammed Y. Khanji [2,3,4], Anwar A. Chahal [2,5,6], Marco Zimarino [1,7], Giulia Renda [1,7], Luigi Sciarra [8], Francesco Pelliccia [9], Sabina Gallina [1,7,*] and Fabrizio Ricci [1,7,10,*]

1. Department of Neuroscience, Imaging and Clinical Sciences, "G. D'Annunzio" University of Chieti-Pescara, 66100 Chieti, Italy
2. Barts Heart Centre, Barts Health NHS Trust, London EC1A 7BE, UK
3. Newham University Hospital, Barts Health NHS Trust, London E13 8SL, UK
4. NIHR Barts Biomedical Research Centre, William Harvey Research Institute, Queen Mary University of London, London EC1A 7BE, UK
5. Inherited Cardiovascular Diseases, WellSpan Health, Lancaster, PA 17605, USA
6. Cardiac Electrophysiology, Cardiovascular Division, Hospital of the University of Pennsylvania, Philadelphia, PA 17605, USA
7. Heart Department, SS. Annunziata Hospital, ASL 2 Abruzzo, 66100 Chieti, Italy
8. Department of Life, Health and Environmental Sciences, University of L'Aquila, 67100 L'Aquila, Italy
9. Department of Cardiovascular Sciences, Sapienza University, 00166 Rome, Italy
10. Department of Clinical Sciences, Lund University, 21428 Malmö, Sweden
* Correspondence: sabina.gallina@unich.it (S.G.); fabrizio.ricci@unich.it (F.R.)
† These authors contributed equally to this work.

Abstract: Sarcomeric hypertrophic cardiomyopathy (HCM) is a prevalent genetic disorder characterised by left ventricular hypertrophy, myocardial disarray, and an increased risk of heart failure and sudden cardiac death. Despite advances in understanding its pathophysiology, treatment options for HCM remain limited. This narrative review aims to provide a comprehensive overview of current clinical practice and explore emerging therapeutic strategies for sarcomeric HCM, with a focus on cardiac myosin inhibitors. We first discuss the conventional management of HCM, including lifestyle modifications, pharmacological therapies, and invasive interventions, emphasizing their limitations and challenges. Next, we highlight recent advances in molecular genetics and their potential applications in refining HCM diagnosis, risk stratification, and treatment. We delve into emerging therapies, such as gene editing, RNA-based therapies, targeted small molecules, and cardiac myosin modulators like mavacamten and aficamten, which hold promise in modulating the underlying molecular mechanisms of HCM. Mavacamten and aficamten, selective modulators of cardiac myosin, have demonstrated encouraging results in clinical trials by reducing left ventricular outflow tract obstruction and improving symptoms in patients with obstructive HCM. We discuss their mechanisms of action, clinical trial outcomes, and potential implications for the future of HCM management. Furthermore, we examine the role of precision medicine in HCM management, exploring how individualised treatment strategies, including exercise prescription as part of the management plan, may optimise patient outcomes. Finally, we underscore the importance of multidisciplinary care and patient-centred approaches to address the complex needs of HCM patients. This review also aims to encourage further research and collaboration in the field of HCM, promoting the development of novel and more effective therapeutic strategies, such as cardiac myosin modulators, to hopefully improve the quality of life and outcome of patients with sarcomeric HCM.

Keywords: hypertrophic cardiomyopathy; treatment; myosin modulators; genetics; cardiovascular imaging

Citation: Ottaviani, A.; Mansour, D.; Molinari, L.V.; Galanti, K.; Mantini, C.; Khanji, M.Y.; Chahal, A.A.; Zimarino, M.; Renda, G.; Sciarra, L.; et al. Revisiting Diagnosis and Treatment of Hypertrophic Cardiomyopathy: Current Practice and Novel Perspectives. *J. Clin. Med.* **2023**, *12*, 5710. https://doi.org/10.3390/jcm12175710

Academic Editor: Thomas H. Schindler

Received: 29 July 2023
Revised: 26 August 2023
Accepted: 29 August 2023
Published: 1 September 2023

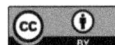

Copyright: © 2023 by the authors. Licensee MDPI, Basel, Switzerland. This article is an open access article distributed under the terms and conditions of the Creative Commons Attribution (CC BY) license (https://creativecommons.org/licenses/by/4.0/).

1. Introduction

Hypertrophic cardiomyopathy (HCM) is a hereditary cardiac condition featuring left ventricular hypertrophy (LVH), which abnormal loading conditions cannot fully explain. It has been traditionally viewed as an uncommon condition with few effective treatment alternatives for controlling the possibility of dangerous disease advancement and malignant ventricular arrhythmias [1]. HCM is a common inheritable cardiac disorder usually following an autosomal dominant inheritance pattern. LVH in the absence of cardiovascular diseases occurs in approximately 1:500 subjects in the general population; when both clinical and genetic diagnoses are considered [2], this prevalence increases to 1 case per 200 [3–5]. HCM stems from multiple mutations that affect at least 14 genes [6] responsible for sarcomeric proteins. Over 1400 distinct variants in at least 11 genes are known to cause HCM; still, nearly 70% occur either in the MYH7 gene, which encodes for the β-myosin heavy chain, or in the MYBPC3 gene, which encodes for the myosin binding protein C. HCM can also occur as part of a syndrome and might exhibit non-sarcomeric genocopies. It is essential that these are identified, as targeted therapies are available for them, whereas treatments for sarcomeric HCM would be inappropriate. Key distinctions include amyloidosis, Fabry disease, glycogen storage diseases, and syndromic disorders, such as RASopathies, Timothy syndrome, and Emery–Dreifuss muscular dystrophy (FHL1).

1.1. Pathophysiology

HCM is characterised by the absence of any abnormal loading conditions while exhibiting LVH. The clinical manifestation of HCM is varied and includes several pathological features, which stem from both the direct functional impacts of the disease-causing mutation and the secondary changes in function that the affected myocardium undergoes in response to it.

HCM features myocardial fibrosis (ranging from microscopic fibrosis within the myocardium to significant macroscopic scarring), abnormalities in small coronary vessels (microvascular remodelling and dysfunction), haphazard organisation of tissue (myocardial disarray), papillary muscle abnormalities (hypertrophy, feathering, apical insertion), and anomalies in the mitral valve (elongated anterior leaflet), as well as ventricular and supraventricular tachyarrhythmias.

The varied genetic makeup of HCM plays a significant role in explaining the wide range of differences seen among patients with HCM. In a study by Beltrami et al., MYBPC3-related HCM showed an increased long-term prevalence of systolic dysfunction compared with MYH7, despite similar outcomes [7]. Such observations suggest different pathophysiology of clinical progression in the two subsets and may prove relevant for understanding of genotype-phenotype correlations in HCM. Additionally, relatives with the same genetic mutation may present with different clinical features. As a result, the management of HCM patients poses a considerable challenge, necessitating tailored and individualised approaches [1].

1.2. Obstructive vs. Nonobstructive HCM

Obstructive HCM (oHCM) features LVOT obstruction (LVOTO), defined by the presence of a peak LVOT gradient of ≥ 30 mmHg by continuous wave Doppler echocardiography, with resting or provoked gradients ≥ 50 mmHg generally considered to be the threshold for septal reduction therapy in those patients with drug-refractory symptoms [3]. LVOTO is a common finding in HCM patients and may be present during rest or provoked by a Valsalva manoeuvre, exercise, or drug. It is a dynamic consequence, dependent on preload conditions and anatomy, in which the LVOT becomes obstructed and typically affects around 50% of individuals diagnosed with HCM at some stage. In addition, individuals with oHCM often experience symptoms of heart failure (HF), such as shortness of breath, difficulty exercising, and angina. They may also experience syncope or pre-syncope, particularly on exertion or lifting. Since its initial discovery, clinical and preclinical research findings have transformed the understanding of HCM from a rare and dangerous condition to a relatively frequent disease with generally stable progression. Compared to other inherited heart muscle disorders, HCM has lower morbidity and mortality (including sudden death) [1]. While some individuals with HCM may have a typical lifespan, LVOTO, atrial fibrillation, or ventricular arrhythmias can considerably impact each person's prognosis and quality of life.

1.3. HCM Phenocopies

HCM is a genetic cause of cardiomyopathy that is widespread worldwide. Genetic testing advancements have improved the detection of sarcomeric mutations responsible for HCM [8]. However, this has also highlighted the importance of identifying inborn errors of metabolism or metabolic storage disorders that can mimic HCM (phenocopies). Distinguishing these conditions can be challenging. HCM phenocopies are common, and it is crucial to differentiate them early due to significant differences in prognosis, management, and natural history compared to sarcomeric HCM (Table 1).

Table 1. Red flags for differential diagnosis between sarcomeric HCM and phenocopies.

	Inheritance Pattern	Ancillary Signs and Symptoms	ECG Abnormalities	Laboratory Findings	Echocardiography	CMR Imaging
Sarcomeric HCM	AD	Uncommon	- High QRS voltages - LV strain pattern - Giant TWI - Q waves of pseudo-necrosis		- Moderate-to-severe LVH (asymmetrical and septal but potentially found at any location) - 10-20% can have RVH - Diastolic dysfunction - LVOT obstruction - Mitral valve abnormalities (mitral SAM, leaflets elongation, chordal elongation, laxity, and hypermobility) - Papillary muscle abnormalities (hypertrophy, splaying and apical displaced insertion) - Atrial enlargement - Apical aneurysm	- LGE at RV insertion points and intramural patchy more frequently observe at sites of hypertrophied segments - Perfusion defects - Increased values of T1 mapping indices - Increased T2 mapping/T2w hyperintensity in hot-phase of disease
Anderson–Fabry disease	X-linked	- Visual impairment - Sensorineural deafness - Paranesthesia/sensory abnormalities - Angiokeratoma - Higher stroke risk - Males > females, but females can be affected (lyonization) from mild conduction disease to overt oHCM	- Short PR interval - Pre-excitation - AV block	- In males, low or undetectable alpha-1-galactosidase - Proteinuria with/without reduced glomerular filtration rate	- Concentric LVH ((but can have LVOTO) - Increased atrioventricular valve thickness - Increased RV free wall thickness - Global hypokinesia (with/without LV dilatation)	- Basal-mid infero-lateral LGE - Low T1 mapping values (accumulation/hypertrophy phases) - T1 pseudonormalisation (advanced stage) - Progressive T1 mapping dispersion
Cardiac amyloidosis	AD (for h-TTR)	- Carpal tunnel syndrome (bilateral) - Visual impairment - Paranesthesia/sensory abnormalities - Autonomic dysfunction	- Low QRS voltage - AV block - Pseudoinfarct pattern - Bundle branch block	Proteinuria with/without reduced glomerular filtration rate	- Ground-glass appearance of myocardium - Thickened interatrial septum, atrioventricular valve thickness, RV free wall - Pericardial effusion - Global hypokinesia (with/without LV dilatation) - relative longitudinal apical sparing (cherry apex)	- Diffuse subendocardial LGE (zebra pattern) - Abnormal T1 nulling - Increased T1 mapping indices - Increased T2 mapping values (AL)
Mitochondrial cardiomyopathies	X-linked or matrilinear inheritance	- Sensorineural deafness - Learning difficulties/mental retardation - Visual impairment - Muscle weakness	- Short PR interval Preexcitation - Abnormal CPET with low VO$_2$ max	- ↑ CK - ↑ AST, ALT - Lactate	Global hypokinesia (with/without LV dilatation)	- Large amount non-ischemic LGE pattern, mostly confined to the basal LV inferolateral wall

Table 1. Cont.

	Inheritance Pattern	Ancillary Signs and Symptoms	ECG Abnormalities	Laboratory Findings	Echocardiography	CMR Imaging
Hypertensive heart disease	None	Uncommon	Isolated LVH	Microalbuminuria	- LVH symmetrical or eccentric (mild to moderate). - Normal systolic and diastolic function	Non-specific findings
Danon disease	X-linked	- Learning difficulties/cognitive impairment - Visual impairment	- Short PR - Pre-excitation - AV block - Extreme LVH (Sokolow > 100)	- ↑ CK - ↑ AST, ALT	- Extreme concentric LVH - Global hypokinesia (with/without LV dilatation)	- Large amount subendocardial or transmural scarring, with typical septal sparing
Athlete's heart	None	Uncommon	Isolated LVH TWI in anterior precordial leads with J point elevation (consider ethnicity)		- LVH (mild to moderate) - Normal systolic function - Normal diastolic function	- Absence of LGE or junctional pattern - Low/normal T1 mapping indices

AD, autosomal dominant; ALT, alanine aminotransferase; AST, aspartate aminotransferase; AV, atrioventricular; CK, creatine kinase; CPET, cardiopulmonary exercise testing; ECG, electrocardiogram; HCM, hypertrophic cardiomyopathy; LGE, late gadolinium enhancement; LV, left ventricle; LVH, left ventricular hypertrophy; LVOTO, left ventricular outflow tract obstruction; RV, right ventricle; RVH, right ventricular hypertrophy; TWI, T-wave inversion.

- **Anderson–Fabry disease:** this is a genetic disorder caused by mutations in the α-galactosidase A (GLA) gene that results in the accumulation of glycosphingolipids in various systems of the body. The disease is known to cause LVH, which can be diagnosed through echocardiography in almost 50% of male patients aged 30–40 [9]. LVH in Anderson–Fabry Disease happens due to an abnormal build-up of glycosphingolipids, leading to reduced α-galactosidase A activity. Most patients also exhibit abnormal ECG results, with voltage criteria for LVH, short PR interval and conduction disorders. Echocardiography shows concentric LVH, diastolic dysfunction, and systolic dysfunction in the later stages of the disease. Cardiovascular magnetic resonance (CMR) scans also show concentric LVH, with a late gadolinium enhancement (LGE) of the basal inferolateral wall being a characteristic feature. Moreover, LGE in these patients increases the risk of major cardiovascular events [10,11]. Most Fabry patients exhibit concentric LVH [12]; however, asymmetrical septal and apical hypertrophy can be observed. Cardiovascular involvement can be highly variable and mutation dependent, also affecting the eligibility of precision therapies such as oral chaperone therapy. Enzyme replacement therapy is dependent on serum alpha-1-galactosidase levels.
- **Cardiac amyloidosis:** this is a cardiomyopathy caused by the deposition of amyloid protein outside of the heart cells, affecting the myocardium. This condition can occur in amyloid light-chain (AL) amyloidosis and transthyretin amyloidosis. Cardiac involvement in amyloidosis is associated with poor prognosis and can lead to various symptoms, including chest pain, HF, arrhythmias, stroke, and signs and symptoms of autonomic dysfunction. The disease also affects other organs, with symptoms such as carpal tunnel syndrome, easy bruising, macroglossia, neuropathy, and hepatomegaly. The ECG in amyloid cardiomyopathy often shows low-voltage QRS complexes. Echocardiography typically reveals bi-ventricular hypertrophy, valve thickening, bi-atrial dilatation, and diastolic dysfunction. Strain and strain rate imaging using speckle tracking can help to differentiate amyloid cardiomyopathy from sarcomeric HCM. In most cases, the pattern of LVH in cardiac amyloid is concentric and non-obstructive, but some cases can present with asymmetric obstructive forms, mimicking sarcomeric forms of HCM. CMR has a central role in the non-invasive diagnosis of cardiac amyloidosis due to its ability to provide tissue characterisation in addition to high-resolution morphologic and functional assessment. While multiple LGE patterns have been described in cardiac amyloidosis, subendocardial and transmural distributions predominate. Both patterns are present to different extents in AL and ATTR cardiac amyloidosis, with subendocardial LGE being more prevalent in

AL and transmural LGE more prevalent in ATTR cardiac amyloidosis. LGE initially appears predominant in the basal segments, but as the disease advances, biventricular transmural involvement occurs [13,14]. Additionally, it's worth noting that wild-type ATTR features almost universal involvement of cardiac structures, while hereditary ATTR involvement varies. Both types of amyloidosis can mimic HCM. On the other hand, AL amyloidosis, the most prevalent form, affects the heart in approximately 50% of cases. It often presents as a non-ischemic dilated phenotype, resulting in global impairment of cardiac function.

- **Mitochondrial cardiomyopathies:** this is a heterogeneous group of conditions that arise due to genetic mutations in the mitochondrial DNA inherited maternally. This leads to impaired energy production and affects various systems in the body, including the central nervous system, heart, and skeletal system. The symptoms of the disease can manifest at any age, from infancy to adulthood. In around 25% of patients, non-obstructive cardiomyopathy with mild concentric hypertrophy is observed, significantly worsening the prognosis. Approximately 50% of these patients develop HF, and the mortality rate reaches 70% before the age of 30. In cases of HF, cardiac transplantation may be considered a treatment option.

- **RAS-HCM:** HCM phenotype can be associated with malformation syndromes, including Noonan syndrome and LEOPARD syndrome. These syndromes belong to a group of developmental disorders called RASopathies caused by mutations in genes involved in the RAS/mitogen-activated protein kinase (RAS/MAPK) pathway. Noonan syndrome is inherited in an autosomal dominant pattern and is characterised by various congenital heart defects, including hypertrophic cardiomyopathy, which can affect up to 25% of patients. Additionally, Noonan syndrome patients may have pulmonary and aortic valve stenosis and atrioventricular septal defects. LEOPARD syndrome is an allelic variant of Noonan syndrome and is characterised by a combination of clinical features, including lentigines, electrocardiographic abnormalities, ocular hypertelorism, pulmonic stenosis, abnormal male genitalia, retardation of growth, and deafness. A recent multi-omics study in myectomy tissue from HCM patients shows activation of the RAS-MAPK signalling, suggesting that RAS-HCM and sarcomeric HCM may, in fact, share some final common pathways. In a multicentre retrospective study aimed to understand the arrhythmic progression of RAS-HCM better and pinpoint shortcomings in its management, RAS-HCM was associated with heightened morbidity and a comparable risk of SCD to sarcomeric HCM [15]. Notably, there was a discernibly low frequency of ICD implantation among RAS-HCM patients, resulting in potentially preventable sudden deaths. Prospective studies are needed to identify risk factors for SCD and develop specific recommendations for ICD implantation in RAS-HCM [16].

- **Hypertensive heart disease:** LVH caused by hypertension can be challenging to differentiate from HCM (Table 2) caused by sarcomeric mutations, as there is a frequent overlap (up to 25%) in the patterns of hypertrophy seen in both conditions. Similarly, features of HCM, such as the systolic anterior motion (SAM) of the mitral valve anterior leaflets, chordal slack, friction or impact lesions (from chronic mitral–septal contact on septum) or dynamic LVOTO due to basal septal hypertrophy can also be observed in patients with LVH caused by hypertension, especially if untreated hypertension is severe and low preload. However, SAM in hypertensive LVH occurs at the end of systole, unlike in HCM, where it occurs earlier. Several echocardiographic techniques have been used to differentiate between the two conditions [17]. Tissue Doppler imaging can show more impairment of diastolic function in HCM and lower early diastolic velocities. Two-dimensional (2D) strain echocardiography can also aid in the diagnosis, as radial strain in the mid and apical short axis segments is commonly reduced in HCM with sarcomeric mutations. Similarly, the systolic longitudinal strain has been found to be reduced in HCM, and it has value in distinguishing between HCM and hypertensive LVH. CMR imaging can identify typical patterns of fibrosis associated with HCM. Serum markers such as norepinephrine, atrial natriuretic peptide, and brain natriuretic peptide tend to be higher in HCM patients than in those with hypertensive LVH. A thorough clinical assessment of relatives may be crucial in making a diagnosis, as the identification of HCM in family members dramatically increases the likelihood that LVH has a genetic basis.

Table 2. Criteria to differentiate HCM from hypertensive heart disease.

Imaging Features (Echo, CMR, CT)	HCM	Hypertensive Heart Disease
LVH	Severe, asymmetric IVS/ILW ratio > 1.3	Mild (<15 mm, except blacks and chronic renal failure), concentric or midly asymmetric
LVOTO	Frequent	Rare
Sigmoid septum	Rare	Frequent
Mitral valve and papillary muscle abnormalities	Frequent	Rare
Crypts	Common	Rare
Basal-apical muscle bundles	Frequent	Rare
Severe longitudinal systolic dysfunction	Frequent	Rare
Severe strain abnormalities	Frequent	Less frequent
LGE	Frequent, RV insertion points, and intramural with patchy enhancement being the most common pattern	Less frequent, non-subendocardial, no specific pattern

CMR, cardiovascular magnetic resonance; HCM, hypertrophic cardiomyopathy; ILW, infero-lateral wall; IVS, interventricular septum; LGE, late gadolinium enhancement; LVH, left ventricular hypertrophy; LVOTO, left ventricular outflow obstruction.

- **Danon disease:** this is a rare X-linked dominant genetic disorder caused by a deficiency in lysosome-associated membrane protein-2 (LAMP2), leading to lysosomal storage. The prevalence of the disease may be underestimated due to difficulties in diagnosis, but LAMP2 mutations have been identified in 1–8% of patients with suspected HCM who underwent genetic testing. The disease manifests in males with severe symptoms at an earlier age, while females may develop later onset and milder symptoms due to X-linked inheritance. Diagnosis is confirmed by molecular genetic screening that reveals a LAMP2 gene mutation. Clinical suspicion of the condition should prompt testing of serum creatine kinase and liver enzyme levels, which are usually raised in this condition. ECG may show ventricular pre-excitation with Wolff–Parkinson–White (WPW)-pattern in up to two-thirds of men and less than a third of women, along with very large voltage complexes in male teenagers, raising suspicion of the condition. Echocardiography typically shows severe concentric LVH, but asymmetric septal hypertrophy has also been observed. Skeletal muscle biopsy may show intra-sarcoplasmic periodic acid-Schiff-positive vacuoles. In late stages, the disease may progress to a dilated cardiomyopathy phenotype [18,19].
- **Pompe disease:** this is a genetic disorder that follows an autosomal recessive pattern of inheritance, resulting from the deficiency of acid maltase (acid alpha [α]-glucosidase) enzyme. The condition is characterised by the deposition of glycogen in multiple organs and can present in three different forms: infantile, juvenile, and adult. The infantile form is the most severe and can lead to death within two years due to extreme LVH, HF, hypotonia, macroglossia, and hepatomegaly. While dilated cardiomyopathy can occur in some patients, the infantile form of the disease often presents with asymmetric LVH and LVOTO. In contrast, later onset forms have milder cardiac involvement and present with proximal myopathy. Diagnosis can be confirmed by demonstrating enzyme deficiency in fibroblasts, lymphocytes, and/or urine, and

skeletal muscle biopsy showing vacuolar glycogen deposition. ECG can show features of LVH as well as short PR interval with pre-excitation or conduction block [20].

- **PRKAG2 cardiomyopathy:** this is a genetic disorder with autosomal dominant inheritance caused by mutations in the PRKAG2 gene, which codes for the regulatory gamma-subunit of AMP-activated protein kinase (AMPK). This condition typically affects adolescents and young adults and is characterised by muscle weakness and imaging showing LVH with global hypokinesia. While the LVH in PRKAG2 cardiomyopathy is often associated with excess glycogen deposition and can be variable in severity, it can also be asymmetric, resembling the pattern seen in HCM caused by mutations in sarcomeric genes. However, PRKAG2 cardiomyopathy is different from sarcomeric HCM in that it progresses early to systolic dysfunction and dilated cardiomyopathy. This condition may also be associated with WPW syndrome and degeneration of the conduction system [21,22]. There are no known precision-based therapies for *PRKAG2* cardiomyopathy.

- **Cori–Forbes cardiomyopathy:** this is a genetic disorder caused by mutations in the glycogen debranching enzyme (amylo-alpha-1, 6-glucosidase [AGL]) gene. It is inherited in an autosomal recessive pattern and can present in infants, adolescents, or young adults. Common clinical features of Forbes disease include muscle weakness, poor growth, and hypoglycemia. In addition, patients may develop concentric LVH, which can progress to dilated cardiomyopathy in later years [23].

- **Athlete's heart:** in response to chronic high-intensity physical activity, the cardiovascular system activates a series of adaptive physiological mechanisms defined as the athlete's heart, including a constellation of changes with increased biventricular mass, volume, and wall thickness. A stepwise approach to the cardiovascular assessment of athletes is essential to make sense of overlapping clinical phenotypes and eventually provide a correct differential diagnosis between HCM and adaptive cardiac response to exercise. Twelve-lead ECG enhances the sensitivity of the screening process by allowing early detection of cardiovascular conditions distinctively manifesting with ECG abnormalities. Echocardiography has a pivotal role in differentiating physiologic and pathologic responses to exercise, namely athlete's heart, from HCM. Combining different methods, such as 2D and 3D measurements of cardiac size, volumes, wall thickness, mass index, tissue velocity, and myocardial strain imaging, cardiac ultrasound allows comprehensive morphologic and functional evaluation of the heart and distinction between physiologic and pathologic remodelling. In the presence of abnormal, uncertain, and/or controversial findings from the upstream diagnostic work up, CMR imaging can help distinguish between exercise-induced cardiac remodelling and cardiovascular pathology. CMR represents the current gold standard in the non-invasive assessment of cardiac morphology and quantification of volumes and flow and offers the opportunity for advanced myocardial tissue characterisation with excellent accuracy and precision [24,25].

2. Clinical Diagnosis and Imaging Tools

Timely detection and effective management are crucial for improving the prognosis of HCM. The 2020 AHA/ACC guidelines [3] recommend a comprehensive approach, starting with a detailed physical examination and thorough medical and family histories for individuals suspected of having HCM. Consideration for clinical evaluation of HCM arises when there is a family history of HCM, the presence of symptoms or cardiac events, detection of a heart murmur during physical examination, findings from echocardiography performed for other reasons, or an abnormal 12-lead ECG. A comprehensive clinical examination for HCM necessitates gathering an extensive personal and familial cardiac history that extends across three generations [26]. Pedigree analysis is particularly valuable as it helps to tease out the genetic origin of the disease and identify at-risk family members. Important attributes to consider in the family history include SCD, unexplained HF, cardiac transplantation, pacemaker and defibrillator implants, and evidence of systemic diseases such as early-onset stroke, skeletal muscle weakness, renal dysfunction, diabetes, and deafness. Pedigree analysis can also help to identify the mode of inheritance, with most genetic forms of HCM being autosomal dominant and showing affected individuals in each generation, regardless of sex. However, the recent finding of a Carter effect suggests a possible multifactorial threshold model of inheritance with sex dimorphism for liability [26]. An in-depth physical examination incorporating specific manoeuvres like the Valsalva, squat to stand, passive leg raising, or walking is also recommended. Neurological examination should be performed for syndromic HCM and myopathies (i.e., *FHL1* with contractures). Following physical examination, initial assessment often includes an ECG, which may appear normal in some cases at the initial presentation. However, it typically reveals a variable combination of LVH, ST- and T-wave abnormalities, and pathological Q-waves. Several patterns are also recognised: (i) widespread and deep T-wave inversion typical of apical and mid cavity HCM; (ii) pre-excitation with PRKAG2 and Danon (LAMP2); (iii) voltage criteria LVH with ST changes and LV strain, seen in HCM; (iv) ST elevation preceding T-wave inversion indicative of apical aneurysm; and (v) inferior Q waves indicative of extensive scarring.

The next step is performing imaging to identify LVH when clinical findings indicate its existence. Cardiac imaging is indeed essential to confirm the diagnosis, understand the underlying pathophysiology, and evaluate the risk of SCD. However, diagnosing HCM can sometimes pose unique challenges. These include patients presenting at advanced stages of the disease, with dilated, hypokinetic and/or thinned left ventricle (LV) (burnt-out phase), athletes with HCM [27], concurrent conditions associated with LVH, or isolated basal septal hypertrophy, particularly in older hypertensive individuals [28].

Echocardiography is pivotal as the primary diagnostic and monitoring tool in HCM [29]. M-mode, 2D, and Doppler transthoracic echocardiography (TTE) are commonly employed techniques, while strain imaging and 3D can help to detect subtle changes in early phenotypes. The ACC/AHA and ESC guidelines recommend the use of TTE, to be performed at rest and during Valsalva, as the initial diagnostic approach in patients with suspected HCM. TTE is also recommended for screening family members of HCM patients. TTE enables a comprehensive assessment of LV wall thickness, as well as the identification of mitral valve abnormalities, systolic anterior motion, LVOTO, left atrial enlargement, LV diastolic and systolic function, right ventricular function, and pulmonary haemodynamics. If initial findings are inconclusive, echocardiography with intravenous contrast, transoesophageal echocardiography (TOE), or cardiovascular magnetic resonance (CMR) imaging can be recommended [30,31]. TTE can also differentiate between different phenotypes of HCM, distinguishing obstructive from non-obstructive types. Tissue Doppler imaging (TDI) is an advanced tool useful to quantify the radial and longitudinal motion of the myocardium. In HCM, TDI can identify isolated reduction of systolic velocities in patients with preserved LVEF, early diagnosis before the development of overt LV hypertrophy, and presence of intraventricular dyssynchrony [32]. Strain measures myocardial deformation in multiple directions throughout the cardiac cycle. In HCM, reduction of LV global longitudinal strain (GLS) does occur in individuals with preserved LVEF and is a marker of subclinical myocardial dysfunction with demonstrated incremental prognostic value [32,33]. However, as strain-based measures are yet to be standardised and adopted into clinical HCM guidelines, GLS should be used to help distinguish HCM from cardiac amyloidosis, and athletic remodelling [31]. Three-dimensional echocardiography can aid further in assessing LV geometry, spiral distribution of hypertrophy, patterns of papillary muscle abnormalities, and recognising septal insertion of the moderator band and apical-basal muscle bundles preventing overestimation of maximal wall thickness [34]. Three-dimensional technology is also valuable in TOE to better detail the abnormalities of the mitral valve apparatus, SAM features, and underlying causes. Stress echocardiography, which involves imaging the heart during controlled exercise using an exercise bike or treadmill, can reveal hidden or latent obstruction in symptomatic patients. This is particularly useful when baseline TTE has failed to show LVOT gradients of ≥ 50 mmHg even when accompanied by the previously described physiological manoeuvres.

In the past, CMR was usually performed when echocardiography yielded inconclusive findings, but its use has become increasingly popular in recent years, and is now recommended in all patients with cardiomyopathy at initial evaluation (Class I, LoE B) [35]. While echocardiography is the first-line imaging modality and considered the standard for diagnosing HCM, it has limitations due to its dependence on adequate acoustic windows and challenges in obtaining cross-sectional images at the correct angles. Doppler assessment of LVOT mid cavity and apical gradients is crucial with echocardiography to guide management. In this regard, CMR complements echocardiography by enabling a complete and accurate assessment of all myocardial segments of the LV, here including the anterolateral wall, apical segments, septal junctions, and of the RV. It also allows evaluation of the papillary muscles (hypertrophy, abnormal insertion, feathering, and apical displacement) and detection of myocardial crypts. This comprehensive evaluation allows for precise reconstruction of cardiac size, morphology, function, and tissue characterisation. CMR with LGE is now recommended in HCM patients for diagnostic work up (Class I, LoE B) and further risk assessment (Class IIa, LoE B) [36]. Gadolinium-enhanced CMR plays a crucial role in precisely identifying myocardial fibrosis. The presence of LGE indicates replacement myocardial fibrosis and helps stratify the risk of ventricular arrhythmias and sudden cardiac death. Numerous studies have investigated the association between LGE and long-term outcomes in HCM and have consistently reported a significant positive relationship between presence of LGE and heightened risk of total and cardiovascular death, and HF. Native T1 mapping and extracellular volume fraction (ECV) are prolonged in HCM, indicating the presence of myocardial disarray and diffuse fibrosis. These values not only correlate with the risk of developing VT but also help differentiate HCM from other conditions. Tissue characterisation with CMR can also help to exclude other causes of LVH such as Fabry's (low myocardial T1) or cardiac amyloidosis (elevated T1 and patterns of LGE). Coronary microvascular dysfunction can be further explored with stress CMR perfusion imaging as a valuable tool to detect perfusion abnormalities that might occur before the development of overt LVH or scarring in HCM gene mutation carriers due to microvascular obstruction, supply–demand mismatch, extravascular compressive forces, and elevated intraventricular pressures (Figure 1). An independent association between microvascular disease electrocardiographic abnormalities has been observed in subclinical HCM, also suggesting the arrhythmogenic potential of small vessel disease [37]. Furthermore, measurable changes in microvascular function and myocardial microstructure by diffusion tensor imaging represent novel early-phenotype biomarkers in the emerging era of disease-modifying therapy [38–40]. Further research is yet to be conducted to establish the role of this novel approaches [38].

Cardiac computed tomography (CCT) is not commonly used in patients with HCM. Its indications arise when there are unclear findings on echocardiography, poor acoustic windows, or contraindications for performing CMR. CCT can be performed for evaluating ischemia in patients with HCM due to its ability to assess cardiac morphology, coronary anatomy, and myocardial perfusion. However, this still needs to be improved in clinical practice as only a few centres offer dynamic perfusion CT imaging. If significant stenosis is identified in the major epicardial artery, it serves as an indication for invasive angiography. This approach facilitated the detection of underlying disease processes and enabled surgeons to develop a clear plan regarding the volume and location of the surgery, ultimately reducing the occurrence of perioperative complications. According to international guidelines [3], there is currently no compelling justification for routine invasive haemodynamic evaluation in the assessment of patients with oHCM or conducting routine coronary angiography in the general population with HCM. These invasive procedures are typically recommended when clinical and noninvasive imaging examinations do not provide sufficient diagnostic information, but obtaining such information would impact patient management. Invasive cardiac catheterisation, while not essential for diagnosis, can be employed to determine the extent of obstruction and evaluate the haemodynamics of blood flow. It is particularly recommended in cases where obstructive HCM coexists with valvular aortic stenosis. This assessment allows for the identification of diastolic abnormalities, such as increased chamber stiffness and impaired LV relaxation. Additionally, invasive angiography provides insight into the characteristics of HCM, including asymmetric hypertrophy, mitral regurgitation, and systolic anterior movement of the anterior leaflet of the mitral valve, subaortic membranes, and subaortic conus. Moreover, coronary angiography is the primary investigative tool in patients with HCM who exhibit symptoms of angina or possess risk factors for coronary atherosclerosis. It is an integral component of alcohol septal ablation and is performed before surgical myectomy. The purpose of coronary angiography in these cases is to assess the septal anatomy and identify the presence of coronary artery disease that may require intervention, beyond the scope of septal ablation.

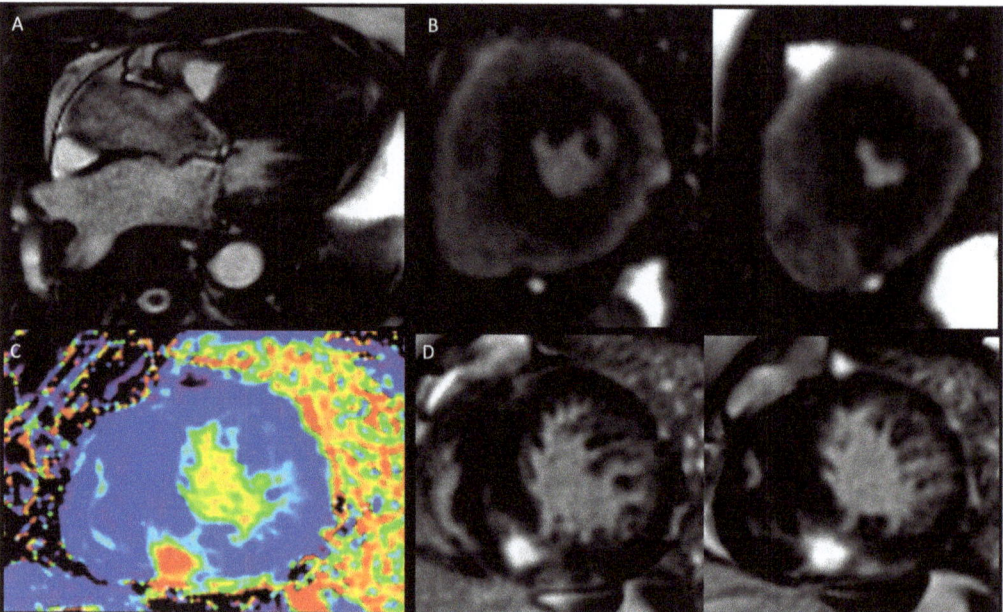

Figure 1. Phenotyping hypertrophic cardiomyopathy by CMR. Panel (**A**): Cine imaging—three chamber view depicting asymmetric left ventricular hypertrophy (LVH) with systolic anterior movement and left ventricular outflow tract turbulence. Panel (**B**): Adenosine stress perfusion imaging with perfusion defect in the areas of LVH and late gadolinium enhancement (LGE). Panel (**C**): extracellular volume mapping. Panel (**D**): LGE module: short-axis views showing right ventricular insertion point LGE and septal diffuse mid-wall LGE.

3. Sudden Cardiac Death Risk Assessment and Prevention

The management of HCM requires a collaborative approach, where the patient and the healthcare team work together harmoniously [29]. This partnership entails the active involvement of the patient and relatives in decision-making processes, ensuring their understanding of the benefits, risks, action plans, and ultimate goals concerning their condition. Patient engagement has proven to enhance confidence in clinical choices and improve health outcomes based on available evidence. The primary objective of shared decision-making is to minimise the risk of new complications, slow disease progression, and improve the quality of life. Shared decision-making involves a comprehensive dialogue among the healthcare team, which includes primary care physicians, cardiologists, paediatricians, internists, nurse practitioners, and patients. Numerous studies highlight the importance of shared decision-making in HCM management, primarily due to the absence of straightforward solutions. Patient treatment options may vary depending on factors such as the need for invasive therapies to address LVOTO, genetic testing, implantation of a cardioverter defibrillator (ICD), or participation in physical activities, particularly for professional athletes. It is crucial to consider that strenuous physical exertion poses a risk of sudden cardiac death in certain individuals with HCM. However, recent evidence suggests that among individuals with HCM or those who are genotype positive/phenotype negative and are treated in experienced centres, those exercising vigorously did not experience a higher rate of death or life-threatening arrhythmias than those exercising moderately or sedentary [41]. Shared decision making holds particular significance for athletes with HCM, especially for those who aspire to resume sports activity. Many international sports organisations have strict guidelines [42] regarding athletes with HCM and other arrhythmogenic disorders. Therefore, shared decision making should not be oversimplified as a process in which athletes have sole decision-making authority. It is essential to avoid limiting shared decision making solely to patient autonomy, even in the context of athletes.

SCD, although rare (overall 1–2% rate), is the most devastating complication of HCM. Therefore, it is crucial to identify and stratify risk factors. The stratification of risk factors is primarily based on clinical symptoms, complaints, and radiological reports. Stratification in paediatric patients is different, and work up includes non-sarcomeric causes, given earlier onset, and checking for biallelic or digenic disease. In adults, both the ACC/AHA and ESC guidelines recommend secondary prevention ICD implantation for patients who meet specific criteria.

According to the AHA/ACC guidelines, established risk markers of SCD in HCM patients include prior cardiac arrest or sustained ventricular tachycardia, family history of HCM-related sudden death in first-degree relatives, unexplained syncope, maximum LV wall thickness over 30 mm, LVEF < 50%, LV apical aneurysm (with or without LGE), non-sustained ventricular tachycardia on Holter monitoring, and extensive LGE ($\geq$15% of LV mass). Importantly, in patients aged $\geq$ 16 years, 5-year risk estimates of SCD can be considered to fully inform patients during shared decision-making discussions. Notably, the evolution of SCD risk assessment, including the addition of new risk markers, has resulted in the removal of abnormal blood pressure response to exercise as a routine part of the SCD risk evaluation.

According to the 2014 ESC guidelines [43] for the diagnosis and management of HCM and the 2023 ESC guidelines for the management of cardiomyopathies [35], the HCM Risk-SCD tool (HCM Risk-Kids for children and adolescents < 16 years) is recommended to assess the 5-year risk of SCD in HCM patients. The ESC risk stratification scheme shares some factors with the ACC/AHA approach, such as left ventricular wall thickness, family history of SCD, and syncope. However, the ESC model includes additional factors like age, LV outflow tract gradient, and left atrial diameter. Using the HCM Risk-SCD tool, patients can be classified as low risk (5-year risk < 4%), intermediate risk (5-year risk $\geq$ 4 to <6%), and high risk (5-year risk $\geq$ 6%) of SCD. For the low-risk group, ICD is usually not recommended. The intermediate-risk group may be considered for ICD, while the high-risk group should be considered for ICD placement. In practice, the presence of extensive LGE ($\geq$15%) and LV systolic dysfunction (LVEF < 50%) can be used may be used in shared decision making with patients about prophylactic ICD implantation in low to intermediate risk categories. Furthermore, while the 2022 ESC Guidelines for the management of patients with ventricular arrhythmias included genetic testing to identify single or multiple sarcomeric pathogenic variants to evaluate the need for ICD implantation in intermediate risk patients [36], the 2023 ESC guidelines for the management of cardiomyopathies [35] now recommend against routine use of the presence of sarcomeric variant(s) to guide decisions around ICD implantation for primary prevention.

4. Therapeutic Approaches

Clinicians usually focus their preventive measures on patients presenting with overt signs and symptoms of disease, particularly in younger patients. Nevertheless, the complications of the disease have a higher chance of affecting individuals who are between the ages of 50 to 70 years old. HCM patients experience a 'honeymoon period', which is the time between the initial detection and the onset of severe clinical signs of the disease [1]. This period can last for over 30 years. Clinicians can exploit this temporal window to actively prevent or delay the adverse progression of the disease through medication or medically necessary procedures that can change the course of the disease. Although empirical therapeutic approaches can currently manage acute complications by reducing symptoms and improving quality of life, there are no drugs or interventions available that have been found to significantly slow the progression of LV systolic or diastolic dysfunction or prevent the transition from subclinical to overt HCM. However, a recent study by Joy et al. revealed that it might be possible to prevent the transition from subclinical to overt HCM in some individuals with genetic variants. Furthermore, positive myocardial remodelling might be more amenable to reversal at the subclinical stage of disease than in overt HCM, when cardiac hypertrophy and fibrosis are challenging to reverse. Studies to explore this possibility would benefit from a comprehensive phenotypic description of subclinical HCM, with the potential for therapeutic targeting of those individuals with early phenotypic changes. An era in which cascade screening is replaced by cascade prevention, enable by novel phenotyping, is a tempting prospect [44].

Despite being a prevalent disease, HCM lacks specific drug treatment, especially in terms of selective disease-modifying drugs. HCM was erroneously regarded as a rare disease, which has hindered the completion of large, randomised trials. As a result, most of the current guidelines are based on small observational studies, case series, or expert consensus. The present recommendations are established using empirical data from non-specific drugs like disopyramide, non-dihydropyridine calcium channel blockers, or β-blockers, administered mainly to oHCM symptomatic patients. Nonetheless, such medications provide complete relief from obstruction in only a small subgroup of patients, implying that most treated individuals are left with lingering LVOT gradients and symptoms.

For patients with oHCM whose gradient remains above 50 mmHg and remain symptomatic despite optimal drug treatment, invasive septal reduction therapies are recommended [3,43]. These therapies include either surgical septal myectomy (where possible and favourable perioperative risk in high volume centres, or, requiring other surgery such as mitral valve surgery), or catheter-based alcohol septal ablation, if not suitable for myectomy and anatomy amenable to septal ablation. However, there are potential risks associated with these treatment options, and the risk of complications is lower in specialised medical centres. Unfortunately, access to these centres may be limited for many people around the world.

Recently, new compounds have been created to treat HCM by directly targeting the hypercontractility and altered energetics of the cardiac muscle. These innovative drugs work through allosteric inhibition of myosin, the primary protein of the heart muscle responsible for generating force [45]. In this review, we will thoroughly examine the use of different categories of medications in patients with HCM (Table 3), including conventional treatment, as well as new disease-modifying treatments and emerging gene modulation approaches.

Table 3. Main drugs used or tested in HCM.

Class of Drug and Mechanism of Action	Drug and Daily Dose	Side Effect	Patients	Notes
BBs Blockade of β-receptors	Metoprolol 25–200 mg Atenolol 25–100 mg Bisoprolol 1.25–10 mg Nadolol 20–80 mg	Hypotension Bradycardia Bronchoconstriction Fatigue Limb ischemia	oHCM, noHCM	To titrate focusing on symptoms to the maximally tolerated dose
CCBs Blockade of L-type calcium channels	Verapamil 120–240 mg Diltiazem 120–240 mg	Headache, dizziness Constipation Flushing HF Conduction disturbances	oHCM, noHCM	Combination of CCBs and BBs is generally not recommended
Disopyramide (Class IA antiarrhythmic) Blockade of INaL. Other minor effects on peak INa, L-type calcium channels, ryanodine receptors and IKr	300–600 mg	Antagonism of muscarinic receptors (dry mouth, constipation, urinary hesitancy, etc.)	Refractory symptomatic oHCM despite BBs or CCBs	It can increase ventricular rate response in patients with atrial fibrillation (use concomitantly with AV blocking agent)
Cibenzoline (Class IA antiarrhythmic) Blockade of INaL and peak INa	100–400 mg	Lower inhibitory activity on muscarinic receptors than disopyramide	oHCM	Used in Japan and Korea. Not listed in ESC or AHA/ACC Guidelines
Late sodium channel blockers Blockade of INaL	Ranolazine Eleclazine	Dizziness Headache Nausea	Not approved	Not listed in ESC or AHA/ACC Guidelines
Potassium channel blockers Dofetilide Sotalol		Caution renal failure, reduce dose Monitor QTc interval as risk of life-threatening QT prolongation and TdP		Particularly useful for AF Sotalol in low doses has beta blocking effects and higher doses class III Singh–Vaughan Williams effects Exhibits reverse use-dependent effects (i.e., more potent when bradycardic)
ARBs Blockade of AT1 receptor	Valsartan 80–320 mg	Hypotension Cough Hyperkalaemia Worsen kidney function	noHCM with HFrEF	Further evidence is desirable in early HCM (VANISH)
ARNIs Blockade of AT1 receptor and neprilysin	Sacubitril/Valsartan 24/26 to 97/103 mg	Hypotension Cough Hyperkalaemia Worsen kidney function	noHCM with HFrEF	Further evidence is desirable in symptomatic noHCM with HFpEF (SILICOFCM study)
Mavacamten (myosin inhibitor) Allosteric inhibition of cardiac myosin ATPase	2.5–15 mg	Decrease in ejection fraction	NYHA II-III oHCM (in America)	Inducer of CYP3A4, CYP2C9, and CYP2C19. Long half-life (7–10 days)
Aficamten (myosin inhibitor) Allosteric inhibition of cardiac Myosin ATPase	Not established	Decrease in ejection fraction	Not yet approved	Absence of interaction with CYP3A4, CYP2C9, and CYP2C19. Short half-life (2 days)

ARB, angiotensin receptor blocker; ARNI, angiotensin receptor neprilysin inhibitor; AT1, angiotensin type 1; ATP, adenosine triphosphate; BBs, beta-blockers; CCBs, calcium channel blockers; HCM, hypertrophic cardiomyopathy; HFpEF, heart failure with preserved ejection fraction; HFrEF, heart failure with reduced ejection fraction; noHCM, nonobstructive HCM; oHCM, obstructive HCM, TdP, torsade de pointes.

4.1. Conventional Treatment

Conventional treatment of HCM includes pharmacological therapy, surgery, and lifestyle modifications [46]. This approach is defined as "non-selective" because it does not target the primary mechanisms of the disease, but it acts on the consequences of the hypertrophic myocardium. Although there is no evidence that conventional drugs are able to prevent disease progression [47], they aim to manage symptoms, improve cardiac function, and reduce the risk of complications. β-blockers, calcium channel blockers, and disopyramide are the most common non-selective drugs used in HCM.

4.1.1. β-Blockers

In the context of HCM, β-blockers (BBs) are commonly prescribed, specifically those without vasodilating effects. Metoprolol and atenolol are among the most widely used BBs, but nadolol and bisoprolol can also be used [48]. Currently, the choice of β-blocker is more influenced by the clinical practice of the single institution rather than specific recommendations guided by randomised evidence.

LVOTO is a common cause of exertional dyspnea, angina, and or fatigue in patients with HCM. These symptoms occur due to myocardial hypercontractility combined with a strong adrenergic drive [1]. Indeed, BBs are very effective in patients with symptomatic LVOTO, and they should be titrated focusing on symptoms to the maximally tolerated dose. On the other hand, BBs could also be very helpful in limiting symptoms in noHCM and preserved ejection fraction. This cohort of patients often complains about angina and shortness of breath, associated with microvascular ischemia, diastolic dysfunction, and elevated filling pressures. BBs help to relieve symptoms through their negative chronotropic and inotropic effects [3,43].

NoHCM is usually well tolerated, and only a small portion of individuals with this condition develop HF with reduced ejection fraction (HFrEF). In these cases, BBs can be prescribed to reduce death and HF hospitalization [49], in addition to ACE inhibitors (ACEIs), angiotensin II receptor antagonists (ARBs), angiotensin receptor-neprilysin inhibitors (ARNIs), SGLT2 inhibitors (iSGLT2s), and mineralocorticoid receptor antagonists (MRAs).

According to the ESC guidelines [35,43], BBs are first-line drugs to improve symptoms in patients with resting or provoked LVOTO (Class I, LoE B), and in patients with symptomatic noHCM and EF > 50% (Class IIa, LoE C). BBs are also recommended in noHCM and EF < 50% (Class IIa, LoE C). The 2020 American guidelines [3] confirm the recommendations and level of evidence for β-blockers in both oHCM and noHCM. Special mention should be made of asymptomatic patients with noHCM and preserved EF; in this case, the benefit of β-blockers is not proven (Class 2b, LoE C-EO).

4.1.2. Calcium Channel Blockers

The CCBs used in HCM are the non-dihydropyridine agents, devoid of vasodilating effects. Dihydropyridine CCBs are generally contraindicated in HCM because systemic vasodilation may increase LVOT gradients and obstructive symptoms [50]. The hypertrophic cardiomyocyte has higher than normal cytosolic calcium concentration, leading to hypercontractility, diastolic dysfunction, and arrhythmias [51]. Non-dihydropyridine CCBs act by inhibiting L-type calcium channels, exerting negative inotropic and chronotropic effects on working myocytes and sinoatrial node cells, respectively.

Diltiazem and verapamil are the most common drugs of this class [29]. Their efficacy is similar to BBs in reducing symptoms [52]. Non-dihydropyridine agents are commonly suggested when BBs are not well tolerated. Side effects of CCBs include headache, dizziness, nausea, constipation, edema, and flushing. They can rarely lead to HF, especially in patients with high resting gradients and advanced HF, or conduction disturbances. The combination of CCBs and BBs is generally not recommended due to the risk of bradycardia and hypotension [1].

The ESC guidelines [35,43] recommend verapamil or diltiazem (Class I, LoE B) in patients with oHCM who are intolerant or have contraindications to BBs, in order to improve symptoms. They are also indicated in symptomatic noHCM with preserved ejection fraction (Class IIa, LoE C). These recommendations are also endorsed by the 2020 American guidelines [3]. Like BBs, using CCBs in asymptomatic patients with noHCM is possible but requires further evidence (Class 2b, LoE C-EO).

4.1.3. Disopyramide

Disopyramide is a class IA antiarrhythmic drug exerting its effects through multiple mechanisms. It primarily acts by blocking the cardiac sodium channel INaL to reduce the influx of sodium ions into cardiac cells during the action potential, while exerting a minor effect on the peak sodium current INa, responsible for the action potential upstroke. In addition to its effect on the sodium channels, disopyramide also has a secondary blocking effect on L-type calcium channels. By blocking these channels, disopyramide reduces the influx of calcium ions into the cardiac cells during the plateau phase of the action potential. This contributes to a decrease in contractility and a reduction in myocardial oxygen consumption. Disopyramide also affects the ryanodine receptors, which are calcium-release channels located on the sarcoplasmic reticulum of cardiac cells. By blocking these channels, disopyramide helps to decrease the release of calcium from the sarcoplasmic reticulum, which leads to a decrease in diastolic calcium concentration. This effect can contribute to the relaxation of the cardiac muscle during diastole [53]. Lastly, disopyramide has a mild blocking effect on the delayed potassium current (IKr). This action prolongs the repolarization phase of the action potential. Due to this effect, disopyramide was historically used in acute coronary syndrome to prevent arrhythmias. Subsequently, this drug has found application in HCM with LVOTO. Its use is justified by its strong negative inotropic effect due to the reduction of intracellular calcium and indirectly to the reduction of sodium, which leads to increased activity of the sodium-calcium exchanger. Furthermore, disopyramide reduces the haemodynamic consequences of the Venturi effect by lowering flow velocities in the LVOT, thereby reducing the pulling force on the anterior mitral leaflet. Side effects of disopyramide are primarily due to its antagonism of muscarinic receptors. They include dry mouth, constipation, and urinary hesitancy. New clinical studies suggest a different effect of disopyramide based on the degree of electrophysiological remodelling of the cell [54]. In hypertrophic cells, the duration of the action potential is pathologically prolonged due to the increase of INaL and L-type calcium current, and the reduction of repolarising potassium currents. By inhibiting the sodium current, disopyramide appears to reduce the duration of the action potential in these cells. Therefore, it may reduce the dispersion of the action potential and prevent the development of re-entrant arrhythmias [55].

The ESC guidelines suggest using disopyramide in addition to BBs (or, if this is not possible, with verapamil) to improve symptoms in patients with resting or provoked LVOTO (Class I, LoE B). It could be used also as monotherapy, although with a lower level of recommendation (Class IIb, LoE C) to improve symptoms in patients with resting or provoked LVOTO (Class IIb, LoE C), taking caution in patient with atrial fibrillation, in whom it can increase ventricular rate response. The 2020 American guidelines also recommend the use of disopyramide in symptomatic oHCM despite treatment with BBs and non-dihydropyridine calcium antagonists (Class 1, LoE B-NR).

4.1.4. Cibenzoline

Cibenzoline is a Class IA antiarrhythmic drug used for the treatment of oHCM in Japan and Korea [56]. It shares some similarities with disopyramide in terms of its mechanism of action. Like disopyramide, cibenzoline blocks sodium channels (peak INa and INaL), which leads to a reduction in intracellular calcium concentration. This effect is responsible for its negative inotropic effect and its use in managing symptoms of oHCM [57]. By reducing the LV pressure gradient and limiting LV remodelling, cibenzoline helps alleviate symptoms associated with oHCM. Cibenzoline is considered safe and well tolerated [58]. It does not significantly alter heart rate, but slightly prolongs the QT interval. In comparison to disopyramide, cibenzoline has lower inhibitory activity on muscarinic receptors. This drug is currently not mentioned in the European or American guidelines.

4.1.5. Late Sodium Channel Blockers

This class of drugs consists of ranolazine and eleclazine. Their mechanism of action involves the inhibition of sodium current INaL, which led to a reduction of intracellular calcium. In hypertrophic cells, the pathologically increased INaL current prolongs the action potential duration, which predisposes to the development of early after-depolarization events. Ranolazine and eleclazine exert an antiarrhythmic function because they reduce the INaL sodium current and, consequently, the development of early after-depolarization events. Moreover, they normalise diastolic calcium, improving the relaxation of myocardium in HCM and probably lowering the incidence of delayed after-depolarizations, which are diastolic calcium-release events.

Two trials have attempted to demonstrate the effect of ranolazine and cibenzoline on symptoms in HCM. In the RESTYLE HCM trial, ranolazine was tested on symptomatic patients with noHCM, but it did not show a significant improvement in functional capacity as measured by cardiopulmonary exercise testing [59]. However, an improvement in the arrhythmic profile and lower levels of BNP were observed. The LIBERTY HCM trial aimed to test eleclazine in symptomatic patients with and without LVOTO. The study was prematurely terminated following the discouraging results seen in other trials [60]. These drugs are currently not mentioned the European or American guidelines.

4.1.6. Angiotensin II Receptor Antagonists

ARBs are among the most used medications for the treatment of hypertension and HF. By binding to the AT1 receptor expressed on cardiomyocytes and fibroblasts, angiotensin II promotes the development of hypertrophy and fibrosis [61]. Therefore, the use of ARBs should slow down the progression of the disease and promote reverse remodelling, particularly by improving diastolic function [62]. However, the available studies on the use of ARBs in HCM have failed to demonstrate a clear benefit in terms of reducing cardiac mass and its fibrotic component [63].

New encouraging perspectives come from the multicentre, double-blind, phase II trial VANISH. This study tested valsartan in a population of patients with early-stage HCM, characterized by limited alterations on echocardiography. Standardized changes from baseline to year 2 in LV wall thickness, mass, and volumes; left atrial volume; tissue Doppler diastolic and systolic velocities; and serum levels of high-sensitivity troponin T and N-terminal pro-B-type natriuretic protein were integrated into a single composite z-score as the primary outcome. The results published at a 2-year follow up showed a reduction in the worsening of diastolic function and in the development of hypertrophy in the group treated with valsartan compared to the placebo. These findings seem to confer a primary importance to early screening, although further evidence is desirable in this regard [64]. According to the current American and European guidelines [3,43], ARBs are recommended in patients with HCM and systolic dysfunction and progression towards end stage. However, caution is advised when considering the early usage of ARBs in cases of obstruction, as they have the potential to affect both preload and afterload, which could worsen the obstruction.

4.1.7. Angiotensin Receptor Neprilysin Inhibitors

ARNIs have been shown to be among the most effective HF drugs, by improving both systolic and diastolic function. New evidence suggests that this class may induce reverse remodelling in a hypertrophic heart [65]. By inhibiting both the RAAS and the natriuretic peptides system, ARNIs block pathways involving calcineurin-NFAT, JNK, ERK1/ERK2, and p38, mediating an anti-hypertrophic signalling [62]. This effect may be less pronounced in the presence of long-standing hypertensive heart disease or ischemic heart disease, which are characterized by the presence of fibrotic tissue. ARNIs are currently used in the context of HCM with HFrEF. New horizons will be outlined by the results of the SILICOFCM study (NCT03832660), aimed at extending the use of ARNIs to symptomatic patients with noHCM and preserved ejection fraction [66].

4.1.8. Septal Reduction Therapy

Septal reduction therapy (SRT) represents an important option for severely symptomatic patients with LVOTO [67]. There are two established techniques: myectomy and alcohol septal ablation. Originally, myectomy involved widening the LVOT by resecting the myocardium at the level of the anterior basal septum. Nowadays, it has evolved to extend beyond the mitral–septal contact point, including the mid-ventricular septum as well. This procedure not only reduces LVOTO gradient and Venturi effect, but also the pushing forces responsible for systolic anterior motion and, therefore, mitral insufficiency. When mitral regurgitation is caused by morphological alterations of the valve apparatus, myectomy can be combined with mitral repair (or, more rarely, replacement). In patients with a history of atrial fibrillation undergoing myectomy, it is possible to perform the Maze procedure to reduce the occurrence of arrhythmic events. Although left atrial appendage ligation is often also performed, this does not protect against thromboembolic events in HCM with AF due to underlying atrial myopathy.

Septal myectomy is considered the current gold standard due to its excellent results in terms of effectiveness and safety [29]. Most patients undergoing myectomy report an improvement in symptoms and quality of life, supported by an increase in peak VO_2 during cardiopulmonary exercise testing. These results are correlated with the immediate abolition of LVOTO and with the reduction in ventricular filling pressures, leading to reverse left atrium remodelling and modest regression of LVH. The main complications are complete heart block requiring a permanent pacemaker, ventricular septal defect, and aortic regurgitation.

Alcohol septal ablation (ASA) involves injecting alcohol into a septal perforator artery: the area supplied by the affected vessel will undergo necrosis and fibrosis, resulting in a reduction in wall thickness. Contrast echocardiography is essential to assess if the coronary anatomy is compatible with the procedure. If the contrast is not localized exclusively in the basal septum and adjacent mitral–septal contact point, the patient is not eligible. This technique is mostly reserved for frail patients with a high surgical risk or contraindications to surgery [68]. ASA is the first alternative to myectomy [69]. Both procedures are associated with an improvement in functional status, although there are no randomized comparison trials available. ASA has the advantage of shorter hospitalization and less invasiveness [70]. The risk of mortality and complications is similar; however, ASA is burdened with a higher incidence of AV blocks, scar-related ventricular arrhythmias, and a slower and less uniform reduction in LVOTO gradient. Finally, it is not indicated in patients with surgically correctable valve abnormalities or in patients with excessively hypertrophied or thinned septum [71].

According to the European guidelines, SRT is reserved for patients with LVOTO peak gradient > 50 mmHg with recurrent exertional syncope (Class IIa, LoE C) or severely symptomatic (NYHA III-IV, Class I, LoE B) despite optimised medical therapy. Myectomy is preferred when surgical repair of other lesions is necessary (Class I, LoE C). Mitral valve repair is indicated in cases of moderate to severe regurgitation not caused by SAM (Class IIa, LoE C). The American guidelines recommend SRT in patients with symptomatic oHCM despite optimised medical therapy (Class 1, LoE B-NR). In presence of associated cardiac disease requiring surgery, myectomy is recommended (Class 1, LoE B-NR); if myectomy is contraindicated, ASA is preferred (Class 1, LoE C-LD). Furthermore, these guidelines open the possibility of early intervention (NYHA II) in case of pulmonary hypertension, atrial enlargement with episodes of atrial fibrillation, low functional capacity, or children/young adults with resting LVOTO > 100 mmHg (Class 2b, LoE B-NR). SRT can also be considered as an alternative to escalating medical therapy in symptomatic and eligible patients, after evaluating and collectively discussing the pros and cons of the choice (Class 2b, LoE C-

LD). Both guidelines emphasize the importance of experienced high-volume HCM centres. A surgeon should perform at least 10 myectomies or ASA procedures per year to ensure adequate expertise and maintain a low level of risk.

4.1.9. Lifestyle Interventions

Patients with HCM need to adopt certain lifestyle adjustments [72]. These include avoiding dehydration, excessive alcohol consumption, extreme temperatures (hot/cold), and heavy meals, as these situations could trigger or worsen LVOTO. For the same reasons, European guidelines also discourage using venous or arterial dilators, nitrates, and phosphodiesterase-5 inhibitors. Digoxin should also be avoided due to its positive inotropic effect. The role and methods of physical activity are highly debated. New evidence highlights the role of aerobic exercise in reverse remodelling of the ventricle. In fact, exercise reduces levels of angiotensin II, BNP, and aldosterone, mimicking the effects of many pharmacological therapies.

Current European guidelines discourage high-intensity physical activity, although they emphasize the importance of a healthy lifestyle [43]. American guidelines recommend physical activity from mild to moderate intensity, as it improves the quality of life and cardiopulmonary fitness (Class 1, LoE B-NR) [3]. They consider physical activity of any intensity reasonable (Class 2a, LoE C-LD) for individuals with a positive genotype and negative phenotype. Finally, the practice of high-intensity sports for patients with HCM can be considered reasonable (Class 2b, LoE C-LD), following a comprehensive evaluation of the risk of sudden cardiac death and a shared discussion to be repeated annually.

Some recently completed or ongoing trials may change the above recommendations in the near future [41]. The LIVE-HCM prospective cohort study compared the outcome associated with vigorous exercise, moderate exercise, or sedentary lifestyle in HCM individuals. This trial enrolled 1660 participants who were followed for three years, excluding participants with NYHA class III or IV symptoms. HCM subjects exercising vigorously did not experience a higher rate of the composite endpoint of death, resuscitated sudden cardiac arrest, arrhythmic syncope, and appropriate shock from an implantable cardioverter defibrillator than those exercising moderately or those who were sedentary [41].

Another trial is the phase II SILICOFCM study (Figure 2). The objective of this ongoing trial is to evaluate the benefits of pharmacological therapy with ARNIs compared to lifestyle interventions in patients with noHCM. Both ARNIs therapy and lifestyle interventions with exercise training and dietary supplementation with inorganic nitrate, could have a potential role in improving symptoms, cardiac performance, and reverse remodelling, although this is still not fully clarified [66].

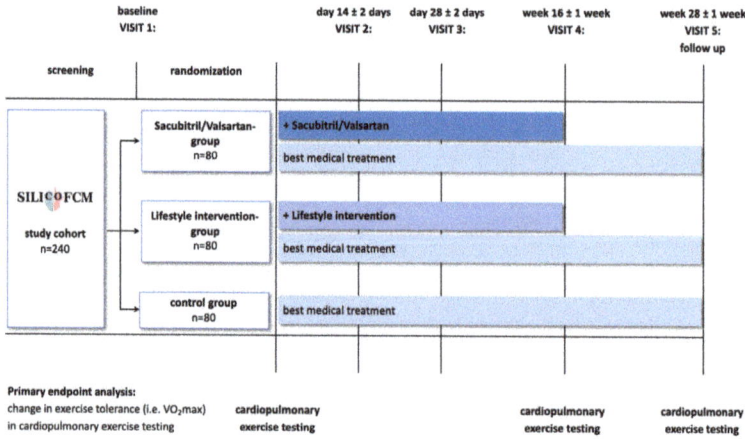

Figure 2. SILICOFCM trial design. Reproduced with permission from Tafelmeier M.et al., 2020 [66].

4.2. Novel Therapeutic Approaches

The myocardium regular contractions are achieved by carefully balancing performance and energy expenditure [73]. Myosin molecule activation state plays a crucial role in both determining and influencing myocardial contraction by being able to shift between two conformations during relaxation: namely a sequestered "super relaxed state" (SRX) and a "disordered relaxed state" (DRX) [56]. The difference lies in ATPase (adenosine triphosphatase) activity: in SRX conformation, myosin has low enzyme activity. On the other hand, in DRX state, more myosin heads are available to interact with actin, with greater enzyme activity (Figure 3).

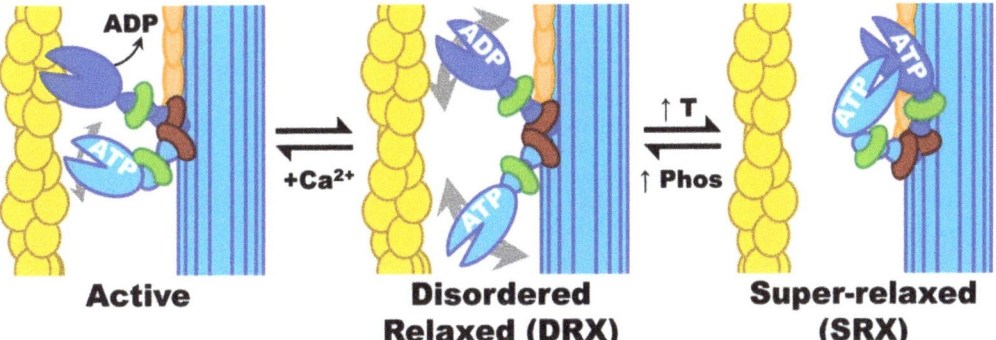

Figure 3. Myosin biochemical and structural states. Actin filaments are activated by Ca^{2+} (which binds to troponin, not shown) allowing myosin heads to be activated by actin binding followed by rapid turnover of ATP and molecular force generation. When Ca^{2+} is removed, and ATP replaces ADP, myosin heads return to DRX, which can then cycle to and from SRX. When myosin heads are not ordered on the thick filament backbone (as in SRX), they are disordered and can rotate about in the interfilament space, as depicted by grey double-headed arrows in DRX. Actin, yellow; myosin heavy chain, blue; essential light chain, green; regulatory light chain, red; myosin binding protein C, orange; DRX, disordered relaxed; SRX, super-relaxed. Reproduced with permission from Phung et al., 2018 [74].

In unaffected patients, energy demand seems to be the main factor influencing the transition between the two states. Energy is in fact conserved in SRX conformation. This can be achieved by preventing the formation of unnecessary cross bridges. The DRX state instead allows a greater performance at the cost of higher energy consumption [75]. Experimental evidence indicates that a pathological shift of the myosin equilibrium towards the DRX state causes impaired relaxation in HCM. This increases the number of myosin heads available to interact with actin, which in turn leads to both an enhanced contraction and higher energy expenditure [76]. Moreover, mutations in R403Q (the first identified mutation in HCM) and various HCM variants in MYBPC3 have been linked to impaired relaxation, hyperdynamic contractions, and increased energy consumption by the sarcomeres [77]. This is therefore linked to the balance between SRX and DRX states of myosin. Interestingly these characteristics often precede the development of LVH.

4.2.1. Mavacamten

Mavacamten is a novel specific myosin inhibitor that has the ability to restore the equilibrium between SRX and DRX conformations of myosin, reducing the myocardial force of contraction and consumption of ATP by myosin [78]. Experimental studies on mouse cardiac myofibrils have shown that mavacamten has a dose-dependent reduction in ATPase activity. This highlights its direct action on myosin, targeting its enzymatic activity. Mavacamten demonstrated an inhibitory effect on the basal rate of ADP release in bovine cardiac myosin, reducing it by 50% without affecting the rate of ADP release when myosin was in an actin-associated state. The number of myosin heads available for interaction with actin during the transition from the weakly to the strongly bound conformation is greatly reduced. Mavacamten effectively prevents these myosin heads from taking part in the actomyosin chemo-mechanical cycle. By decreasing ATPase activity, mavacamten leads to a reduction in the power generated by the sarcomere [79]. Furthermore, after 20–26 weeks of treatment, histological analysis of the myocardium highlighted a decrease of 80% of fibrosis. This raises mavacamten to a disease-modifying drug status, as fibrosis is a characteristic feature of the disease. However, this effect is not seen after the onset of hypertrophy [80]. As follows, Mavacamten maximum effect is exerted at the early stages of disease progression.

Experimental studies on Mavacamten administration (10 µM) to Yucatan minipigs carrying R403Q mutation showed a significant restored the percentage of SRX, shifting SRX/DRX ratio back to wild-type animals. Mavacamten stabilizes myosin heads in the closed SRX states and reduces the available myosin molecules for interaction with actin, preventing unnecessary actomyosin interaction, preserving myocardial physiological performance. Mavacamten can therefore restore the normal expression of genes involved in contractility and metabolism in HCM, restoring the physiological transcription pathways. The improvement in functional parameters resulting from mavacamten treatment correlates with the normalization of the SRX/DRX balance. This suggests that hyperdynamic contractility seen in HCM is likely promoted by an increased proportion of myosin in the DRX conformation, while delayed relaxation is mediated by a reduction of myosin heads in the SRX state [81].

4.2.2. Mavacamten Trials

Mavacamten improves performance in patients with oHCM by reducing LVOTO. Several studies have been conducted in this area, with some still ongoing. One notable study is the PIONEER-HCM trial, which was a phase II, multicentre, open-label trial involving 21 patients with oHCM [82]. The participants were divided into two cohorts (A and B) and each participant underwent a 12-week treatment cycle with once-daily oral mavacamten, followed by a 4-week post-treatment phase. In cohort A, the patients were treated with mavacamten to gain insights into the pharmacokinetic and pharmacodynamic relationship of the compound. The starting dose was based on the patient's weight, with a dose of 10 mg/day for patients weighing 60 kg or less and 15 mg/day for those weighing more than 60 kg. On the other hand, cohort B received lower concentrations of mavacamten, with a dose of 2 mg/day for all patients. The dosage variation aimed to evaluate whether different doses could influence the expected effect [83]. The study results indicate that 12 weeks of mavacamten treatment had beneficial effects on patients with oHCM, by significantly reducing the degree of post-exercise LVOTO. This correlated with improvement in exertional capacity and symptom relief. The effect on LVOTO reduction was more prominent in cohort A, with a mean reduction of 82% compared to 29% in cohort B. Higher doses of mavacamten may therefore yield better outcomes for patients. Mavacamten administration was not exempt from adverse effects although most of them were reported as mild (80%). Most commonly, it caused a reduction in LVEF below 50% and atrial fibrillation [83]. The PIO-NEER-OLE study (NCT03496168), an ongoing 5-year extension of the PIONEER-HCM trial, is currently being conducted. This prospective, open-label, multicentre trial aims to assess the long-term effects of mavacamten. Interim analysis conducted after the first year indicates sustained efficacy of mavacamten throughout 156 weeks of follow up [84]. The PIOONER-OLE study is anticipated to conclude in November 2023 [85].

MAVERICK-HCM (Mavacamten in adults with symptomatic non-obstructive hypertrophic cardiomyopathy) was a phase II, multicentre, double-blind, randomized, placebo-controlled study that enrolled 59 patients with symptomatic noHCM, preserved left ventricular ejection fraction (LVEF $\geq$ 55%), increased NT-proBNP ($\geq$300 pg/mL), and exertional symptoms classified as New York Heart Association (NYHA) functional class II/III. The patients were randomly assigned to three different cohorts [86]. Cohort 1 consisted of 19 patients who received a pharmacokinetic-adjusted dose of mavacamten, with a target serum drug concentration of approximately 200 ng/mL. Patients in Cohort 2 were instead treated with higher doses of mavacamten to achieve serum drug concentrations averaging around 500 ng/mL. Finally, Cohort 3 received a placebo. The treatment duration for all cohorts was 16 weeks. Results showed that NT-proBNP decreased by 53% in the mavacamten group compared to 1% in the placebo group. Additionally, cardiac Troponin-I decreased by 34% in the mavacamten group, whereas there was a 4% increase in the placebo group. Further analyses demonstrated that Mavacamten improved echo parameters of diastolic function [86].

EXPLORER-HCM was a phase III, multicentre, randomized, double-blind, placebo-controlled trial conducted in 68 clinical cardiovascular centres across 13 countries [87]. The study aimed to evaluate the efficacy and safety profile of mavacamten, which proved to be superior to placebo in both primary and secondary endpoints. For the primary endpoint, 45 out of 123 patients (37%) in the mavacamten group experienced a 1.5 mL/kg per min or greater increase in peak oxygen consumption (pVO$_2$) with at least one-point reduction in NYHA class or an increase of over 30 mL/kg per min in pVO$_2$ with no changes in NYHA class. In contrast, only 22 out of 128 patients (17%) in the placebo group achieved the primary endpoint. Additionally, patients receiving mavacamten showed improvements in post-exercise LVOT gradient, pVO$_2$, and patient-reported health status. Significantly, almost 30% of patients (32 out of 117) treated with mavacamten achieved a complete pharmacological response, defined as a reduction in LVOT gradient to less than 30 mmHg with marked improvement in symptoms. This response was observed in less than 1% of patients (one out of 126) in the placebo group. Notably, the greatest benefit was observed in patients who were not receiving BBs. Treatment with mavacamten also resulted in consistent improvements in patients' reported health status, with greater symptom relief and improved quality of life compared to the placebo group. There was a strong correlation between the magnitude of improvement in health status and the extent of improvement in pVO$_2$, emphasizing the association between mavacamten treatment and enhancements in patient well-being and quality of life. Improvement in health status was reversed 8 weeks after the completion of treatment. A reduction in LVOT was associated with a significant decrease in LVEF. However, the normalization of LVEF after the conclusion of therapy was not immediate, suggesting that, although rare, the improvement in the health status of oHCM patients could be counteracted by the slow reversal of the drug's effect due to its long half-life.

VALOR-HCM was a randomized controlled trial conducted by Desai et al. [88], which investigated whether the addition of mavacamten to maximally tolerated background medical therapy could reduce guideline eligibility for SRT in highly symptomatic oHCM patients. The trial included 112 highly symptomatic patients with oHCM who met the guideline criteria for SRT. These patients had a mean age of 60 ± 12 years, with 51% being male, and 93% classified as NYHA functional class III. The study was conducted between July 2020 and October 2021 at 19 sites in the United States. After 16 weeks of treatment, the results showed that 77% of the patients randomized to placebo (43 out of 56) continued to meet the guideline criteria for SRT or chose to undergo the procedure. Only 7.9% of the mavacamten-treated patients (10 out of 56) met the guideline criteria or elected to undergo SRT (treatment difference of 58.9% [95% CI: 44.0–73.9%]; $p < 0.001$). The addition of mavacamten significantly reduced the eligibility for SRT in these highly symptomatic oHCM patients. Furthermore, this study demonstrated that mavacamten treatment resulted in a significant reduction in LVOT gradients. As in other trials, there were improvements observed in NYHA functional classification and quality-of-life measures among the mavacamten-treated patients. VALOR-HCM was not able to provide long-term safety outcomes due to its focus on a 16-week treatment period. To assess long-term safety, efficacy, and clinically guided dosing, the ongoing 5-year extension study, MAVA-LTE (Mavacamten Long Term Extension; NCT03723655), is currently underway.

An interim analysis has already been performed for this study. During the 36-week follow up evaluated, mavacamten has been shown to achieve significant reduction in both resting and Valsalva-induced LVOTO gradients, with changes reported as -27.4 ± 33 mmHg and -45.7 ± 39.9 mmHg, respectively [89].

ODISSEY-HCM (NCT05582395) is an ongoing randomized, double-blind, phase III study to evaluate mavacamten in adults with symptomatic noHCM compared to placebo. The composite primary endpoints include change from baseline in Kansas City Cardiomyopathy Questionnaire (23 item) Clinical Summary Score and change from baseline in peak oxygen consumption (pVO_2) at week 48. The recruitment phase is ongoing [90].

Overall, trial results for mavacamten have showcased positive safety and efficacy profile. As a result of these findings, the Food and Drug Administration, on April 2022, and the European Commission, on June 2023, have approved this drug for the treatment of symptomatic (NYHA, class II-III) oHCM in adult patients. Furthermore, on 15 June 2023, FDA approved a revised label for mavacamten to reflect drug ability to reduce the need or eligibility for SRT in patients with obstructive HCM as evidenced by the VALOR-HCM trial. Importantly, since mavacamten was initially approved, its prescription details have carried a "Boxed Warning" about the potential risk of HF. This warning stems from data indicating that its use might lead to a reduction in LVEF, which could potentially result in HF due to systolic dysfunction. Of note, mavacamten, as primarily metabolized by CYP2C19, exhibits a wide-ranging elimination half-life dependent on the CYP2C19 phenotype, spanning from 72 to 533 h. For poor metabolisers or patients awaiting genotyping results, the recommended starting dose is 2.5 mg. The dose can only be increased beyond 5 mg once genotyping has confirmed that the patient is not a poor metabolizer [91]. For all other phenotypes, the starting dose is 5 mg. Dose adjustments throughout the treatment, initially at 4-week intervals and subsequently at 12-week intervals, are directed by LVOT gradient and LVEF, as detailed in decision trees in the summary of product characteristics.

New ESC guidelines [35] delivered class IIa recommendation for mavacamten in addition to a beta blocker (or, if this is not possible, with verapamil or diltiazem), or as monotherapy, to improve symptoms in adult patients with resting or provoked LVOTO.

4.2.3. Aficamten

A second myosin inhibitor/allosteric modulator currently under development for the treatment of HCM is CK-274, also known as Aficamten [92]. While Aficamten shares a similar molecular effect with mavacamten, it binds to a different regulatory site on the myosin heads. Aficamten possesses certain pharmacokinetic advantages over mavacamten. It exhibits a shorter half-life of approximately 2 days, allowing for a faster washout in the presence of side effects. Additionally, aficamten does not interact with the enzymes CYP2C19 and CYP3A4, reducing the likelihood of drug–drug interactions. These characteristics contribute to the potential clinical benefits of aficamten in the management of HCM [1].

4.2.4. Aficamten Trials

Phase II REDWOOD-HCM study evaluated the efficacy of aficamten in oHCM patients. Patients with oHCM and LVOT gradients ≥ 30 mmHg at rest or ≥ 50 mmHg with Valsalva were randomized 2:1 to receive aficamten ($n = 28$) or placebo ($n = 13$) in two dose-finding cohorts. Most patients treated with aficamten (78.6% in Cohort 1 and 92.9% in Cohort 2) achieved the treatment target of reducing the resting gradient below 30 mmHg and the post-Valsalva gradient below 50 mmHg by week 10. The mean differences were -40 ± 27 mmHg and -43 ± 37 mmHg in Cohorts 1 and 2, respectively, at rest ($p = 0.0003$ and $p = 0.0004$ versus placebo, respectively). During Valsalva, mean differences were -36 ± 27 mmHg and -53 ± 44 mmHg in the two cohorts, respectively ($p = 0.001$ and $p < 0.0001$ versus placebo, respectively). The incidence of adverse events was similar between the treatment arms, with a negligible reduction in LVEF observed in patients who were administered aficamten. LVEF was transiently reduced below 50% in only one treated patient [93]. FOREST-HCM (previously known as REDWOOD-OLE; NCT04848506) is the 5-year extension study of REDWOOD-HCM [94]. At 48 weeks, aficamten was shown to be safe and well tolerated in patients with oHCM. This trial highlighted a substantial reduction in peak resting and Valsalva LVOT-gradients from baseline to week 48 (resting mean ± SD: −32 ± 28 mmHg; Valsalva mean ± SD: −47 ± 28 mmHg). There was a modest reduction in LVEF from baseline to week 48 (−5 ± 3%) and no patients experienced an aficamten-related reduction in LV ejection fraction < 50%. There was a substantial improvement in functional class, as by week 48, 88% of patients experienced ≥1 NYHA functional class improvement while none had functional worsening.

These data support the continued development of aficamten, which is currently being investigated in the large randomized, placebo-controlled, phase III clinical trial SEQUOIA-HCM (NCT05186818). This study aims to recruit a total of 270 symptomatic oHCM patients. The primary endpoint is the change in pVO$_2$ measured by cardiopulmonary exercise testing from baseline to week 24 (Figure 4). Following the positive results from Cohort 3 of REDWOOD-HCM, patients whose background therapy includes disopyramide, are eligible for enrolment [95]. The recruitment phase is ongoing [96].

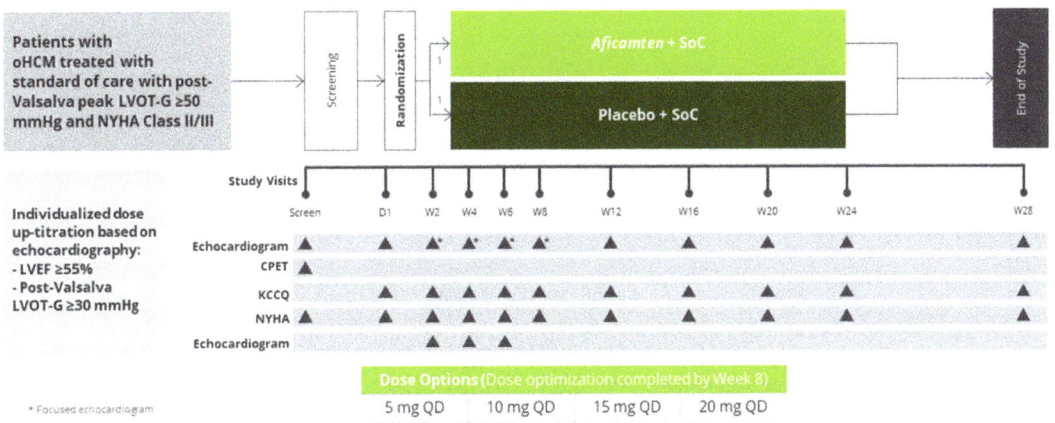

Figure 4. SEQUOIA-HCM trial design. Reproduced with permission from Incorporated, C. 2021 [97].

MAPLE HCM (NCT04349072) is phase 3 multicentre, randomized, double blind active-comparator clinical trial of aficamten compared to metoprolol in patients with symptomatic oHCM. A summary of completed trials is reported in Table 4.

Table 4. Completed studies on Mavacamten and Aficamten treatment in HCM patients.

Trial	Study Design	Study Population	Dose and Timeline	Sample Size	Results
EXPLORER-HCM [76]	Randomized double blind placebo control	Obstructive HCM NYHA II–III	Mavacamten 2.5–15 mg 30 weeks	251	Primary endpoint achieved in 37% of mavacamten patients vs. 17% placebo patients
MAVERICK-HCM [75]	Randomized double blind placebo control	Non-obstructive HCM NYHA class II–III	Mavacamten 16 weeks	59	Median NT-proBNP reduced by 53% in mavacamten group vs. 1% in placebo group. Median TnI reduced by 34% in mavacamten group vs. 4% in placebo group

Table 4. Cont.

Trial	Study Design	Study Population	Dose and Timeline	Sample Size	Results
REDWOOD-HCM [81] Cohorts 1 and 2	Randomized double blind placebo control	Obstructive HCM NYHA II–III	Aficamten 5–15 mg (Cohort 1) 10–30 mg (Cohort 2) 10 weeks	41	Resting LVOTO gradient reduction: median difference of -40 ± 27 mmHg -43 ± 37 mmHg Post-Valsalva LVOTO gradient reduction: -36 ± 27 mmHg -53 ± 44 mmHg
REDWOOD-HCM Cohort 3 [84]	Open label	Obstructive HCM NYHA I–III On disopyramide	Aficamten 5–15 mg 10 weeks	13	Resting LVOTO gradient reduction: -28 ± 3.2 mmHg Post-Valsalva LVOTO gradient reduction: -27 ± 5.9 mmHg
REDWOOD-HCM Cohort 4 [83]	Open label	Non-obstructive HCM NYHA II–III	Aficamten 5–15 mg 10 weeks	41	NT-proBNP reduction (mean reduction by 66%, $p < 0.0001$), TnI reduction (-21%, $p < 0.01$)
VALOR-HCM [77]	Randomized double blind placebo control	Obstructive HCM, referred or under active consideration for SRT	Mavacamten 2.5–15 mg 32 weeks	112	After 16 weeks, 17.9% of mavacamten patients eligible to SRT vs. 76.8% in placebo group ($p < 0.001$)
PIONEER-HCM [71] Cohort A	Open label	Diagnosed with HCM, resting LVOT gradient ≥ 30 mmHg and post-exercise peak LVOTO gradient ≥ 50 mmHg	Mavacamten 10–15 mg 12 weeks	11	pVO$_2$ improvement: +3.5 mL/kg/min, (95%CI:1.2;5.9); Peak exercise LVOTO gradient reduction: -90 mmHg (95%CI: -138; -41)
PIONEER-HCM [71] Cohort B	Open label	Obstructive HCM NYHA II–III	Mavacamten 2–5 mg/die 12 weeks	10	pVO$_2$ improvement +1.7 mL/kg/min, (95%CI: 0.0–3.3) Peak exercise LVOTO gradient reduction: -25 mmHg (95%CI: -47; -3.0)
FOREST-HCM [82]	Open label	Obstructive HCM	Aficamten 5–20 mg 48 weeks	38	Resting LVOTO gradient reduction: -32 ± 28 Resting LVOTO gradient reduction: -47 ± 28
MAVA-LTE [78]	Open label	Obstructive HCM	Mavacamten 2.5–15 mg 36 weeks	137	Resting LVOTO gradient reduction: -27.4 ± 33 Resting LVOTO gradient reduction: -45.7 ± 39.9

HCM, hypertrophic cardiomyopathy; NYHA, New York Heart Association; LVOTO, left ventricular outflow obstruction.

5. Personalized Therapy

The management of HCM represents a major challenge due to the substantial genotypical variability observed in this disease. To better assess the efficacy of pharmacological therapies, human-based computational methodologies have emerged as powerful tools in recent years. By integrating experimental and clinical data, simulation studies have shed light on HCM pathophysiology, phenotypic expression, arrhythmic risk, and response to pharmacological interventions. These advancements have enhanced our mechanistic understanding of the disease and paved the way for personalized therapy in HCM [98].

Passini et al. utilized human experimental data on HCM to develop and calibrate an electrophysiological model of HCM cardiomyocytes [99]. This model successfully elucidated key mechanisms contributing to arrhythmia development in HCM and identified potential pharmacological targets. Reactivation of the overexpressed ICaL (L-type calcium current) was identified as a crucial factor driving repolarization abnormalities in HCM. Through simulated human drug trials, the researchers investigated anti-arrhythmic strategies tailored to the HCM phenotype. Selective ICaL block demonstrated high efficacy in suppressing pro-arrhythmic abnormalities but compromised calcium transient amplitude. Conversely, multichannel blockage of sodium–calcium exchanger, late sodium current INaL, and ICaL exhibited a more favourable efficacy profile without negative effects on systolic calcium.

In the majority of HCM cases, the disease is caused by genetic mutations affecting sarcomeric proteins. In silico studies have explored the primary effects of point mutations on sarcomere contractility and their propensity for arrhythmogenesis [100]. Computational techniques ranging from molecular dynamics to spatially explicit sarcomere modelling have been employed. By focusing on early human pathophysiology associated with HCM mutations, independent of compensatory responses and long-term remodelling, effective targets can be identified. Modulating these targets pharmacologically could aid in resolving the disease phenotype. Leveraging information on the impact of myosin mutations on cellular contractility, Margara et al. employed an in silico model of human electromechanical cardiomyocytes to simulate the effects of the novel myosin inhibitor mavacamten and investigate its mutation-specific efficacy in HCM [101].

Germline editing is a promising strategy for addressing monogenic diseases by preventing the transmission of mutations to future generations. The development of genome editing technologies, such as CRISPR/Cas9, has generated considerable enthusiasm for their therapeutic potential in cardiovascular diseases. However, several challenges are still ahead before a clinical implementation can be realized [102].

Current techniques, including CRISPR/Cas9, induce double-stranded DNA breaks at specific genetic loci, which triggers the cell's intrinsic repair mechanisms. Recent advancements have demonstrated the feasibility of high-fidelity gene repair in human embryos carrying HCM mutations. In a study, oocytes from healthy women were inseminated with sperm from a male patient carrying a heterozygous MYBPC3 mutation. By simultaneously injecting a mutation-specific CRISPR/Cas9 system during early metaphase, the mutation was successfully edited in 100% of cases. Importantly, this technique also eliminated mosaicism, a phenomenon where sister cells within the same embryo possess different genotypes [103]. However, off-target effects remain a significant concern.

Another promising gene-based therapeutic approach for monogenic diseases is allele-specific gene silencing. This technique typically involves the transduction of an adenovirus vector containing short-interfering ribonucleic acid (siRNA) segments designed to suppress the expression of a specific pathogenic allele. This method, known as ribonucleic acid interference (RNAi), has shown efficacy in pre-clinical models for attenuating the phenotype of mutations associated with conditions such as catecholaminergic polymorphic ventricular tachycardia, HCM, and restrictive cardiomyopathy [104]. However, this approach is better suited for conditions caused by gain-of-function mutations (e.g., MYH7) and may not apply to the entire spectrum of HCM (e.g., MYBPC3).

Reichard et al. [105] explored the efficacy of two distinct genetic therapies in mice carrying the heterozygous HCM pathogenic variant myosin R403Q. Their approach focused on both a genetic therapy approach involving an adenine base editor (ABE8e, allowing for precise modification of the genomic DNA sequence) and delivery of RNA-guided Cas9 nuclease using AAV9. In the first case, a single dose of this dual-AAV9 system successfully corrected the pathogenic variant in over 70% of ventricular cardiomyocytes, leading to the restoration of normal cardiac structure and function. Furthermore, this correction remained durable over time. The second genetic therapy using RNA-guided Cas9 nuclease aimed to inactivate the pathogenic allele entirely. Although effective, it exhibited dose-dependent toxicities. This study highlighted the substantial potential of single-dose genetic therapies to correct or silence pathogenic variants, thus preventing the development of HCM. In fact, they achieved a long-lasting in vivo base editing of the pathogenic single-nucleotide variant in myosin, which is highly and selectively expressed in cardiomyocytes. Moving forward, the further development and translation of this approach hold significant promise for correcting the most severe human pathogenic variants.

6. Artificial Intelligence: Hype or Hope?

In a study conducted by Tison et al. [106] use of artificial intelligence-enhanced electrocardiogram (AI-ECG) readings was investigated for assessing disease status and treatment response in patients with oHCM. The two algorithms used were independently created by UCSF and Mayo Clinic [107]. The study was based on data from the PIONEER-OLE trial and revealed a significant correlation between AI-ECG HCM scores and disease status, as measured by reductions in LVOT gradients and NT-proBNP levels over time in patients receiving mavacamten. The observed longitudinal associations between the AI-ECG HCM score and disease parameters likely reflect changes in the raw ECG waveform that can be detected by AI-ECG and are indicative of the pathophysiology and severity of HCM. This study presents a novel paradigm in which AI-ECG, which can be conveniently implemented remotely using smartphone-enabled electrodes, may enable the assessment of disease status and treatment response [108,109]. Future investigations can further evaluate the utility of this approach in guiding drug titration to improve patient safety and outcomes.

7. Conclusions

Just a few years ago, treatment for HCM was restricted to symptomatic management. The use of non-selective medications like β blockers and calcium channel blockers, alongside septal reduction surgery, ICDs for primary and secondary prevention of SCD, and lifestyle modifications, constituted the mainstays of HCM treatment for a considerable period. However, advancements in our understanding of the pathophysiological processes and molecular foundations of the disease have led to the development of specific new drug classes. These have the potential to impact not just symptoms, but also the progression of the disease itself. Emblematic of this shift in paradigm are myosin modulators, such as mavacamten and aficamten. In addition, significant breakthroughs may arise from the fields of genetics and biotechnology, heralding a transformation as captivating as it was previously unthinkable. One such example is the use of genome-editing technologies like CRISPR/Cas9, which can potentially repair the genome of embryos, exploiting the monogenic nature of HCM. Other possibilities encompass the modulation of gene expression by siRNAs that inhibit the expression of the disease-causing allele. In the future, artificial intelligence could also play a significant role in this field, contributing to minimally invasive and remote monitoring tools that could enhance risk stratification schemes and facilitate early therapeutic interventions. In summary, we are witnessing a true revolution in the therapeutic approach to HCM. HCM patients will soon benefit from an entirely new range of more specific and efficacious drugs. The dawn of precision medicine has indeed truly arrived.

Author Contributions: Conceptualization, A.O., F.R., L.V.M., D.M., F.P. and S.G.; methodology, A.O., L.V.M. and D.M.; writing—original draft preparation, A.O., L.V.M., D.M., K.G. and M.Y.K.; writing—review and editing, F.R., M.Y.K., G.R., F.P., A.A.C., S.G., C.M., L.S. and M.Z.; supervision, L.S., S.G., F.P. and A.A.C.; funding acquisition, F.R. and S.G. All authors have read and agreed to the published version of the manuscript.

Funding: 2019 Search for Excellence Starting Grant, G.d'Annunzio University of Chieti-Pescara.

Institutional Review Board Statement: Not applicable.

Informed Consent Statement: Not applicable.

Data Availability Statement: Not applicable.

Conflicts of Interest: F.R. declares lecture fees from Takeda, Menarini and PIAM pharma, travel/accommodation/meeting expenses from Bayer and Daichii-Sankyo. The other authors declare no conflict of interest.

References

1. Palandri, C.; Santini, L.; Argirò, A.; Margara, F.; Doste, R.; Bueno-Orovio, A.; Olivotto, I.; Coppini, R. Pharmacological Management of Hypertrophic Cardiomyopathy: From Bench to Bedside. *Drugs* **2022**, *82*, 889–912. [CrossRef] [PubMed]
2. Autore, C.; Francia, P.; Tini, G.; Musumeci, B. Old and New Therapeutic Solutions in the Treatment of Hypertrophic Cardiomyopathy. *Eur. Heart J. Suppl.* **2023**, *25* (Suppl. B), B12–B15. [CrossRef] [PubMed]
3. Ommen, S.R.; Mital, S.; Burke, M.A.; Day, S.M.; Deswal, A.; Elliott, P.; Evanovich, L.L.; Hung, J.; Joglar, J.A.; Kantor, P.; et al. 2020 AHA/ACC Guideline for the Diagnosis and Treatment of Patients with Hypertrophic Cardiomyopathy: A Report of the American College of Cardiology/American Heart Association Joint Committee on Clinical Practice Guidelines. *Circulation* **2020**, *142*, e558–e631. [CrossRef]
4. Todde, G.; Canciello, G.; Borrelli, F.; Perillo, E.F.; Esposito, G.; Lombardi, R.; Losi, M.A. Diagnosis and Treatment of Obstructive Hypertrophic Cardiomyopathy. *Cardiogenetics* **2023**, *13*, 75–91. [CrossRef]
5. Maron, B.J.; Desai, M.Y.; Nishimura, R.A.; Spirito, P.; Rakowski, H.; Towbin, J.A.; Rowin, E.J.; Maron, M.S.; Sherrid, M.V. Diagnosis and Evaluation of Hypertrophic Cardiomyopathy. *J. Am. Coll. Cardiol.* **2022**, *79*, 372–389. [CrossRef] [PubMed]
6. Biddinger, K.J.; Jurgens, S.J.; Maamari, D.; Gaziano, L.; Choi, S.H.; Morrill, V.N.; Halford, J.L.; Khera, A.V.; Lubitz, S.A.; Ellinor, P.T.; et al. Rare and Common Genetic Variation Underlying the Risk of Hypertrophic Cardiomyopathy in a National Biobank. *JAMA Cardiol.* **2022**, *7*, 715–722. [CrossRef] [PubMed]
7. Beltrami, M.; Fedele, E.; Fumagalli, C.; Mazzarotto, F.; Girolami, F.; Ferrantini, C.; Coppini, R.; Tofani, L.; Bertaccini, B.; Poggesi, C.; et al. Long-Term Prevalence of Systolic Dysfunction in MYBPC3 Versus MYH7-Related Hypertrophic Cardiomyopathy. *Circ. Genomic. Precis. Med.* **2023**, *16*, 363–371. [CrossRef] [PubMed]
8. Sankaranarayanan, R.; Fleming, J.E.; Garratt, J.C. Mimics of Hypertrophic Cardiomyopathy—Diagnostic Clues to Aid Early Identification of Phenocopies. *Arrhythmia Electrophysiol. Rev.* **2013**, *2*, 36–40. [CrossRef]
9. Sachdev, B.; Takenaka, T.; Teraguchi, H.; Tei, C.; Lee, P.; McKenna, W.J.; Elliott, P.M. Prevalence of Anderson-Fabry Disease in Male Patients with Late Onset Hypertrophic Cardiomyopathy. *Circulation* **2002**, *105*, 1407–1411. [CrossRef]
10. Ricci, F.; Bisaccia, G.; Mansour, D.; Molinari, L.V.; Di Mauro, M.; Renda, G.; Khanji, M.Y.; Gallina, S. Prognostic Significance of Late Gadolinium Enhancement in Fabry Disease—A Systematic Review and Meta-Analysis. *Am. J. Cardiol.* **2023**, *202*, 4–5. [CrossRef]
11. Gange, C.A.; Link, M.S.; Maron, M.S. Utility of Cardiovascular Magnetic Resonance in the Diagnosis of Anderson-Fabry Disease. *Circulation* **2009**, *120*, e96–e97. [CrossRef] [PubMed]
12. Linhart, A.; Elliott, P.M. The Heart in Anderson-Fabry Disease and Other Lysosomal Storage Disorders. *Heart Br. Card. Soc.* **2007**, *93*, 528–535. [CrossRef] [PubMed]
13. Dorbala, S.; Ando, Y.; Bokhari, S.; Dispenzieri, A.; Falk, R.H.; Ferrari, V.A.; Fontana, M.; Gheysens, O.; Gillmore, J.D.; Glaudemans, A.W.J.M.; et al. ASNC/AHA/ASE/EANM/HFSA/ISA/SCMR/SNMMI Expert Consensus Recommendations for Multimodality Imaging in Cardiac Amyloidosis: Part 1 of 2-Evidence Base and Standardized Methods of Imaging. *J. Nucl. Cardiol.* **2019**, *26*, 2065–2123. [CrossRef] [PubMed]
14. Dorbala, S.; Ando, Y.; Bokhari, S.; Dispenzieri, A.; Falk, R.H.; Ferrari, V.A.; Fontana, M.; Gheysens, O.; Gillmore, J.D.; Glaudemans, A.W.J.M.; et al. ASNC/AHA/ASE/EANM/HFSA/ISA/SCMR/SNMMI Expert Consensus Recommendations for Multimodality Imaging in Cardiac Amyloidosis: Part 2 of 2-Diagnostic Criteria and Appropriate Utilization. *J. Nucl. Cardiol.* **2020**, *27*, 659–673. [CrossRef] [PubMed]
15. Lynch, A.; Tatangelo, M.; Ahuja, S.; Steve Fan, C.-P.; Min, S.; Lafreniere-Roula, M.; Papaz, T.; Zhou, V.; Armstrong, K.; Aziz, P.F.; et al. Risk of Sudden Death in Patients with RASopathy Hypertrophic Cardiomyopathy. *J. Am. Coll. Cardiol.* **2023**, *81*, 1035–1045. [CrossRef] [PubMed]
16. Ackerman, M.J.; Garmany, R. RASopathy-Associated Cardiac Hypertrophy: A Shocking Gap in Care. *J. Am. Coll. Cardiol.* **2023**, *81*, 1046–1048. [CrossRef] [PubMed]
17. Nagakura, T.; Takeuchi, M.; Yoshitani, H.; Nakai, H.; Nishikage, T.; Kokumai, T.; Otani, S.; Yoshiyama, M.; Yoshikawa, J. Hypertrophic Cardiomyopathy Is Associated with More Severe Left Ventricular Dyssynchrony than Is Hypertensive Left Ventricular Hypertrophy. *Echocardiography* **2007**, *24*, 677–684. [CrossRef]
18. Bourek, D.; Jirikowic, J.; Taylor, M. Natural History of Danon Disease. *Genet. Med.* **2011**, *13*, 563–568. [CrossRef]
19. Charron, P.; Villard, E.; Sébillon, P.; Laforêt, P.; Maisonobe, T.; Duboscq-Bidot, L.; Romero, N.; Drouin-Garraud, V.; Frébourg, T.; Richard, P.; et al. Danon's Disease as a Cause of Hypertrophic Cardiomyopathy: A Systematic Survey. *Heart Br. Card. Soc.* **2004**, *90*, 842–846. [CrossRef]
20. Fayssoil, A. Cardiomyopathy in Pompe's Disease. *Eur. J. Intern. Med.* **2008**, *19*, 57–59. [CrossRef]
21. Kelly, B.P.; Russell, M.W.; Hennessy, J.R.; Ensing, G.J. Severe Hypertrophic Cardiomyopathy in an Infant with a Novel PRKAG2 Gene Mutation: Potential Differences between Infantile and Adult Onset Presentation. *Pediatr. Cardiol.* **2009**, *30*, 1176–1179. [CrossRef] [PubMed]

22. Wolf, C.M.; Arad, M.; Ahmad, F.; Sanbe, A.; Bernstein, S.A.; Toka, O.; Konno, T.; Morley, G.; Robbins, J.; Seidman, J.G.; et al. Reversibility of PRKAG2 Glycogen-Storage Cardiomyopathy and Electrophysiological Manifestations. *Circulation* **2008**, *117*, 144–154. [CrossRef] [PubMed]
23. Galanti, K.; Di Marino, M.; Mantini, C.; Gallina, S.; Ricci, F. Burnt-out Cori-Forbes Cardiomyopathy. *Eur. Heart J. Case Rep.* **2023**, *7*, ytad326. [CrossRef] [PubMed]
24. Maron, B.J. Distinguishing Hypertrophic Cardiomyopathy from Athlete's Heart: A Clinical Problem of Increasing Magnitude and Significance. *Heart Br. Card. Soc.* **2005**, *91*, 1380–1382. [CrossRef] [PubMed]
25. De Innocentiis, C.; Ricci, F.; Khanji, M.Y.; Aung, N.; Tana, C.; Verrengia, E.; Petersen, S.E.; Gallina, S. Athlete's Heart: Diagnostic Challenges and Future Perspectives. *Sports Med.* **2018**, *48*, 2463–2477. [CrossRef] [PubMed]
26. Ricci, F.; Banihashemi, B.; Pirouzifard, M.; Sundquist, J.; Sundquist, K.; Sutton, R.; Fedorowski, A.; Zöller, B. Familial Risk of Dilated and Hypertrophic Cardiomyopathy: A National Family Study in Sweden. *ESC Heart Fail.* **2023**, *10*, 121–132. [CrossRef] [PubMed]
27. Malhotra, A.; Sharma, S. Hypertrophic Cardiomyopathy in Athletes. *Eur. Cardiol.* **2017**, *12*, 80–82. [CrossRef] [PubMed]
28. Canepa, M.; Pozios, I.; Vianello, P.F.; Ameri, P.; Brunelli, C.; Ferrucci, L.; Abraham, T.P. Distinguishing Ventricular Septal Bulge versus Hypertrophic Cardiomyopathy in the Elderly. *Heart Br. Card. Soc.* **2016**, *102*, 1087–1094. [CrossRef]
29. Sebastian, S.A.; Panthangi, V.; Singh, K.; Rayaroth, R.; Gupta, A.; Shantharam, D.; Rasool, B.Q.; Padda, I.; Co, E.L.; Johal, G. Hypertrophic Cardiomyopathy: Current Treatment and Future Options. *Curr. Probl. Cardiol.* **2023**, *48*, 101552. [CrossRef]
30. Nagueh, S.F.; Phelan, D.; Abraham, T.; Armour, A.; Desai, M.Y.; Dragulescu, A.; Gilliland, Y.; Lester, S.J.; Maldonado, Y.; Mohiddin, S.; et al. Recommendations for Multimodality Cardiovascular Imaging of Patients with Hypertrophic Cardiomyopathy: An Update from the American Society of Echocardiography, in Collaboration with the American Society of Nuclear Cardiology, the Society for Cardiovascular Magnetic Resonance, and the Society of Cardiovascular Computed Tomography. *J. Am. Soc. Echocardiogr.* **2022**, *35*, 533–569. [CrossRef]
31. Turvey, L.; Augustine, D.X.; Robinson, S.; Oxborough, D.; Stout, M.; Smith, N.; Harkness, A.; Williams, L.; Steeds, R.P.; Bradlow, W. Transthoracic Echocardiography of Hypertrophic Cardiomyopathy in Adults: A Practical Guideline from the British Society of Echocardiography. *Echo Res. Pract.* **2021**, *8*, G61–G86. [CrossRef] [PubMed]
32. D'Andrea, A.; Caso, P.; Cuomo, S.; Salerno, G.; Scarafile, R.; Mita, C.; De Corato, G.; Sarubbi, B.; Scherillo, M.; Calabrò, R. Prognostic Value of Intra-Left Ventricular Electromechanical Asynchrony in Patients with Mild Hypertrophic Cardiomyopathy Compared with Power Athletes. *Br. J. Sports Med.* **2006**, *40*, 244–250; discussion 244–250. [CrossRef] [PubMed]
33. Haland, T.F.; Almaas, V.M.; Hasselberg, N.E.; Saberniak, J.; Leren, I.S.; Hopp, E.; Edvardsen, T.; Haugaa, K.H. Strain Echocardiography Is Related to Fibrosis and Ventricular Arrhythmias in Hypertrophic Cardiomyopathy. *Eur. Heart J. Cardiovasc. Imaging* **2016**, *17*, 613–621. [CrossRef]
34. Erden, M.; van Velzen, H.G.; Menting, M.E.; van den Bosch, A.E.; Ren, B.; Michels, M.; Vletter, W.B.; van Domburg, R.T.; Schinkel, A.F.L. Three-Dimensional Echocardiography for the Assessment of Left Ventricular Geometry and Papillary Muscle Morphology in Hypertrophic Cardiomyopathy. *J. Ultrasound* **2018**, *21*, 17–24. [CrossRef] [PubMed]
35. Arbelo, E.; Protonotarios, A.; Gimeno, J.R.; Arbustini, E.; Barriales-Villa, R.; Basso, C.; Bezzina, C.R.; Biagini, E.; Blom, N.A.; de Boer, R.A.; et al. 2023 ESC Guidelines for the Management of Cardiomyopathies: Developed by the Task Force on the Management of Cardiomyopathies of the European Society of Cardiology (ESC). *Eur. Heart J.* **2023**, ehad194, *online ahead of print*. [CrossRef] [PubMed]
36. Zeppenfeld, K.; Tfelt-Hansen, J.; De Riva, M.; Winkel, B.G.; Behr, E.R.; Blom, N.A.; Charron, P.; Corrado, D.; Dagres, N.; De Chillou, C. 2022 ESC Guidelines for the Management of Patients with Ventricular Arrhythmias and the Prevention of Sudden Cardiac Death. *Eur. Heart J.* **2022**, *43*, 3997–4126. [CrossRef] [PubMed]
37. Penetrance of Hypertrophic Cardiomyopathy in Sarcomere Protein Mutation Carriers. Available online: https://pubmed.ncbi.nlm.nih.gov/32731933/ (accessed on 21 July 2023).
38. Joy, G.; Kelly, C.I.; Webber, M.; Pierce, I.; Teh, I.; McGrath, L.; Velazquez, P.; Hughes, R.K.; Kotwal, H.; Das, A.; et al. Microstructural and Microvascular Phenotype of Sarcomere Mutation Carriers and Overt Hypertrophic Cardiomyopathy. *Circulation* **2023**, *ahead of print*. [CrossRef] [PubMed]
39. Lillo, R.; Graziani, F.; Franceschi, F.; Iannaccone, G.; Massetti, M.; Olivotto, I.; Crea, F.; Liuzzo, G. Inflammation across the Spectrum of Hypertrophic Cardiac Phenotypes. *Heart Fail. Rev.* **2023**, *28*, 1065–1075. [CrossRef]
40. Matthia, E.L.; Setteducato, M.L.; Elzeneini, M.; Vernace, N.; Salerno, M.; Kramer, C.M.; Keeley, E.C. Circulating Biomarkers in Hypertrophic Cardiomyopathy. *J. Am. Heart Assoc.* **2022**, *11*, e027618. [CrossRef]
41. Lampert, R.; Ackerman, M.J.; Marino, B.S.; Burg, M.; Ainsworth, B.; Salberg, L.; Tome Esteban, M.T.; Ho, C.Y.; Abraham, R.; Balaji, S.; et al. Vigorous Exercise in Patients with Hypertrophic Cardiomyopathy. *JAMA Cardiol.* **2023**, *8*, 595–605. [CrossRef]
42. Delise, P.; Mos, L.; Sciarra, L.; Basso, C.; Biffi, A.; Cecchi, F.; Colivicchi, F.; Corrado, D.; D'Andrea, A.; Di Cesare, E.; et al. Italian Cardiological Guidelines (COCIS) for Competitive Sport Eligibility in Athletes with Heart Disease: Update 2020. *J. Cardiovasc. Med.* **2021**, *22*, 874–891. [CrossRef] [PubMed]
43. 2014 ESC Guidelines on Diagnosis and Management of Hypertrophic Cardiomyopathy: The Task Force for the Diagnosis and Management of Hypertrophic Cardiomyopathy of the European Society of Cardiology (ESC). *Eur. Heart J.* **2014**, *35*, 2733–2779. [CrossRef]

44. Joy, G.; Moon, J.C.; Lopes, L.R. Detection of Subclinical Hypertrophic Cardiomyopathy. *Nat. Rev. Cardiol.* **2023**, *20*, 369–370. [CrossRef] [PubMed]
45. Rapezzi, C. EXPLORER-HCM: Il mavacamten nel trattamento della cardiomiopatia ipertrofica ostruttiva sintomatica. *G. Ital. Cardiol.* **2021**, *22*, 30–32.
46. Argirò, A.; Zampieri, M.; Marchi, A.; Franco, A.D.; Pàlinkàs, E.D.; Biagioni, G.; Chiti, C.; Mazzoni, C.; Fornaro, A.; Targetti, M.; et al. Approcci terapeutici nella cardiomiopatia ipertrofica: Dal controllo dei sintomi alla terapia di precisione. *G. Ital. Cardiol.* **2023**, *24*, 1–8.
47. Rosenzveig, A.; Garg, N.; Rao, S.J.; Kanwal, A.K.; Kanwal, S.; Aronow, W.S.; Martinez, M.W. Current and Emerging Pharmacotherapy for the Management of Hypertrophic Cardiomyopathy. *Expert Opin. Pharmacother.* **2023**, *24*, 1349–1360. [CrossRef] [PubMed]
48. Ammirati, E.; Contri, R.; Coppini, R.; Cecchi, F.; Frigerio, M.; Olivotto, I. Pharmacological Treatment of Hypertrophic Cardiomyopathy: Current Practice and Novel Perspectives: Pharmacological Treatment of HCM. *Eur. J. Heart Fail.* **2016**, *18*, 1106–1118. [CrossRef]
49. McDonagh, T.A.; Metra, M.; Adamo, M.; Gardner, R.S.; Baumbach, A.; Böhm, M.; Burri, H.; Butler, J.; Čelutkienė, J.; Chioncel, O.; et al. 2021 ESC Guidelines for the Diagnosis and Treatment of Acute and Chronic Heart Failure. *Eur. Heart J.* **2021**, *42*, 3599–3726. [CrossRef]
50. Frishman, W.H. Calcium Channel Blockers: Differences between Subclasses. *Am. J. Cardiovasc. Drugs* **2007**, *7* (Suppl. S1), 17–23. [CrossRef]
51. Coppini, R.; Santini, L.; Olivotto, I.; Ackerman, M.J.; Cerbai, E. Abnormalities in Sodium Current and Calcium Homoeostasis as Drivers of Arrhythmogenesis in Hypertrophic Cardiomyopathy. *Cardiovasc. Res.* **2020**, *116*, 1585–1599. [CrossRef]
52. Gilligan, D.M.; Chan, W.L.; Joshi, J.; Clarke, P.; Fletcher, A.; Krikler, S.; Oakley, C.M. A Double-Blind, Placebo-Controlled Crossover Trial of Nadolol and Verapamil in Mild and Moderately Symptomatic Hypertrophic Cardiomyopathy. *J. Am. Coll. Cardiol.* **1993**, *21*, 1672–1679. [CrossRef] [PubMed]
53. Sherrid, M.V.; Barac, I.; McKenna, W.J.; Elliott, P.M.; Dickie, S.; Chojnowska, L.; Casey, S.; Maron, B.J. Multicenter Study of the Efficacy and Safety of Disopyramide in Obstructive Hypertrophic Cardiomyopathy. *J. Am. Coll. Cardiol.* **2005**, *45*, 1251–1258. [CrossRef] [PubMed]
54. Coppini, R.; Ferrantini, C.; Pioner, J.M.; Santini, L.; Wang, Z.J.; Palandri, C.; Scardigli, M.; Vitale, G.; Sacconi, L.; Stefàno, P.; et al. Electrophysiological and Contractile Effects of Disopyramide in Patients with Obstructive Hypertrophic Cardiomyopathy: A Translational Study. *JACC Basic Transl. Sci.* **2019**, *4*, 795–813. [CrossRef] [PubMed]
55. Maurizi, N.; Chiriatti, C.; Fumagalli, C.; Targetti, M.; Passantino, S.; Antiochos, P.; Skalidis, I.; Chiti, C.; Biagioni, G.; Tomberli, A.; et al. Real-World Use and Predictors of Response to Disopyramide in Patients with Obstructive Hypertrophic Cardiomyopathy. *J. Clin. Med.* **2023**, *12*, 2725. [CrossRef] [PubMed]
56. Morady, F.; Scheinman, M.M.; Desai, J. Disopyramide. *Ann. Intern. Med.* **1982**, *96*, 337–343. [CrossRef] [PubMed]
57. Hamada, M.; Shigematsu, Y.; Ikeda, S.; Hara, Y.; Okayama, H.; Kodama, K.; Ochi, T.; Hiwada, K. Class Ia Antiarrhythmic Drug Cibenzoline: A New Approach to the Medical Treatment of Hypertrophic Obstructive Cardiomyopathy. *Circulation* **1997**, *96*, 1520–1524. [CrossRef]
58. Anan, R. Editorial: Cibenzoline for Left Ventricular Outflow Tract Obstruction in Tako-Tsubo Cardiomyopathy and Hypertrophic Cardiomyopathy. *J. Cardiol. Cases* **2015**, *11*, 158–159. [CrossRef]
59. Olivotto, I.; Camici, P.G.; Merlini, P.A.; Rapezzi, C.; Patten, M.; Climent, V.; Sinagra, G.; Tomberli, B.; Marin, F.; Ehlermann, P.; et al. Efficacy of Ranolazine in Patients with Symptomatic Hypertrophic Cardiomyopathy: The RESTYLE-HCM Randomized, Double-Blind, Placebo-Controlled Study. *Circ. Heart Fail.* **2018**, *11*, e004124. [CrossRef]
60. Olivotto, I.; Hellawell, J.L.; Farzaneh-Far, R.; Blair, C.; Coppini, R.; Myers, J.; Belardinelli, L.; Maron, M.S. Novel Approach Targeting the Complex Pathophysiology of Hypertrophic Cardiomyopathy: The Impact of Late Sodium Current Inhibition on Exercise Capacity in Subjects with Symptomatic Hypertrophic Cardiomyopathy (LIBERTY-HCM) Trial. *Circ. Heart Fail.* **2016**, *9*, e002764. [CrossRef]
61. Axelsson, A.; Iversen, K.; Vejlstrup, N.; Ho, C.; Norsk, J.; Langhoff, L.; Ahtarovski, K.; Corell, P.; Havndrup, O.; Jensen, M.; et al. Efficacy and Safety of the Angiotensin II Receptor Blocker Losartan for Hypertrophic Cardiomyopathy: The INHERIT Randomised, Double-Blind, Placebo-Controlled Trial. *Lancet Diabetes Endocrinol.* **2015**, *3*, 123–131. [CrossRef]
62. Martin, T.G.; Juarros, M.A.; Leinwand, L.A. Regression of Cardiac Hypertrophy in Health and Disease: Mechanisms and Therapeutic Potential. *Nat. Rev. Cardiol.* **2023**, *20*, 347–363. [CrossRef] [PubMed]
63. Olivotto, I.; Ashley, E.A. INHERIT (INHibition of the Renin Angiotensin System in Hypertrophic Cardiomyopathy and the Effect on Hypertrophy—A Randomised Intervention Trial with Losartan). *Glob. Cardiol. Sci. Pract.* **2015**, *2015*, 7. [CrossRef] [PubMed]
64. Ho, C.Y.; Day, S.M.; Axelsson, A.; Russell, M.W.; Zahka, K.; Lever, H.M.; Pereira, A.C.; Colan, S.D.; Margossian, R.; Murphy, A.M.; et al. Valsartan in Early-Stage Hypertrophic Cardiomyopathy: A Randomized Phase 2 Trial. *Nat. Med.* **2021**, *27*, 1818–1824. [CrossRef] [PubMed]
65. Packer, M.; McMurray, J.J.; Desai, A.S.; Gong, J.; Lefkowitz, M.P.; Rizkala, A.R.; Rouleau, J.L.; Shi, V.C.; Solomon, S.D.; Swedberg, K.; et al. Angiotensin Receptor Neprilysin Inhibition Compared with Enalapril on the Risk of Clinical Progression in Surviving Patients with Heart Failure. *Circulation* **2015**, *131*, 54–61. [CrossRef]

66. Tafelmeier, M.; Baessler, A.; Wagner, S.; Unsoeld, B.; Preveden, A.; Barlocco, F.; Tomberli, A.; Popovic, D.; Brennan, P.; MacGowan, G.A.; et al. Design of the SILICOFCM Study: Effect of Sacubitril/Valsartan vs Lifestyle Intervention on Functional Capacity in Patients with Hypertrophic Cardiomyopathy. *Clin. Cardiol.* **2020**, *43*, 430–440. [CrossRef]
67. Nishimura, R.A.; Ommen, S.R. Septal Reduction Therapy for Obstructive Hypertrophic Cardiomyopathy and Sudden Death. *Circ. Cardiovasc. Interv.* **2010**, *3*, 91–93. [CrossRef]
68. Ommen, S.R.; Mital, S.; Burke, M.A.; Day, S.M.; Deswal, A.; Elliott, P.; Evanovich, L.L.; Hung, J.; Joglar, J.A.; Kantor, P.; et al. 2020 AHA/ACC Guideline for the Diagnosis and Treatment of Patients with Hypertrophic Cardiomyopathy: A Report of the American College of Cardiology/American Heart Association Joint Committee on Clinical Practice Guidelines. *J. Am. Coll. Cardiol.* **2020**, *76*, e159–e240. [CrossRef] [PubMed]
69. Maron, B.J.; Desai, M.Y.; Nishimura, R.A.; Spirito, P.; Rakowski, H.; Towbin, J.A.; Dearani, J.A.; Rowin, E.J.; Maron, M.S.; Sherrid, M.V. Management of Hypertrophic Cardiomyopathy. *J. Am. Coll. Cardiol.* **2022**, *79*, 390–414. [CrossRef]
70. Pelliccia, F.; Niccoli, G.; Gragnano, F.; Limongelli, G.; Moscarella, E.; Andò, G.; Esposito, A.; Stabile, E.; Ussia, G.P.; Tarantini, G.; et al. Alcohol Septal Ablation for Hypertrophic Obstructive Cardiomyopathy: A Contemporary Reappraisal. *EuroIntervention* **2019**, *15*, 411–417. [CrossRef]
71. Gersh, B.J.; Maron, B.J.; Bonow, R.O.; Dearani, J.A.; Fifer, M.A.; Link, M.S.; Naidu, S.S.; Nishimura, R.A.; Ommen, S.R.; Rakowski, H.; et al. 2011 ACCF/AHA Guideline for the Diagnosis and Treatment of Hypertrophic Cardiomyopathy: A Report of the American College of Cardiology Foundation/American Heart Association Task Force on Practice Guidelines. Developed in Collaboration with the American Association for Thoracic Surgery, American Society of Echocardiography, American Society of Nuclear Cardiology, Heart Failure Society of America, Heart Rhythm Society, Society for Cardiovascular Angiography and Interventions, and Society of Thoracic Surgeons. *J. Am. Coll. Cardiol.* **2011**, *58*, e212–e260. [CrossRef]
72. Pelliccia, A. New Evidences Recommend an Active Lifestyle in Young HCM Patients. *Int. J. Cardiol.* **2022**, *369*, 82–83. [CrossRef] [PubMed]
73. Stewart, S.; Mason, D.T.; Braunwald, E. Impaired Rate of Left Ventricular Filling in Idiopathic Hypertrophic Subaortic Stenosis and Valvular Aortic Stenosis. *Circulation* **1968**, *37*, 8–14. [CrossRef] [PubMed]
74. Phung, L.; Karvinen, S.; Colson, B.; Thomas, D.; Lowe, D. Age Affects Myosin Relaxation States in Skeletal Muscle Fibers of Female but Not Male Mice. *PLoS ONE* **2018**, *13*, e0199062. [CrossRef] [PubMed]
75. Toepfer, C.N.; Garfinkel, A.C.; Venturini, G.; Wakimoto, H.; Repetti, G.; Alamo, L.; Sharma, A.; Agarwal, R.; Ewoldt, J.F.; Cloonan, P.; et al. Myosin Sequestration Regulates Sarcomere Function, Cardiomyocyte Energetics, and Metabolism, Informing the Pathogenesis of Hypertrophic Cardiomyopathy. *Circulation* **2020**, *141*, 828–842. [CrossRef] [PubMed]
76. Toepfer, C.N.; Wakimoto, H.; Garfinkel, A.C.; McDonough, B.; Liao, D.; Jiang, J.; Tai, A.C.; Gorham, J.M.; Lunde, I.G.; Lun, M.; et al. Hypertrophic Cardiomyopathy Mutations in MYBPC3 Dysregulate Myosin. *Sci. Transl. Med.* **2019**, *11*, eaat1199. [CrossRef] [PubMed]
77. Volkmann, N.; Lui, H.; Hazelwood, L.; Trybus, K.M.; Lowey, S.; Hanein, D. The R403Q Myosin Mutation Implicated in Familial Hypertrophic Cardiomyopathy Causes Disorder at the Actomyosin Interface. *PLoS ONE* **2007**, *2*, e1123. [CrossRef] [PubMed]
78. Green, E.M.; Wakimoto, H.; Anderson, R.L.; Evanchik, M.J.; Gorham, J.M.; Harrison, B.C.; Henze, M.; Kawas, R.; Oslob, J.D.; Rodriguez, H.M.; et al. A Small-Molecule Inhibitor of Sarcomere Contractility Suppresses Hypertrophic Cardiomyopathy in Mice. *Science* **2016**, *351*, 617–621. [CrossRef]
79. Spudich, J.A. Hypertrophic and Dilated Cardiomyopathy: Four Decades of Basic Research on Muscle Lead to Potential Therapeutic Approaches to These Devastating Genetic Diseases. *Biophys. J.* **2014**, *106*, 1236–1249. [CrossRef]
80. Ashrafian, H.; Redwood, C.; Blair, E.; Watkins, H. Hypertrophic Cardiomyopathy:A Paradigm for Myocardial Energy Depletion. *Trends Genet. TIG* **2003**, *19*, 263–268. [CrossRef]
81. Schenk, A.; Fields, N. Mavacamten-A Targeted Therapy for Hypertrophic Cardiomyopathy. *J. Cardiovasc. Pharmacol.* **2023**, *81*, 317–326. [CrossRef]
82. MyoKardia, Inc. A Phase 2 Open-Label Pilot Study to Evaluate Efficacy, Pharmacokinetics, Pharmacodynamics, Safety, and Tolerability of MYK-461 in Subjects with Symptomatic Hypertrophic Cardiomyopathy and Left Ventricular Outflow Tract Obstruction; Clinical Trial Registration NCT02842242. clinicaltrials.gov. 2021. Available online: https://clinicaltrials.gov/study/NCT02842242 (accessed on 12 July 2023).
83. Heitner, S.B.; Jacoby, D.; Lester, S.J.; Owens, A.; Wang, A.; Zhang, D.; Lambing, J.; Lee, J.; Semigran, M.; Sehnert, A.J. Mavacamten Treatment for Obstructive Hypertrophic Cardiomyopathy: A Clinical Trial. *Ann. Intern. Med.* **2019**, *170*, 741–748. [CrossRef] [PubMed]
84. Masri, A.; Lester, S.J.; Stendahl, J.; Hegde, S.M.; Sehnert, A.; Balaratnam, G.; Fox, S.; Wang, A. Long-Term Safety and Efficacy of Mavacamten in Patients (Pts) with Symptomatic Obstructive Hypertrophic Cardiomyopathy (Hcm): Updated Results from the Pioneer-Ole Study. *J. Am. Coll. Cardiol.* **2023**, *81* (Suppl. S8), 346. [CrossRef]
85. Heitner, S.B.; Lester, S.; Wang, A.; Hegde, S.M.; Fang, L.; Balaratnam, G.; Sehnert, A.J.; Jacoby, D. Abstract 13962: Precision Pharmacological Treatment for Obstructive Hypertrophic Cardiomyopathy with Mavacamten: One-Year Results From PIONEER-OLE. *Circulation* **2019**, *140* (Suppl. S1), A13962. [CrossRef]
86. Ho, C.Y.; Mealiffe, M.E.; Bach, R.G.; Bhattacharya, M.; Choudhury, L.; Edelberg, J.M.; Hegde, S.M.; Jacoby, D.; Lakdawala, N.K.; Lester, S.J.; et al. Evaluation of Mavacamten in Symptomatic Patients with Nonobstructive Hypertrophic Cardiomyopathy. *J. Am. Coll. Cardiol.* **2020**, *75*, 2649–2660. [CrossRef] [PubMed]

87. Olivotto, I.; Oreziak, A.; Barriales-Villa, R.; Abraham, T.P.; Masri, A.; Garcia-Pavia, P.; Saberi, S.; Lakdawala, N.K.; Wheeler, M.T.; Owens, A.; et al. Mavacamten for Treatment of Symptomatic Obstructive Hypertrophic Cardiomyopathy (EXPLORER-HCM): A Randomised, Double-Blind, Placebo-Controlled, Phase 3 Trial. *Lancet* **2020**, *396*, 759–769. [CrossRef] [PubMed]
88. Desai, M.Y.; Owens, A.; Geske, J.B.; Wolski, K.; Naidu, S.S.; Smedira, N.G.; Cremer, P.C.; Schaff, H.; McErlean, E.; Sewell, C.; et al. Myosin Inhibition in Patients with Obstructive Hypertrophic Cardiomyopathy Referred for Septal Reduction Therapy. *J. Am. Coll. Cardiol.* **2022**, *80*, 95–108. [CrossRef]
89. Rader, F.; Choudhury, L.; Saberi, S.; Fermin, D.; Wheeler, M.T.; Abraham, T.P.; Oreziak, A.; Garcia, P.P.; Zwas, D.; Sehnert, A.J.; et al. Long-Term Safety of Mavacamten in Patients with Obstructive Hypertrophic Cardiomyopathy: Interim Results of the Mava-Long Term Extension (Lte) Study. *J. Am. Coll. Cardiol.* **2021**, *77* (Suppl. S1), 532. [CrossRef]
90. Bristol-Myers Squibb. A Randomized, Double-Blind, Placebo-Controlled Clinical Study to Evaluate Mavacamten in Adults with Symptomatic Non-Obstructive Hypertrophic Cardiomyopathy; Clinical Trial Registration NCT05582395. Available online: https://clinicaltrials.gov/study/NCT05582395 (accessed on 16 July 2023).
91. DeVries, J.H.; Irs, A.; Hillege, H.L. The European Medicines Agency Assessment of Mavacamten as Treatment of Symptomatic Obstructive Hypertrophic Cardiomyopathy in Adult Patients. *Eur. Heart J.* **2023**, ehad429. [CrossRef]
92. Chuang, C.; Collibee, S.; Ashcraft, L.; Wang, W.; Vander Wal, M.; Wang, X.; Hwee, D.T.; Wu, Y.; Wang, J.; Chin, E.R.; et al. Discovery of Aficamten (CK-274), a Next-Generation Cardiac Myosin Inhibitor for the Treatment of Hypertrophic Cardiomyopathy. *J. Med. Chem.* **2021**, *64*, 14142–14152. [CrossRef]
93. Maron, M.S.; Masri, A.; Choudhury, L.; Olivotto, I.; Saberi, S.; Wang, A.; Garcia, P.P.; Lakdawala, N.K.; Nagueh, S.F.; Rader, F.; et al. Phase 2 Study of Aficamten in Patients with Obstructive Hypertrophic Cardiomyopathy. *J. Am. Coll. Cardiol.* **2023**, *81*, 34–45. [CrossRef]
94. REDWOOD-HCM OLE: Aficamten Improves Patient-Measured Health Status. TCTMD.com. Available online: https://www.tctmd.com/news/redwood-hcm-ole-aficamten-improves-patient-measured-health-status (accessed on 18 July 2023).
95. Owens, A.T.; Masri, A.; Abraham, T.P.; Choudhury, L.; Rader, F.; Symanski, J.D.; Turer, A.T.; Wong, T.C.; Tower-Rader, A.; Coats, C.J.; et al. Aficamten for Drug-Refractory Severe Obstructive Hypertrophic Cardiomyopathy in Patients Receiving Disopyramide: REDWOOD-HCM Cohort 3. *J. Card. Fail.* **2023**. [CrossRef] [PubMed]
96. Cytokinetics. A Phase 3, Multi-Center, Randomized, Double-Blind, Placebo-Controlled Trial to Evaluate the Efficacy and Safety of CK-3773274 in Adults with Symptomatic Hypertrophic Cardiomyopathy and Left Ventricular Outflow Tract Obstruction; Clinical Trial Registration NCT05186818. clinicaltrials.gov. 2023. Available online: https://clinicaltrials.gov/study/NCT05186818 (accessed on 16 July 2023).
97. Cytokinetics, Incorporated. Cytokinetics Outlines Go-To-Market Strategy for Omecamtiv Mecarbil and Provides Updates on Cardiovascular Pipeline at Today's Analyst & Investor Day. GlobeNewswire News Room. Available online: https://www.globenewswire.com/en/news-release/2021/10/07/2310261/35409/en/Cytokinetics-Outlines-Go-To-Market-Strategy-for-Omecamtiv-Mecarbil-and-Provides-Updates-on-Cardiovascular-Pipeline-at-Today-s-Analyst-Investor-Day.html (accessed on 18 July 2023).
98. Corral-Acero, J.; Margara, F.; Marciniak, M.; Rodero, C.; Loncaric, F.; Feng, Y.; Gilbert, Y.; Fernandes, J.F.; Bukhari, H.A.; Wajdan, A.; et al. The 'Digital Twin' to enable the vision of precision cardiology. *Eur. Heart J.* **2020**, *41*, 4556–4564. [CrossRef] [PubMed]
99. Passini, E.; Mincholé, A.; Coppini, R.; Cerbai, E.; Rodriguez, B.; Severi, S.; Bueno-Orovio, A. Mechanisms of Pro-Arrhythmic Abnormalities in Ventricular Repolarisation and Anti-Arrhythmic Therapies in Human Hypertrophic Cardiomyopathy. *J. Mol. Cell. Cardiol.* **2016**, *96*, 72–81. [CrossRef] [PubMed]
100. Sewanan, L.R.; Moore, J.R.; Lehman, W.; Campbell, S.G. Predicting Effects of Tropomyosin Mutations on Cardiac Muscle Contraction through Myofilament Modeling. *Front. Physiol.* **2016**, *7*, 473. [CrossRef] [PubMed]
101. Margara, F.; Wang, Z.J.; Levrero-Florencio, F.; Santiago, A.; Vázquez, M.; Bueno-Orovio, A.; Rodriguez, B. In-Silico Human Electro-Mechanical Ventricular Modelling and Simulation for Drug-Induced pro-Arrhythmia and Inotropic Risk Assessment. *Prog. Biophys. Mol. Biol.* **2021**, *159*, 58–74. [CrossRef] [PubMed]
102. Musunuru, K. Genome Editing: The Recent History and Perspective in Cardiovascular Diseases. *J. Am. Coll. Cardiol.* **2017**, *70*, 2808–2821. [CrossRef] [PubMed]
103. Ma, H.; Marti-Gutierrez, N.; Park, S.-W.; Wu, J.; Lee, Y.; Suzuki, K.; Koski, A.; Ji, D.; Hayama, T.; Ahmed, R.; et al. Correction of a Pathogenic Gene Mutation in Human Embryos. *Nature* **2017**, *548*, 413–419. [CrossRef]
104. Bongianino, R.; Denegri, M.; Mazzanti, A.; Lodola, F.; Vollero, A.; Boncompagni, S.; Fasciano, S.; Rizzo, G.; Mangione, D.; Barbaro, S.; et al. Allele-Specific Silencing of Mutant MRNA Rescues Ultrastructural and Arrhythmic Phenotype in Mice Carriers of the R4496C Mutation in the Ryanodine Receptor Gene (RYR2). *Circ. Res.* **2017**, *121*, 525–536. [CrossRef]
105. Reichart, D.; Newby, G.A.; Wakimoto, H.; Lun, M.; Gorham, J.M.; Curran, J.J.; Raguram, A.; DeLaughter, D.M.; Conner, D.A.; Marsiglia, J.D.C.; et al. Efficient in Vivo Genome Editing Prevents Hypertrophic Cardiomyopathy in Mice. *Nat. Med.* **2023**, *29*, 412–421. [CrossRef]
106. Tison, G.H.; Siontis, K.C.; Abreau, S.; Attia, Z.; Agarwal, P.; Balasubramanyam, A.; Li, Y.; Sehnert, A.J.; Edelberg, J.M.; Friedman, P.A.; et al. Assessment of Disease Status and Treatment Response with Artificial Intelligence—Enhanced Electrocardiography in Obstructive Hypertrophic Cardiomyopathy. *J. Am. Coll. Cardiol.* **2022**, *79*, 1032–1034. [CrossRef]
107. Tison, G.H.; Zhang, J.; Delling, F.N.; Deo, R.C. Automated and Interpretable Patient ECG Profiles for Disease Detection, Tracking, and Discovery. *Circ. Cardiovasc. Qual. Outcomes* **2019**, *12*, e005289. [CrossRef] [PubMed]

108. Carrington, M.; Providência, R.; Chahal, C.A.A.; Ricci, F.; Epstein, A.E.; Gallina, S.; Fedorowski, A.; Sutton, R.; Khanji, M.Y. Monitoring and Diagnosis of Intermittent Arrhythmias: Evidence-Based Guidance and Role of Novel Monitoring Strategies. *Eur. Heart J. Open* **2022**, *2*, oeac072. [CrossRef] [PubMed]
109. Carrington, M.; Providência, R.; Chahal, C.A.A.; Ricci, F.; Epstein, A.E.; Gallina, S.; Fedorowski, A.; Sutton, R.; Khanji, M.Y. Clinical Applications of Heart Rhythm Monitoring Tools in Symptomatic Patients and for Screening in High-Risk Groups. *EP Eur.* **2022**, *24*, 1721–1729. [CrossRef] [PubMed]

Disclaimer/Publisher's Note: The statements, opinions and data contained in all publications are solely those of the individual author(s) and contributor(s) and not of MDPI and/or the editor(s). MDPI and/or the editor(s) disclaim responsibility for any injury to people or property resulting from any ideas, methods, instructions or products referred to in the content.

MDPI
St. Alban-Anlage 66
4052 Basel
Switzerland
www.mdpi.com

Journal of Clinical Medicine Editorial Office
E-mail: jcm@mdpi.com
www.mdpi.com/journal/jcm

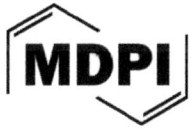

Disclaimer/Publisher's Note: The statements, opinions and data contained in all publications are solely those of the individual author(s) and contributor(s) and not of MDPI and/or the editor(s). MDPI and/or the editor(s) disclaim responsibility for any injury to people or property resulting from any ideas, methods, instructions or products referred to in the content.